Severe Pulmonary Emphysema

Chronic obstructive pulmonary disease is, as of 2024, one of the three main causes of death in the world, affecting around 12% of the world's population. Its incidence is estimated to increase in the coming decades due to continuous exposure to risk factors and an aging population.

Pulmonary emphysema is one of its most serious phenotypes, with chronic and inexorable progression, and in the most severe stages, it is highly disabling and lethal.

This book reviews the current knowledge about the pathophysiology of severe pulmonary emphysema and also the current innovative interventional and minimally invasive therapeutic concepts for the management of these advanced stages of emphysema, based on the best scientific evidence.

This guide provides, to multidisciplinary pulmonary boards of experts in advanced lung diseases, current criteria for the choice of precision therapeutic options and beyond to maintaining optimized medical treatment, controlling lung hyperinflation, and alleviating patients' symptoms.

This book is a valuable resource for clinicians dealing with critically ill patients with COPD.

T0313055

Severe Pulmonary Emphysema

A Comprehensive Guide to Precision Interventional Procedures

Edited by

Luis C. Losso, Pallav L. Shah, Gerard J. Criner,
Walter Weder, and José R. Jardim

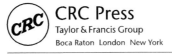

CRC Press
Taylor & Francis Group
Boca Raton London New York

CRC Press is an imprint of the
Taylor & Francis Group, an **informa** business

Designed cover image: created by Didu Losso and Felipe Innocente

First edition published 2025
by CRC Press
2385 NW Executive Center Drive, Suite 320, Boca Raton FL 33431

and by CRC Press
4 Park Square, Milton Park, Abingdon, Oxon, OX14 4RN

CRC Press is an imprint of Taylor & Francis Group, LLC

© 2025 selection and editorial matter Luis C. Losso, Pallav L. Shah, Gerard J. Criner, Walter Weder and José R. Jardim individual chapters, the contributors

ISBN: 9781032170244 (hbk)
ISBN: 9781032170237 (pbk)
ISBN: 9781003251439 (ebk)

DOI: 10.1201/9781003251439

Typeset in Times
by Deanta Global Publishing Services, Chennai, India

Contents

Foreword I

The progress of medicine is achieved by detailed thinkers, who, observing patients with specific morbidities, plan and conduct studies designed to establish the causes and mechanisms responsible for the observed manifestations of those diseases.

Since the seminal observations of Renne Laennec, who close to 200 years ago made the first anatomo-pathological description of the hyperinflated lung of patients dying from a then obscure respiratory ailment, many have been the contributors who not only have described the causes and reasons for the symptoms and signs associated with emphysema, but who based on those observations have approached therapeutic interventions capable of improving the outcomes of those patients.

During the two centuries since Laennec's description, studies have shown that there are different types and extensions of emphysematous lesions, with the physiological consequence that a great deal of the impairments suffered by the emphysematous patient are caused by the hyperinflation associated with this anatomical destruction. The presence of progressive air-trapping, which worsens as increased ventilation is needed by increased ventilatory demand, such as during exercise or an exacerbation, not only worsens the perceived dyspnea by the individual but can further compromise the function of the heart, thereby decreasing badly needed oxygen uptake and delivery to peripheral tissues. Indeed, the very hyperinflated COPD patient is crippled by this ventilatory trap, which in the end is a harbinger of ventilator insufficiency and death. Multiple therapies have been tried over the years. There is no question that the appropriate use of bronchodilators that also decrease hyperinflation, pulmonary rehabilitation that decreases iso-volume ventilation at the same work intensity, and supplemental oxygen in hypoxemic patients, which decrease ventilation, all help to "buy" time in the natural course of these patients. However, most have failed to improve the most important outcome, which is a decrease in the risk of death while offering an improvement in quality of life.

It seems rather contradictory that the most effective therapy for some of these patients, actually, the most functionally limited, with in-homogenous distribution of the emphysema, was developed by surgeons, who thought it possible that by reducing lung volume, it would be possible to provide a better physiological position to the breathing cycle of the neuro-pulmonary-cardiac complex. Furthermore, that by doing so, it would be possible to improve not only how those patients felt, but also how function would improve and ultimately also prolong their life. The journey has been long, and it is unfortunate that some of the initial surgical studies were completed with poor outcomes, which decreased the interest in the general public and the physicians caring for them.

Due to the tenacity of many surgeons and pulmonologists who had a deep understanding of the potential benefits of lung volume reduction (LVR) in better-selected patients, the last three decades not only allowed the establishment of those optimal criteria, but also the study of other forms of therapy different from surgical resection with its potential complications. In that way, different bronchoscopic techniques to achieve lung volume reduction, utilization of the superb capacity of modern imaging techniques to better define the anatomic characteristics that identify optimal candidates for the different procedures, and improvements in the prevention and management of complications have resulted in the advancements that make LVR a life-changing resource for many patients who would otherwise remain crippled by their disease.

This book, edited by Professor Luis C. Losso and his associates Pallav L. Shah, Gerard J. Criner, Walter Weder, and José R. Jardim, gathers a large number of authorities in the field, a no small achievement in the era of virtual information. The book is a great practical resource in one single volume, as it covers not only the actual details of the procedures, but importantly, the different elements that improve the overall outcomes, including candidate selection, optimization of medical therapy including pulmonary rehabilitation, the singular value of precise imaging techniques, peri-intervention management, and a view to the future of the field.

Every medical environment could benefit from having this resource available to the professionals caring for patients with COPD. It is important that they understand that even the most symptomatic of those patients could be a candidate for this therapy that not only improves the duration but also the quality of their life.

A nihilistic approach to patients with COPD is not justified.

Bartolome R. Celli, MD
Professor of Medicine, Harvard Medical School

Foreword II

The editors and authors are to be congratulated for producing this timely and comprehensive update on the current status of surgical and endoscopic interventions for end-stage emphysema.

It is over 200 years since Baillie (in 1795), and subsequently Laennac (in 1825), described the pathologic findings in emphysematous lungs removed at autopsy. Laennac furthermore described the physical and auscultatory findings on clinical examination and correctly recognized how the loss of lung elastic recoil in emphysematous lungs results in diminished expiratory flow rates in small airways. Stokes (in 1837) described the dynamic hyperinflation that occurs in emphysematous patients with initiation of rapid respiration.

In spite of great advances in radiologic examination describing the morphologic variance found in emphysema, the pathophysiologic changes that produce the crippling respiratory mechanics and associated dyspnea have been poorly understood until the latter part of the 20th century. During the interval, multiple surgical interventions have been introduced, highly touted, and soon discarded. These include unilateral/bilateral costochondrectomy, thoracoplasty, phrenicectomy, radical hilar stripping, and glomectomy.

But now is the time to go back to the future – which is now. There needs to be uniform, objective standards for classifying and selecting appropriate emphysema candidates for a proposed intervention procedure, as well as uniform, pre-specified, objective outcome measures by which the results of surgical, endoscopic, or other often competing proposed interventions can be compared in an unbiased fashion. Such standards would allow investigators, clinicians, patients, and insurers to better evaluate the risks and benefits of proposed interventions.

The experience and multidisciplinary contributions contained in this monograph might well foster the universal adoption of such standards.

Joel D. Cooper, MD
Professor of Medicine, University of Pennsylvania

Preface

In the scenario of continuous evolution of pulmonary medicine, innovative minimally invasive treatment modalities for patients with advanced pulmonary emphysema have witnessed significant advances.

Lung hyperinflation treatment, a treatable trait of the pulmonary emphysema phenotype, is undergoing a paradigm shift. Lung volume reduction, through interventional and personalized approaches, has emerged as a precision therapeutic option, offering new hope to individuals struggling with this serious disabling respiratory condition.

This book discusses the knowledge of the characteristics of this complex and heterogeneous disease, clarifying the pathophysiological principles, its clinical manifestation and functional repercussions, and the new personalized medical and interventional treatments for pulmonary hyperinflation, the most severe expression phenotype of advanced emphysema, promoting a patient-centered approach by multidisciplinary teams and prioritizing precision individualized care and optimal therapeutic outcomes.

Topics of this guide range from patient selection criteria and imaging modalities to diverse interventional strategies such as minimally invasive surgical resection, endobronchial valves, coils, and bronchoscopic thermal vapor ablation. By elucidating the nuances of each technique, this book strives to offer readers the knowledge and skills necessary to effectively navigate the complexities of personalized lung volume reduction procedures. Clinical results and future directions in this field are also discussed.

Through insights presented by renowned experts and leaders in the field and cutting-edge research, it aims to serve as a comprehensive guide for clinicians, researchers, and healthcare professionals involved in treating patients with severe emphysema to chart a course toward better patient outcomes and greater quality of life.

It is imperative to embrace innovation, collaboration, and understanding of the individual needs of each patient. This book stands as a testament to collective efforts to advance the frontiers of personalized interventional treatment while heralding a future where precision medicine holds the promise of better outcomes and improved quality of life for those affected by this challenging respiratory condition.

The Editors

Acknowledgments

GRATITUDE TO THE ARTISTS

Didu Losso and Felipe Innocente,

We would like to express our sincere gratitude for the incredible work you did in developing the cover art for this book.

Your creativity and talent were fundamental in conveying the essence and importance of the content of this work. It's admirable to see how you were able to visually capture the complexity and seriousness of this topic in such an impactful way.

We hope that you continue to inspire and impact the world with your unique and powerful art.

The Editors

GRATITUDE TO THE AUTHORS

Dear Authors,

We would like to express our deepest gratitude for the invaluable contribution you all have made to this book.

Your participation is proof of your dedication, competence, and wealth of experience in this relevant field.

Your experience shines through in every paragraph, offering readers an in-depth understanding of the topics. Your meticulous research, insightful analysis, and eloquent prose have undoubtedly enriched the overall quality of the book. The commitment to excellence is evident and has truly elevated the collective work.

In addition to your professional competence, we are sincerely grateful for your belief in this project.

Your willingness to share your knowledge and insights speaks volumes about your generosity and passion for advancing the field. It is authors like yourselves who inspire and drive progress, and we feel privileged to have collaborated with physicians of your caliber.

We are truly honored to have had the opportunity to work alongside you.

With deepest appreciation,

The Editors

About the Editors

Luis C. Losso, MD, PhD

Director, Center for Thoracic Medicine and Minimally Invasive Thoracic Surgery, Hospital Edmundo Vasconcelos, São Paulo, Brazil

Head, Pulmonary Emphysema Precision Treatment Unit

COPD Foundation, Brazilian Captain, USA

Latin American Advisory Board for Minimally Invasive Thoracic Surgery, Professional Education, Johnson & Johnson MedTech

Philosophical Degree in Medicine, Postgraduate Program in Operative Technique and Experimental Surgery at the Escola Paulista de Medicine at the Federal University of São Paulo, Brazil

Certification of Specialist in Thoracic Surgery, Brazilian Society of Thoracic Surgery

Certification of Specialist in Pulmonology, Brazilian Society of Pulmonology

1972 Graduation in Medicine, Faculty of Medicine of Marília

Professor Luis C. Losso's interests include advanced lung disease, severe pulmonary emphysema, and interventional treatments to reduce lung volume; he was involved in trials into the bronchoscopic treatment of pulmonary emphysema with drug-eluting stents.

Professor Losso is active in publishing scientific papers in national and international medical journals; he has edited thoracic surgery books and authored chapters for them; he has been a speaker at international and national lectures on thoracic surgery. Professor Losso is a former president of the South American Chapter of the International Minimally Invasive Thoracic Surgery Group (USA); founder of the Brazilian Society of Thoracic Surgery; founder of the Brazilian Society of Pulmonology; a member of the Ibero-American Association of Thoracic Surgery; and a member of the Latin American Thoracic Association.

Pallav Shah, MD, MBBS, FERS, FRCP

Professor Pallav Shah is currently professor of respiratory medicine at Imperial College, London. He is a senior consultant physician at the Royal Brompton Hospital, and Chelsea and Westminster Hospital. He qualified in medicine at Guy's Hospital Medical School, London, and trained in pulmonology at the Royal Brompton Hospital.

Professor Shah is active in both the research and the development of new treatments. He has over 250 papers and several books to his credit – including his contribution as sectional editor of the thoracic section of *Gray's Anatomy* (39th and 40th editions) and as sectional editor for the respiratory section of the *Oxford Textbook of Medicine* (6th edition). He is also the author of *Atlas of Flexible Bronchoscopy* and chief editor of *Essentials of Clinical Pulmonology*. He has also been involved in the HERMES education program for the European Respiratory Society

Professor Shah pioneered bronchoscopic lung volume reduction for emphysema with devices such as Zephyr endobronchial valves, endobronchial coils, vapor treatment, and intrabronchial valves. More recently he has focused on the treatment of COPD with vapor therapy, targeted nerve ablation, and the novel RejuvenAir (cryospray) procedure for chronic bronchitis.

Gerard J. Criner, MD

Gerard J. Criner, MD, is Professor and Founding Chair of the Department of Thoracic Medicine and Surgery and Temple Lung Center at the Lewis Katz School of Medicine at Temple University in

Philadelphia, Pennsylvania. His research interests include respiratory failure, lung volume reduction surgery, bronchoscopic lung reduction, and the prevention and treatment of acute COPD exacerbations.

Walter Weder, MD

Walter Weder, MD, is professor of surgery and former director of the Department of Thoracic Surgery at the University Hospital Zurich (USZ), Switzerland. He currently works at the Thoracic Surgery Clinic Bethanien, Zurich. He was educated at the Medical School of the University of Zurich and at Stanford University, graduated in Zürich, and became a thoracic surgeon after his surgical training at USZ and a Research Fellowship in Lung Transplantation at Washington University (Joel D. Cooper), St. Louis, USA. He is member of many national and international medical societies, including AATS, ESTS, IASLC, EACTS, ESMO, STS, ISHLT, and ERS.

Professor Weder is also the founding president of the Swiss Society of Thoracic Surgery, the Lung transplant group of Swiss transplants, the former president of the European Society of Thoracic Surgery (ESTS), and board member of ETOP. He was a visiting professor at Harvard University in Boston, MSKCC in NYC, and Shanghai Chest Hospital. In 1992, Professor Walter performed the first lung transplant in Switzerland and in 1994 the first thoracoscopic lung volume reduction procedure worldwide. In 2004, he started a robotic surgery program for mediastinal disease and lung cancer. Over the years, his research activity has focused on thoracic malignancies, especially malignant mesothelioma, and locally advanced lung cancer, as well as emphysema surgery and lung transplantation. He is an author of over 500 peer-reviewed scientific publications.

José R. Jardim, MD

José R. Jardim, MD, graduated in Medicine in 1970 from the Escola Paulista de Medicina, Federal University of São Paulo, Brazil, where he was later awarded his PhD in Medical Sciences. He has also completed a two-year fellowship in respiratory pathophysiology from the McGill University in Montreal, Canada.

Dr. Jardim is a senior professor of respiratory diseases and the former director of the Pulmonary Rehabilitation Centre at Escola Paulista de Medicina of Federal University of São Paulo, Brazil, for over 30 years.

He was chairman of the Education Department twice and served three times as chairman of the COPD Committee at the Brazilian Thoracic Society (SBPT). Dr. Jardim was a member of the Planning Committee of the Rehabilitation Assembly of the American Thoracic Society (ATS) for five years and served at the Nominating Committee of the same assembly. He served on the Board of Directors of ATS representing the International Community. He was president of the Latin American Thoracic Society (ALAT) for two terms and one term for the Brazilian Association for Asthmatic Patients. Currently, he is on the editorial boards for several Brazilian and international journals and has published a book on rehabilitation as well as over 250 peer-reviewed papers and 90 chapters. His main interests are asthma, COPD, and pulmonary rehabilitation.

Contributors

Alexey Abramov, MD
Columbia University Medical Centre
New York, NY, USA

Andrew Akcelik, MD
Department of Surgery
University of California San Francisco
San Francisco, CA, USA

Charles T. Bakhos, MD, MBA MS, FACS
Professor, Department of Thoracic Medicine and
    Surgery
Lewis Katz School of Medicine
Temple University Hospital
Vice-Chief of Thoracic Surgery
Philadelphia, PA, USA

Sean I. Bolet
Lewis Katz School of Medicine
Temple University
Philadelphia, PA, USA

Marina-Dornfeld C. Castro
Professor of Medicine by São Paulo School of
    Medicine
São Paulo Federal University
Head of the Department of Chronic Obstructive
    Pulmonary Diseases of Servidor Público
    Estadual Hospital "Francisco Morato Oliveira"
São Paulo, Brazil

Claudio Caviezel
Department of Thoracic Surgery
University Hospitals Zurich
Zurich, Switzerland

Laurens J. Ceulemans
Department of Thoracic Surgery
University Hospitals Leuven
Leuven, Belgium
Department of Chronic Diseases and Metabolism
    Laboratory of Pneumology and Thoracic
    Surgery (BREATHE)
KU Leuven, Leuven, Belgium

Simin Dadparvar
Division of Nuclear Medicine and Molecular
    Imaging, Department of Radiology
Temple University Hospital
Philadelphia, PA, USA

Kaid Darwiche
Department of Interventional Pneumology
Ruhrland Clinic – University Medicine
    Essen
North Rhine-Westphalia, Germany

Chandra Dass, MBBS, DMRD
Professor of Radiology, Director Thoracic Section
Lewis Katz School of Medicine
Temple University Hospital
Philadelphia, PA, USA

Justin L. Garner, BSc, MBBS, MRCP, PhD
Royal Brompton Hospital
London, UK
National Heart and Lung Institute
Imperial College London
London, UK

Mario C. Ghefter
Director of the Department of Thoracic Surgery
    of the Servidor Público Estadual Hospital
    "Francisco Morato Oliveira"
Thoracic Surgeon at Albert Einstein
    Hospital
São Paulo, Brazil

Mark E. Ginsburg, MD
Columbia University Medical Center
New York, NY, USA

Yogesh Gupta, MD
Department of Radiology
Lewis Katz School of Medicine
Temple University
Philadelphia, PA, USA

Jin Sun Kim
Department of Thoracic Medicine and Surgery
Temple University Hospital
Philadelphia, PA, USA

T. David Koster
Department of Pulmonary Diseases
University of Groningen
University Medical Center Groningen
Groningen, the Netherlands

Maruti Kumaran, MBBS, MD
Associate Professor
Department of Radiology
Thoracic Section
Lewis Katz School of Medicine
Temple University
Philadelphia, PA, USA

Nathaniel Marchetti
Temple University Hospital,
Philadelphia, PA, USA

Hugo G. Oliveira
Department of Pulmonology
Hospital de Clínicas de Porto Alegre
Universidade Federal do Rio Grande do Sul
Porto Alegre, RS, Brazil

Marcel M. Sandrini
Head of Oncological Thoracic Surgery Team
    at Beneficencia Portuguesa and BP Mirante
    Hospitals;
Preceptor of Minimally Invasive Thoracic Surgery
    Training Courses at Johnson & Johnson
    Institute
Full member of the Brazilian Society of Thoracic
    Surgery
São Paulo, Brazil

Dirk-Jan Slebos
Department of Pulmonary Diseases
University of Groningen
University Medical Center Groningen
Groningen, the Netherlands

Bryan P. Stanifer, MD, MPH
Assistant Professor of Surgery
Columbia University Medical Center
New York, NY, USA

Christelle M. Vandervelde
Department of Thoracic Surgery
University Hospitals Leuven
Leuven, Belgium
Department of Chronic Diseases and Metabolism
Laboratory of Pneumology and Thoracic Surgery
(BREATHE)
KU Leuven
Leuven, Belgium

Johannes Wienker
West German Lung Center
Ruhrland Clinic
University Medicine Essen
North Rhine-Westphalia, Germany

Pathophysiology of Emphysema

1

José R. Jardim

INTRODUCTION

Chronic obstructive pulmonary disease (COPD) is considered a heterogeneous disease comprising small and large airway abnormalities and is associated with alveoli destruction. Clinically, patients with COPD are characterized by breathlessness and limitations to physical activities evolving to dyspnea to simple activities of daily life. A forced expiratory maneuver has usually been the most used method to assess pulmonary function registering the expired volume as a function of time.[1] Patients are asked to take a deep breath up to the total lung capacity and then expire as forcefully as possible to the residual volume. GOLD criteria diagnose COPD as the ratio forced expiratory volume in the 1st second over forced volume capacity <0.70. However, patients have been seen with a fixed ratio >0.70 with lung diffusion lower than normal, which may be a reflex of starting alveolar destruction and possibly small airways disease. A study following two groups of smokers with normal spirometry and normal or abnormal lung diffusion for over 40 months showed that the group with lower diffusion developed more COPD (22% vs. 3%).[2]

INFLAMMATORY PROCESS

Several risk factors are associated with the development of the inflammatory pathological process in COPD, including most importantly, tobacco smoking, air pollution, fumes, toxic gases, pesticides, and occupational exposure.[3] However, not all exposed individuals develop COPD, which makes us believe that some of them must have one or more conditions that predispose them to the disease.[4] An inflammatory reaction is a natural response of the body to an injury. It acts to remove harmful stimuli such as pathogens, irritants, and damaged cells and initiates the healing process. Initially, those stimuli are recognized by a group of pattern recognition receptors (PRRs) that exist either on the membrane surface or inside the cytoplasm.[5] At this point, a resolution process evolves, involving apoptosis and subsequent clearance of activated inflammatory cells.[6,7] The inflammatory process starts with the membrane superficial receptor

DOI: 10.1201/9781003251439-1

Toll-like receptors (TLRs), recognizing the pathogen molecules and activating inflammatory cells like nuclear factor kappa-light-chain-enhancer of activated B-cells (NF-κB), produce growth factors, chemokines, pro-inflammatory cytokines interleukin 8 (IL-8), and tumor necrosis factor-alpha (TNF-α) to start the resolution process. IL-8 evokes neutrophils and TNF-α raises the expression of endothelial cell adhesion molecules from lung capillaries. Moreover, many of the known inflammatory target proteins, such as matrix metalloproteinase-9 (MMP-9), intercellular adhesion molecule-1 (ICAM-1), vascular cell adhesion molecule-1 (VCAM-1), cyclooxygenase-2 (COX-2), and cytosolic phospholipase A2 (cPLA2), are specifically associated with airway inflammation in response to various stimuli.[8] The following step is the process of retrieving damaged tissue. A failure in the repair mechanism will turn this initial inflammation into a continuous ongoing process characterizing a chronic persistent inflammatory response. What is not known is why, even with the individual stopping smoking, once the inflammatory response has started, what keeps it as a persistent and progressive process. Factors like oxidative stress, genetic background susceptibility, disturbed macrophage clearance, chronic bronchial colonization, and repeated infections are some of the possible mechanisms involved with this ongoing inflammation.[9]

EVALUATION OF SMALL AIRWAYS AND EMPHYSEMA

Computed tomography (CT) has lately been extensively used as a tool to understand the pathophysiologic natural history of COPD. Studies have shown that initial abnormalities in COPD start on the small airways and only later will there be parenchymal alterations. This abnormalities sequence is associated with the clinical symptoms of patients. While the disease is predominantly bronchial, patients present with cough and sputum, and when emphysema develops, breathlessness will associate with the initial clinical symptoms.

Small airways are considered as having a diameter of <2 mm and are the major sites of obstruction in COPD. In 1978, one of the first studies was published to show a relation between lesions in small airways and inflammatory reactions leading to fibrosis with connective tissue deposition and lung function tests that detected small airways impairment.[10] More recently, the same group showed in a comparison of micro-CT measurements of the number of terminal bronchioles per milliliter of lung volume with the alveolar dimensions (mean linear intercept) that loss of terminal bronchioles preceded the appearance of microscopical emphysematous destruction in the centrilobular emphysematous phenotype of COPD. These results suggest that the narrowing and destruction of terminal bronchioles start before the onset of emphysematous destruction.[11]

Until very recently, a chest CT was not a required tool for COPD diagnosis, however, with a further understanding of COPD pathophysiology, phenotyping the airways and structural parenchyma abnormalities have played an important role in COPD diagnosis, treatment, and intervention. The COPD Gene Study proposed to redefine the diagnosis of COPD by associating chest CT with environmental exposure, clinical symptoms, and spirometry. In a 5-year longitudinal assessment in a cohort of over 10,000 individuals, they showed significant differences in physiological, symptomatic, and CT structural imaging abnormalities despite similar cigarette smoke exposure.[12] The standard procedures for airway CT analysis still need some further refining. However, CT use has proved to be very useful for airway wall thickness measurement, which provides some insight into the small airway involvement in COPD. Moreover, by comparing inspiratory and expiratory areas of gas trapping, CT analysis may help to define small airway involvement in the disease. Fortunately, CT emphysema analysis is a few steps ahead of airway analysis, and it may be quantified by different measurements including loss of tissue in grams per liter or percent of emphysema. Evaluation of emphysema distribution and severity is particularly important for endobronchial valve placement or lung reduction surgery decisions.

A Canadian prospective study evaluated respiratory bronchiolitis (RB), emphysema (E), bronchial-wall thickening (BWT), expiratory air-trapping (AT), and bronchiectasis (B) in thoracic CT scans data from over 1000 participants aged ≥40 years comprising healthy never-smokers, healthy ever-smokers, and individuals with spirometry evidence of COPD; 11% of the never-smoked group and 30% of smokers with normal lung function had evidence of emphysema on CT scans. Emphysema on CT was associated with chronic cough, wheeze, dyspnea, COPD Assessment Test score ≥10, and risk of ≥2 exacerbations over 12 months.[13]

HYPERINFLATION AND FORCED EXPIRATION

A lung is considered hyperinflated when there is a larger gas volume at the end of a spontaneous expiration in comparison with normal values. Hyperinflation is a common occurrence in COPD patients, particularly in emphysematous patients. Expired airflow is dependent on elastic recoil and bronchial permeability. Elastic recoil presents a direct association with lung volume, so the larger the inspiratory volume, the higher the elastic recoil. At the same time the lungs are inflating, the chest wall is being displaced outward. Relaxation after the inspiratory tidal volume will make both the alveoli and chest wall return to their resting position and expiratory tidal volume occur.

Considering the atmosphere pressure (Patm) as zero, there will be two driving pressures in the lungs, the pleural surface (Ppl) and alveoli (Palv) (created by lung elastic recoil). Thus, $Ppl = - Pst(L) + Palv$. In case there is a pull of the lungs on the pleura surface, i.e., a larger Pst, there will be a reduction on the Ppl, becoming more negative. As Pst depends on lung volume, at any time that the relation between Pst and volume is known, Ppl may be determined. Emphysematous lungs are largely characterized by the loss of elastic lung recoil and a pressure-volume curve steeper than the one of normal lungs, determining increased lung compliance. Lesions like human emphysema can be produced experimentally in animals with proteolytic enzymes. With the decrease of lung elastic recoil, the chest wall is not pulled inward as before, and it is displaced outward, increasing the chest wall volume, causing a static hyperinflation.[14]

Static hyperinflation is associated with dyspnea, hospitalizations, respiratory failure, and increased mortality.[15] Dynamic hyperinflation occurs when the patient accomplishes any activity demanding an increase in pulmonary ventilation. As the breathing frequency increases and the elastic recoil is not enough to expire the previous tidal volume before the next tidal volume, an extra volume will be retained in the lungs. Dynamic hyperinflation causes discomfort and shortening of the activity.[16]

During a forced expiratory maneuver, the pleura pressure increases, compressing the alveoli to increase the alveolar pressure and make the air flow out of the alveoli. However, at the same time, the high pleura pressure is also compressing the bronchi, characterizing a dynamic compression. As air flows along the bronchi, there is a progressive pressure loss and there will be a point in the bronchi segment that the pleura space and bronchi pressure are equal. From that point on, the pleura pressure is higher than in the bronchi and dynamic compression occurs. This point is called the equal pressure point (EPP). As air keeps flowing out of the alveoli, its volume decreases and the Pst decreases, and so the Palv makes the EPP displace toward the alveoli. The closer the EPP is to the alveoli, the lower the expired airflow. Bronchial contraction, bronchial-wall damage as in emphysematous patients, or the presence of secretion lead to a substantial intrabronchial pressure drop and EPP displacement toward the alveoli, explaining low airflow in COPD patients. Therefore, maximal bronchodilation and secretion elimination are central in the treatment of emphysematous COPD patients. Another possible strategy to avoid early EPP occurrence is teaching the huffing cough technique to patients.[14]

REFERENCES

1. Global Initiative for Obstructive Lung Disease – GOLD 2024. www.goldcopd.org. Accessed December 20th, 2023.

2. Harvey BG, Strulovici-Barel Y, Kaner RK, Sanders A, Vincent TL, Mezey JG, Crystal RG. Risk for COPD with obstruction of active smokers with normal spirometry and reduced diffusion capacity. *Eur Respir J.* 2015;46(6):1589–1597. doi: 10.1183/13993003.02377-2014.

3. Papi A, Magnoni MS, Muzzio CC, Benso G, Tizzi A. Phenomenology of COPD: interpreting phenotypes with the eclipse study. *Monaldi Arch Chest Dis.* 2016;83:1–8.

4. Hogg JC, Timens W. The pathology of chronic obstructive pulmonary disease: mechanisms of disease. *Ann Rev Pathol.* 2009;4:435–459.

5. Takeuchi O, Akira S. Pattern recognition receptors and inflammation. *Cell.* 2010;140(6):805–820.

6. Ortega-Gómez A, Perretti M, Soehnlein O. Resolution of inflammation: an integrated view. *EMBO Mol Med.* 2013;5(5):661–674.

7. Maskrey BH, Megson IL, Whitfield PD, Rossi AG. Mechanisms of resolution of inflammation. *Arterioscler Thromb Vasc Biol.* 2011;31(5):1001–1006.

8. Aghasafari P, George U, Pidaparti R. A review of inflammatory mechanism in airway diseases. *Inflamm Res.* 2019;68:59–74. doi: 10.1007/s00011-018-1191-2.

9. Brusselle GG, Joos GF, Bracke KR. New insights into the immunology of chronic obstructive pulmonary disease. *Lancet.* 2011;378(9795):1015–1026.

10. Cosio M, Ghezzo H, Hogg JC, Corbin R, Loveland M, Dosman J, Maclkem PT. The relation between structural changes in small airways and pulmonary-function tests. *New Eng J Med.* 1977:1277–1281.

11. McDonough JE, Yuan R, Suzuki M, Seyednejad N, Elliott MW, Sanchez PG, et al. Small-airway obstruction and emphysema in chronic obstructive pulmonary disease. *N Engl J Med.* 2011;365(17):1567–1575. doi: 10.1056/NEJMoa1106955.

12. Lowe KE, Regan EA, Anzueto A, Austin E, Austin JHM, Beaty TH, et al. COPDGene® 2019: redefining the diagnosis of chronic obstructive pulmonary disease. *Chronic Obstr Pulm Dis Foundation.* 2019;6(5):384–399. doi: 10.15326/jcopdf.6.5.2019.0149.

13. Tan WC, Hague CJ, Leipsic J, Bourbeau J, Zheng L, Li PZ, et al. Findings on thoracic computed tomography scans and respiratory outcomes in persons with and without chronic obstructive pulmonary disease: a population-based cohort study. *PLOS ONE.* 2016. doi: 10.1371/journal.pone.0166745.

14. Bouhuys A. *The physiology of breathing. A textbook for medical students.* Grune & Stratton, New York, San Francisco, London.

15. Casanova C, Cote C, de Torres JP, et al. Inspiratory to total lung capacity ratio predicts mortality in patients with chronic obstructive pulmonary disease. *Am J Respir Crit Care Med.* 2005;171:591–597.

16. O´Donnell DE, Revill SM, Webb KA. Dynamic hyperinflation and exercise intolerancein chronic obstructive pulmonary disease. *Am J Respir Crit Care Med.* 2001;164:770–777. https://pubmed.ncbi.nlm.nih.gov/11549531.

Pulmonary Functional Evaluation for the Safe Performance of Lung Volume Reduction

2

Jin Sun Kim and Gerard J. Criner

INTRODUCTION

Bronchoscopic lung volume reduction (BLVR) is a minimally invasive procedure for the management of severe emphysema. Currently, only the Food and Drug Administration (FDA) approved BLVR intervention is the placement of one-way endobronchial valves (EBV) implanted in targeted bronchi of hyperinflated lobes to allow air to exit diseased lobes during exhalation and prevent inspiratory flow during inhalation. This procedure has been shown to reduce hyperinflation and air trapping, improve lung function, and provide symptom relief [1]. Alternative techniques including sealants, coils, and thermal ablation are under investigation. This chapter aims to provide a comprehensive overview of the key considerations in patient selection for BLVR with a focus on selection criteria for EBV placement.

PATIENT SELECTION

Patient selection for BLVR trials historically drew from conditions established in lung volume reduction surgery (LVRS) and data from the National Emphysema Treatment Trial (NETT). Inclusion criteria for LVRS included forced expiratory volume in the first second (FEV_1) ≤45% predicted, residual volume (RV) ≥150% predicted, and total lung capacity (TLC) ≥100% predicted. Patients with diffusing capacity for carbon monoxide (DLCO) <20% were excluded from BLVR trials due to elevated mortality risk seen in this high-risk subgroup in the NETT data [2].

DOI: 10.1201/9781003251439-2

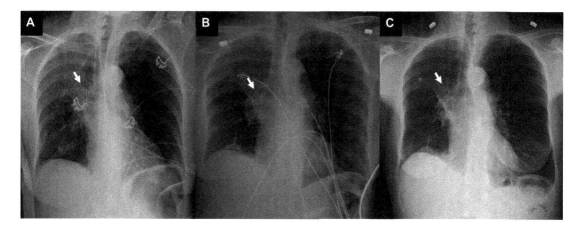

FIGURE 2.1   CXR of hyperinflated lungs, coarse interstitial markings, and bronchiectasis s/p endobronchial valve placement (arrows) in right upper lobe on POD 0 (A), POD 1 (B), and POD 3 (C), subsequent right upper lobe atelectasis and right-sided mediastinal shift.

Over time, the lessons learned from various BLVR trials helped to shape the inclusion and exclusion criteria, targeting optimal patients to treat with EBV placement (Figure 2.1). The VENT study in 2010 was the first prospective randomized controlled trial in patients with severe emphysema. It compared the safety and efficacy of EBV (Zephyr®, PulmonX™ Corporation, Redwood City, CA, USA) to medical therapies in heterogeneous emphysema and found that patients had modest but statistically significant group mean improvements in FEV_1 and 6-minute walk distance (6MWD) after EBV placement. Higher values were seen in patients with greater interlobar heterogeneity of emphysema and complete interlobar fissures [3]. Fissure completeness is considered a surrogate marker for collateral ventilation and can be challenging due to interobserver variability on HRCT [4].

Other studies, including the BeLieVeR-HIFi trial, found that unilateral lobar occlusion with EBV using Chartis™ (PulmonX, Redwood City, CA, USA) measurements of collateral ventilation could identify the absence of collateral ventilation and improve lung function [5, 6]. The STELVIO trial then compared patients with advanced emphysema and absent collateral ventilation who received EBV or medical treatment, and showed that EBV had improvements in lung function, exercise capacity, and quality of life as assessed by St. George's Respiratory Questionnaire (SGRQ) [7]. Post-hoc analysis of high-resolution computed tomography (HRCT) findings found that patients with heterogeneous emphysema as opposed to homogeneous emphysema had larger significant differences in lung function, exercise capacity, and quality of life [7] Subsequently, the IMPACT trial found that EBV placement in patients with homogeneous emphysema and absent collateral ventilation had significant improvements in FEV_1, 6MWD, and SGRQ [8]. The LIBERATE trial was a multicenter prospective randomized controlled clinical trial that found EBV treatment in patients with heterogeneous distribution of emphysema with absent collateral ventilation had benefits in lung function, quality of life, and exercise capacity to at least 12 months after procedure [9].

The EMPROVE trial, a prospective open-label randomized controlled multicenter trial, found improved lung function and survival in patients with severe heterogeneous emphysema treated with the Spiration® Valve System (SVS, Olympus Corporation, Center Valley, PA, USA) [10]. The SVS is a one-way valve using a flexible umbrella shape that restricts airflow to distal portions of the lungs, causing targeted lobar atelectasis [10]. A prior SVS trial found that EBV treatment causing bilateral partial occlusion of the target lobe was safe but did not yield consistent improvement in volumetric change and SGRQ total in all patients [11]. The EMPROVE trial showed that patients with single-lobe total occlusion experience marked persistent benefits in lung function, dyspnea, and quality of life at six, 12, and 24 months, comparable to other randomized clinical trials using EBV in a unilateral single-lung treatment approach [7, 9, 10, 12, 13].

The insights gained from studies like VENT, BeLieVER-HIFi, STELVIO, IMPACT, LIBERATE, and EMPROVE have been instrumental in refining patient selection for EBV placement. These trials highlight the significance of interlobar heterogeneity, collateral ventilation, and fissure completeness in the selection of EBV candidates.

In general, all patients undergoing assessment for BLVR require a thorough review of past medical and surgical history, assessment of clinical symptoms, pulmonary function testing, cardiac evaluation including echocardiogram and cardiac stress tests, cardiopulmonary exercise tests, and imaging including HRCT and ventilation-perfusion scans. Candidates require a clinical diagnosis of COPD with emphysema. Table 2.1 provides a list of inclusion criteria for consideration of BLVR. They must endorse persistent dyspnea despite optimal medical therapy and maximal pulmonary rehabilitation with a modified Medical Research Council dyspnea scale (mMRC) of two or more (Table 2.2). They must be clinically stable on 20 mg prednisone equivalent or less. They must have quit smoking for four or more months and have a body mass index (BMI) of less than 35 kg/m². They must also have little or no collateral ventilation assessed by Chartis™ and/or have fissure integrity identified on quantitative analyses of HRCT (discussed further below under "Fissure Analysis and Collateral Ventilation").

Contraindications for EBV therapies include smoking within four months prior to evaluation, BMI greater than 35 kg/m², the presence of large bullae greater than 30% in either lung, or active pulmonary infections. Incidental pulmonary nodules on evaluation may be a relative contraindication to BLVR as post-procedural atelectasis can distort parenchymal changes, affecting CT follow-up of nodules over time. In addition, patients with comorbid cardiovascular illnesses that would increase surgical mortality including significant coronary heart disease, unstable arrhythmia, myocardial infarction (MI), stroke, and congestive heart failure (CHF) with ejection fraction (EF) less than 40% are excluded. Patients unable to undergo a bronchoscopy, considered to have high postoperative morbidity and mortality, and unable to complete a six-to-ten-week pulmonary rehabilitation program are excluded as well. Patients with prior cardiothoracic surgery including lung transplantation, LVRS, lobectomy, and median sternotomy are not candidates for EBV placement [6, 16]. Table 2.3 provides a list of exclusion criteria for consideration of BLVR.

TABLE 2.1   Inclusion criteria for BLVR

History and physical examination
- A clinical diagnosis of COPD with emphysema
- Persistent dyspnea despite medical therapy (mMRC ≥2)
- Clinically stability on prednisone less than 20 mg/day (or equivalent)
- Nonsmoking for ≥4 months
- BMI <35 kg/m²

Pulmonary function testing
- Post-bronchodilator FEV_1 ≥15% and ≤45% predicted
- RV ≥150% predicted
- TLC ≥100% predicted
- 6MWD ≥100m and <500m
- DLCO >20% predicted

Arterial blood gas
- PaCO2 <55 mmHg on ambient air

Imaging
- Complete fissure on qualitative assessment of HRCT
- Emphysema on imaging

Chartis™ assessment
- Collateral ventilation negative assessed by Chartis™

TABLE 2.2   Modified Medical Research Council (mMRC) Scale [14, 15]

GRADE	DESCRIPTION
0	Endorses breathlessness with strenuous exercise
1	Endorses breathlessness when hurrying on level ground or walking up a slight hill
2	Walks slower than people of the same age on level ground or having to stop for breath when walking at own pace
3	Stops for breath after walking about 100 meters or a few minutes on level ground
4	Endorses breathlessness when dressing or too breathless to leave the house

Historically, individuals diagnosed with alpha-1 antitrypsin deficiency and pulmonary hypertension were deemed ineligible for participation in clinical trials focused on BLVR. Despite this exclusion, recent case series on emphysema patients with alpha-1 antitrypsin deficiency have found promising outcomes, with a retrospective single-center study finding significant improvements in pulmonary function, exercise capacity, and quality of life in patients after EBV placement [17–19]. Moreover, a limited case series has presented evidence suggesting the feasibility of EBV placement in patients with group 3 pulmonary hypertension, demonstrating positive improvement in clinical and hemodynamic markers [20]. These findings suggest the potential for broadening the application of BLVR interventions to a wider range of patients. However, additional larger, multicenter, prospective, controlled studies are essential to ensure its safety and efficacy in these extended patient populations.

TABLE 2.3   Exclusion criteria for BLVR

History and physical examination
- Active smoking or smoking within four months prior to evaluation
- Significant coronary heart disease, unstable arrhythmia, MI within six months, CHF with EF <40%
- Active pulmonary infections
- Severe pulmonary hypertension
- Recent hospitalization for COPD or pulmonary infection three months prior to evaluation
- BMI ≥35 kg/m^2
- Unable to undergo bronchoscopy
- Unable to complete a six-to-ten-week pulmonary rehabilitation
- Prior cardiothoracic surgery including lung transplantation, LVRS, lobectomy, or median sternotomy

Pulmonary function testing
- Post-bronchodilator FEV_1 <15% predicted
- 6MWD <100m and >500m
- DLCO <20% predicted

Arterial blood gas
- PaO2 <45 mmHg on ambient air
- PaCO2 >55 mmHg on ambient air

Imaging
- Incomplete fissure on qualitative assessment of HRCT
- Large bullae >30% in either lung
- Incidental pulmonary nodules

Chartis™ assessment
- Collateral ventilation positive assessed by Chartis™

PULMONARY FUNCTION TESTING AND EXERCISE CAPACITY

Eligible patients with advanced COPD for BLVR on PFT include post-bronchodilator FEV_1 ≤45% predicted, RV ≥150% predicted, TLC ≥100%, and 6MWD ≥100m and <500m (Table 2.1). Contraindications to EBV placement include evidence of end-stage pulmonary disease including resting hypoxemia (arterial partial pressure of oxygen [PaO2] <45 mmHg], hypercapnia (arterial partial pressure of carbon dioxide [PaCO2] >55 mmHg], FEV_1 <15% predicted, DLCO <20%, and 6MWD <100m (Table 2.3).

Surgical NETT data found that a high-risk subgroup included patients with diffuse emphysema on HRCT and FEV_1 levels below 20% predicted or DLCO below 20% [21]. These patients were excluded from studies mentioned above. Yet, a retrospective study conducted at a single center observed positive clinical outcomes, including improvements in lung function, exercise capacity, and quality of life, following EBV treatment in patients with DLCO below 20%, without an associated increase in mortality or adverse effects [22]. Additionally, two small-scale single-center studies reported clinical enhancements in lung function and exercise tolerance after EBV placement in patients with FEV_1 levels below 20%, albeit with varying rates of improvement [23, 24]. In light of these varying findings on the inclusion of high-risk patients in EBV trials, the complex interplay between factors such as FEV_1, DLCO, and emphysema heterogeneity emphasizes the need for continued research and approach in tailoring interventions for patients with severe emphysema.

Patients suffering from emphysema encounter a limitation to exercise linked to the extent of obstruction, static and dynamic hyperinflation, and impact on respiratory muscle function (Figure 2.2) [25]. Some studies indicate a correlation between reduced exercise capacity during CPET and static and dynamic hyperinflation, attributable to the severity of ventilatory restriction [26, 27]. Following LVRS treatment, patients experienced improved elastic recoil, pulmonary function, and dyspnea. Data from NETT revealed that a 6MWD exceeding 140m after completion of pulmonary rehabilitation served as an indicator for higher endurance and functional reserve, and these patients experienced reduced perioperative and postoperative mortality [2]. In a post-hoc analysis, individuals with upper lobe emphysema and low exercise capacity after eight weeks of rehabilitation (defined as <25 W for women and <40 W for men)

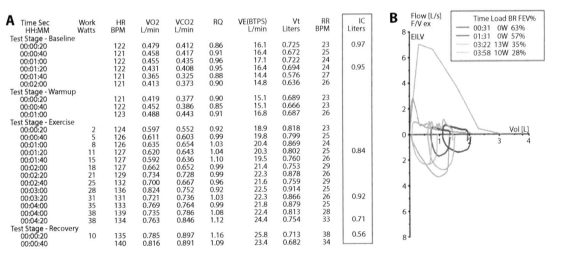

A

Time Sec HH:MM	Work Watts	HR BPM	VO2 L/min	VCO2 L/min	RQ	VE(BTPS) L/min	Vt Liters	RR BPM	IC Liters
Test Stage - Baseline									
00:00:20		122	0.479	0.412	0.86	16.1	0.725	23	0.97
00:00:40		121	0.458	0.417	0.91	16.4	0.672	25	
00:01:00		122	0.455	0.435	0.96	17.1	0.722	24	
00:01:20		122	0.431	0.408	0.95	16.4	0.694	24	0.95
00:01:40		121	0.365	0.325	0.88	14.4	0.576	27	
00:02:00		121	0.413	0.373	0.90	14.8	0.636	26	
Test Stage - Warmup									
00:00:20		121	0.419	0.377	0.90	15.1	0.689	23	
00:00:40		122	0.452	0.386	0.85	15.1	0.666	23	
00:01:00		123	0.488	0.443	0.91	16.8	0.687	26	
Test Stage - Exercise									
00:00:20	2	124	0.597	0.552	0.92	18.9	0.818	23	
00:00:40	5	126	0.611	0.603	0.99	19.8	0.799	25	
00:01:00	8	126	0.635	0.654	1.03	20.4	0.869	24	
00:01:20	11	127	0.620	0.643	1.04	20.3	0.802	25	0.84
00:01:40	15	127	0.592	0.636	1.10	19.5	0.760	26	
00:02:00	18	127	0.662	0.652	0.99	21.4	0.753	29	
00:02:20	21	129	0.734	0.728	0.99	22.3	0.878	26	
00:02:40	25	132	0.700	0.667	0.96	21.6	0.759	29	
00:03:00	28	136	0.824	0.752	0.92	22.5	0.914	25	
00:03:20	31	131	0.721	0.736	1.03	22.3	0.866	26	0.92
00:04:00	35	133	0.769	0.764	0.99	21.8	0.879	25	
00:04:00	38	139	0.735	0.786	1.08	22.4	0.813	28	
00:04:20	38	134	0.763	0.846	1.12	24.4	0.754	33	0.71
Test Stage - Recovery									
00:00:20	10	135	0.785	0.897	1.16	25.8	0.713	38	0.56
00:00:40		140	0.816	0.891	1.09	23.4	0.682	34	

B

Flow [L/s] F/V ex

EILV

Vol [L]

Time Load BR FEV%
— 00:31 0W 63%
— 01:31 0W 57%
03:22 13W 35%
03:58 10W 28%

FIGURE 2.2 Cardiopulmonary exercise test of (A) patient 1 with decreasing inspiratory capacity (box) with exercise indicative of dynamic hyperinflation and (B) patient 2 with flow-volume curves depicting increasing end-expiratory lung volume, decreasing end-inspiratory lung volume (EILV), and worsening expiratory flow limitation (FEV%) with exercise duration at 00:31, 01:31, 3:22, and 3:56.

exhibited decreased mortality, improved exercise capacity, and symptom relief in contrast with those with homogeneous emphysema and high exercise capacity. This latter group experienced increased mortality without changes in exercise capacity or symptoms following LVRS [2]. The implications of these findings for BLVR remain uncertain, emphasizing the need for research on the relevance of exercise tolerance parameters in the context of BLVR.

HIGH-RESOLUTION COMPUTED TOMOGRAPHY

High-resolution computed tomography (HRCT) provides essential information on the distribution and severity of emphysema, fissure integrity, lung volumes, and potential indications of other pulmonary diseases such as bronchiectasis, bronchitis, and pulmonary nodules, which may require further assessment [6, 16]. Software analyses for quantitative emphysema assessment on HRCT utilize low attenuation area (LAA%) at different thresholds to visualize the extent of lung tissue destruction [28]. It is important to note that thresholds are not yet standardized and applying different software programs may yield different results (Figures 2.3 and 2.4). Prior studies including the LIBERATE trial used a target lobe selection greater than 50–60% destruction score (percentage of voxels less than −910 Hounsfield units) on CT as part of the inclusion criteria for EBV placement [7, 9].

Quantitative programming enables the identification of lobes with the highest degree of destruction, serving as one method to identify potential targets for intervention. The distribution of interlobar and intralobar emphysema can also be more precisely characterized as either heterogeneous or homogeneous. The heterogeneity index, derived from LAA% scores, is defined as the absolute difference between emphysema scores in the target and adjacent lobes [3, 9]. An index score of 15% or greater has been used to indicate heterogeneous emphysema, while a value 15% or less indicates homogenous emphysema [3, 9].

FISSURE ANALYSIS AND COLLATERAL VENTILATION

Imaging offers a noninvasive method for evaluating the completeness of interlobar fissures to predict the presence or absence of collateral ventilation (Figure 2.5). Intact fissures are believed to limit collateral ventilation between lobes, leading to increased atelectasis. Both collateral ventilation and fissure integrity are pivotal factors that influence the success of EBV interventions [29]. Incomplete interlobar fissures have been identified as predictive indicators of collateral ventilation [30–32]. Ideal candidates for EBV are those with intact lobar fissures (defined as >90% complete on at least one axis on HRCT) (Figures 2.3 and 2.4) and minimal collateral ventilation, as assessed by the Chartis™ system. Such candidates are more likely to achieve the desired outcomes of lobar occlusion and reduction in hyperinflation [6, 33].

Quantitative imaging demonstrates a 92.9% negative predictive rate in patients with incomplete interlobar fissures (<80% interlobar fissure completeness score) and an 88.1% positive predictive value of complete fissures (>95% fissure completeness score) [16]. HRCT serves as a prescreening tool to rule out patients for EBV treatments or additional invasive diagnostic testing in patients with incomplete fissures [16].

The Chartis™ Pulmonary Assessment System employs an endobronchial catheter-based measurement to quantify fissure analysis. A catheter with an inflatable balloon at the distal tip through the working channel of a bronchoscopy is used to isolate the lung compartment and measure airflow and pressure to quantify collateral ventilation [34]. Patients with no significant interlobar ventilation benefit from valve implantation and are categorized as collateral ventilation negative. Chartis™ as a tool for collateral ventilation assessment entails the need for a bronchoscopic procedure, potentially extending the total

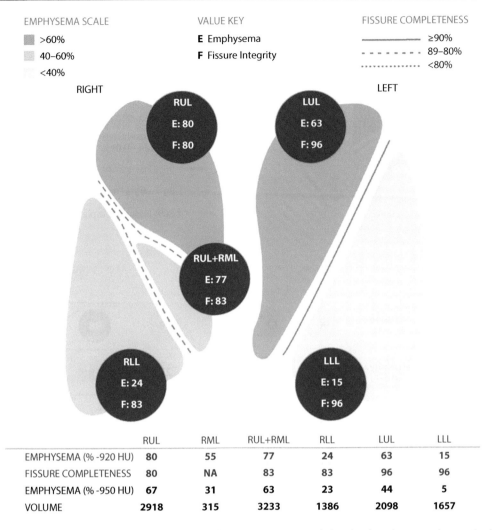

	RUL	RML	RUL+RML	RLL	LUL	LLL
EMPHYSEMA (% -920 HU)	80	55	77	24	63	15
FISSURE COMPLETENESS	80	NA	83	83	96	96
EMPHYSEMA (% -950 HU)	67	31	63	23	44	5
VOLUME	2918	315	3233	1386	2098	1657

FIGURE 2.3 SeleCT report (Olympus™) displaying percentage voxel density (emphysema destruction) less than −920 HU and −950 HU, percentage fissure completeness, and inspiratory lobar volume. Fissure completeness depicted as a percentage and fissure lines (dotted/dashed/solid).

procedural time and increasing procedural costs. Additionally, there is a risk of obtaining false positives in the presence of secretions, apposition of the catheter against an airway wall, or anatomical factors [35–37]. However, the Chartis™ assessment provides important information regarding the likelihood of success of EBV and can be done right before the planned EBV procedure and takes only three to four minutes to perform. The combined use of both diagnostic tools enhances the accuracy of evaluating interlobar fissure completeness and identifying the absence of collateral ventilation.

NUCLEAR PERFUSION/VENTILATION SCANS

Target lobes are also determined by evaluating the percentage of perfusion through ventilation and perfusion (VQ) single-photon emission computed tomography (SPECT)-computed tomography (CT) analysis

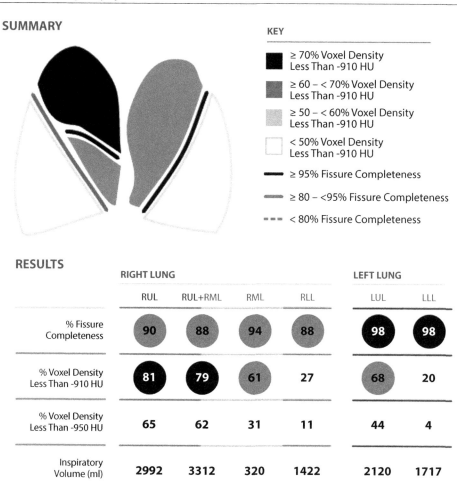

FIGURE 2.4   StratX lung report (PulmonX®) displaying % fissure completeness, % voxel density (emphysema destruction) less than -910 HU and -950 HU, and inspiratory lobar volume. Fissure completeness depicted as a percentage and fissure lines (gray/black, dotted/solid).

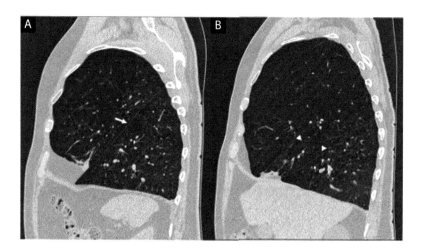

FIGURE 2.5   Sagittal plane of CT chest demonstrating (A) complete interlobar fissure of left lung (arrow) and (B) incomplete minor and major fissure of right lung (arrowheads). On Chartis™ assessment, patient was CV+ in the right upper lobe and right lower lobe.

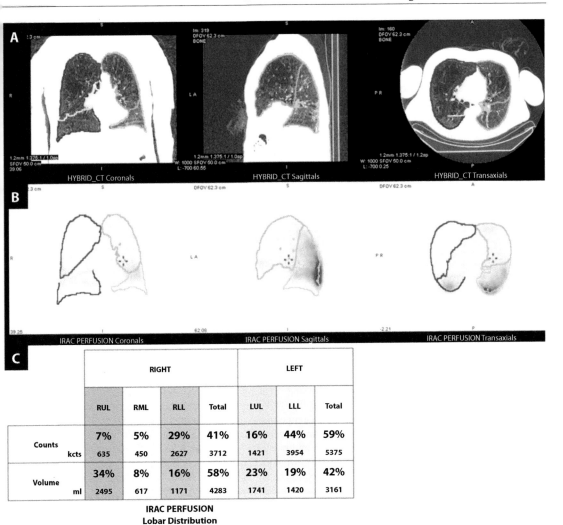

FIGURE 2.6 Nuclear medicine lung quantitative ventilation and perfusion SPECT-CT; (A) CT images with fissures delineated; (B) perfusion images with superimposed fissures from CT; (C) table with relative lobar perfusion based on radionuclide counts (kct and lobar percentage distribution) and volume (ml and lobar percentage distribution).

(Figure 2.6). In the NETT, patients that had LVRS performed in the emphysematous regions that were most oligemic had the greatest magnitude of improvements in FEV_1, exercise performance reduction in dyspnea, quality of life, and survival [38]. Similar data has been preliminarily generated with using perfusion assessment in planning for target lobe selection with BLVR. Patients with low target lobe regional perfusion exhibit significant improvements in exercise capacity and symptom relief compared with those with higher baseline target lobe regional perfusion [39–41]. While the distribution of lobar perfusion may contribute to differences in clinical outcomes post-valve placement, further research is essential to comprehensively grasp the physiologic and functional implications [41]. Interestingly, one study using data from the VENT trial showed that patients with heterogeneous emphysema and low baseline target lobe perfusion had a significant improvement in exercise capacity when compared with those with a high baseline regional perfusion and independent of the extent of emphysematous destruction [39]. In cases where multiple lobes are eligible for treatment based on CT findings, perfusion scans may function as a crucial tool in identifying the optimal target lobe for intervention.

CONCLUSION

In summary, careful selection of patients and target lobes in BLVR procedures are essential in influencing the overall success of the intervention. A thorough assessment, encompassing a detailed analysis of patient history, clinical examination, functional testing, and various imaging modalities, serves as a comprehensive strategy to enhance the efficacy of BLVR. This approach not only aids in refining patient selection but also contributes to the overall improvement in quality of life for individuals grappling with advanced COPD and emphysema.

REFERENCES

1. Valipour, A. and O. C. Burghuber. "An update on the efficacy of endobronchial valve therapy in the management of hyperinflation in patients with chronic obstructive pulmonary disease." *Ther Adv Respir Dis* 9 (2015): 294–301. 10.1177/1753465815599693. https://www.ncbi.nlm.nih.gov/pubmed/26294417.
2. Fishman, A., F. Martinez, K. Naunheim, S. Piantadosi, R. Wise, A. Ries, G. Weinmann, D. E. Wood and G. National Emphysema Treatment Trial Research. "A randomized trial comparing lung-volume-reduction surgery with medical therapy for severe emphysema." *N Engl J Med* 348 (2003): 2059–73. 10.1056/NEJMoa030287. https://www.ncbi.nlm.nih.gov/pubmed/12759479.
3. Sciurba, F. C., A. Ernst, F. J. Herth, C. Strange, G. J. Criner, C. H. Marquette, K. L. Kovitz, R. P. Chiacchierini, J. Goldin, G. McLennan, *et al.* "A randomized study of endobronchial valves for advanced emphysema." *N Engl J Med* 363 (2010): 1233–44. 10.1056/NEJMoa0900928. https://www.ncbi.nlm.nih.gov/pubmed/20860505.
4. Koenigkam-Santos, M., M. Puderbach, D. Gompelmann, R. Eberhardt, F. Herth, H. U. Kauczor and C. P. Heussel. "Incomplete fissures in severe emphysematous patients evaluated with MDCT: Incidence and interobserver agreement among radiologists and pneumologists." *Eur J Radiol* 81 (2012): 4161–6. 10.1016/j.ejrad.2012.06.006. https://www.ncbi.nlm.nih.gov/pubmed/22770581.
5. Davey, C., Z. Zoumot, S. Jordan, W. H. McNulty, D. H. Carr, M. D. Hind, D. M. Hansell, M. B. Rubens, W. Banya, M. I. Polkey, *et al.* "Bronchoscopic lung volume reduction with endobronchial valves for patients with heterogeneous emphysema and intact interlobar fissures (the believer-hifi study): A randomised controlled trial." *Lancet* 386 (2015): 1066–73. 10.1016/S0140-6736(15)60001-0. https://www.ncbi.nlm.nih.gov/pubmed/26116485.
6. Herth, F. J., R. Eberhardt, D. Gompelmann, J. H. Ficker, M. Wagner, L. Ek, B. Schmidt and D. J. Slebos. "Radiological and clinical outcomes of using chartis to plan endobronchial valve treatment." *Eur Respir J* 41 (2013): 302–8. 10.1183/09031936.00015312. https://www.ncbi.nlm.nih.gov/pubmed/22556025.
7. Klooster, K., N. H. ten Hacken, J. E. Hartman, H. A. Kerstjens, E. M. van Rikxoort and D. J. Slebos. "Endobronchial valves for emphysema without interlobar collateral ventilation." *N Engl J Med* 373 (2015): 2325–35. 10.1056/NEJMoa1507807. https://www.ncbi.nlm.nih.gov/pubmed/26650153.
8. Valipour, A., D. J. Slebos, F. Herth, K. Darwiche, M. Wagner, J. H. Ficker, C. Petermann, R. H. Hubner, F. Stanzel, R. Eberhardt, *et al.* "Endobronchial valve therapy in patients with homogeneous emphysema. Results from the impact study." *Am J Respir Crit Care Med* 194 (2016): 1073–82. 10.1164/rccm.201607-1383OC. https://www.ncbi.nlm.nih.gov/pubmed/27580428.
9. Criner, G. J., R. Sue, S. Wright, M. Dransfield, H. Rivas-Perez, T. Wiese, F. C. Sciurba, P. L. Shah, M. M. Wahidi, H. G. de Oliveira, *et al.* "A multicenter randomized controlled trial of zephyr endobronchial valve treatment in heterogeneous emphysema (liberate)." *Am J Respir Crit Care Med* 198 (2018): 1151–64. 10.1164/rccm.201803-0590OC. https://www.ncbi.nlm.nih.gov/pubmed/29787288.
10. Criner, G. J., A. Delage, K. Voelker, D. K. Hogarth, A. Majid, M. Zgoda, D. R. Lazarus, R. Casal, S. B. Benzaquen, R. C. Holladay, *et al.* "Improving lung function in severe heterogenous emphysema with the spiration valve system (EMPROVE). A multicenter, open-label randomized controlled clinical trial." *Am J Respir Crit Care Med* 200 (2019): 1354–62. 10.1164/rccm.201902-0383OC. https://www.ncbi.nlm.nih.gov/pubmed/31365298.

11. Ninane, V., C. Geltner, M. Bezzi, P. Foccoli, J. Gottlieb, T. Welte, L. Seijo, J. J. Zulueta, M. Munavvar, A. Rosell, et al. "Multicentre European study for the treatment of advanced emphysema with bronchial valves." *Eur Respir J* 39 (2012): 1319–25. 10.1183/09031936.00019711. https://www.ncbi.nlm.nih.gov/pubmed/22654006.

12. Criner, G. J., J. M. Mallea, M. Abu-Hijleh, A. Sachdeva, R. Kalhan, C. A. Hergott, D. R. Lazarus, R. A. Mularski, K. Calero, M. F. Reed, et al. "Sustained clinical benefits of spiration valve system in severe emphysema patients: 24-month follow-up of EMPROVE." *Ann Am Thorac Soc* (2023): 10.1513/AnnalsATS.202306-520OC. https://www.ncbi.nlm.nih.gov/pubmed/37948704.

13. Kemp, S. V., D. J. Slebos, A. Kirk, M. Kornaszewska, K. Carron, L. Ek, G. Broman, G. Hillerdal, H. Mal, C. Pison, et al. "A multicenter randomized controlled trial of zephyr endobronchial valve treatment in heterogeneous emphysema (transform)." *Am J Respir Crit Care Med* 196 (2017): 1535–43. 10.1164/rccm.201707-1327OC. https://www.ncbi.nlm.nih.gov/pubmed/28885054.

14. Fletcher, C. M., P. C. Elmes, A. S. Fairbairn and C. H. Wood. "The significance of respiratory symptoms and the diagnosis of chronic bronchitis in a working population." *Br Med J* 2 (1959): 257–66. 10.1136/bmj.2.5147.257. https://www.ncbi.nlm.nih.gov/pubmed/13823475.

15. Mahler, D. A. and C. K. Wells. "Evaluation of clinical methods for rating dyspnea." *Chest* 93 (1988): 580–6. 10.1378/chest.93.3.580. https://www.ncbi.nlm.nih.gov/pubmed/3342669.

16. Koster, T. D., E. M. van Rikxoort, R. H. Huebner, F. Doellinger, K. Klooster, J. P. Charbonnier, S. Radhakrishnan, F. J. Herth and D. J. Slebos. "Predicting lung volume reduction after endobronchial valve therapy is maximized using a combination of diagnostic tools." *Respiration* 92 (2016): 150–7. 10.1159/000448849. https://www.ncbi.nlm.nih.gov/pubmed/27577190.

17. Tuohy, M. M., K. F. Remund, R. Hilfiker, D. T. Murphy, J. G. Murray and J. J. Egan. "Endobronchial valve deployment in severe alpha-1 antitrypsin deficiency emphysema: A case series." *Clin Respir J* 7 (2013): 45–52. 10.1111/j.1752-699X.2012.00280.x. https://www.ncbi.nlm.nih.gov/pubmed/22236390.

18. Hillerdal, G. and S. Mindus. "One- to four-year follow-up of endobronchial lung volume reduction in alpha-1-antitrypsin deficiency patients: A case series." *Respiration* 88 (2014): 320–8. 10.1159/000365662. https://www.ncbi.nlm.nih.gov/pubmed/25227936.

19. Everaerts, S., J. E. Hartman, M. Van Dijk, T. D. Koster, D. J. Slebos and K. Klooster. "Bronchoscopic lung volume reduction in patients with emphysema due to alpha-1 antitrypsin deficiency." *Respiration* 102 (2023): 134–42. 10.1159/000528182. https://www.ncbi.nlm.nih.gov/pubmed/36549279.

20. Eberhardt, R., V. Gerovasili, K. Kontogianni, D. Gompelmann, N. Ehlken, F. J. Herth, E. Grunig and C. Nagel. "Endoscopic lung volume reduction with endobronchial valves in patients with severe emphysema and established pulmonary hypertension." *Respiration* 89 (2015): 41–8. 10.1159/000368369. https://www.ncbi.nlm.nih.gov/pubmed/25502235.

21. National Emphysema Treatment Trial Research, G., A. Fishman, H. Fessler, F. Martinez, R. J. McKenna, Jr., K. Naunheim, S. Piantadosi, G. Weinmann and R. Wise. "Patients at high risk of death after lung-volume-reduction surgery." *N Engl J Med* 345 (2001): 1075–83. 10.1056/NEJMoa11798. https://www.ncbi.nlm.nih.gov/pubmed/11596586.

22. van Dijk, M., J. E. Hartman, K. Klooster, N. H. T. Ten Hacken, H. A. M. Kerstjens and D. J. Slebos. "Endobronchial valve treatment in emphysema patients with a very low dlco." *Respiration* 99 (2020): 163–70. 10.1159/000505428. https://www.ncbi.nlm.nih.gov/pubmed/31962325.

23. Darwiche, K., R. Karpf-Wissel, S. Eisenmann, C. Aigner, S. Welter, P. Zarogoulidis, W. Hohenforst-Schmidt, L. Freitag and F. Oezkan. "Bronchoscopic lung volume reduction with endobronchial valves in low-fevl patients." *Respiration* 92 (2016): 414–19. 10.1159/000452629. https://www.ncbi.nlm.nih.gov/pubmed/27838695.

24. Trudzinski, F. C., A. J. Hoink, D. Leppert, S. Fahndrich, H. Wilkens, T. P. Graeter, F. Langer, R. Bals, P. Minko and P. M. Lepper. "Endoscopic lung volume reduction using endobronchial valves in patients with severe emphysema and very low fevl." *Respiration* 92 (2016): 258–65. 10.1159/000448761. https://www.ncbi.nlm.nih.gov/pubmed/27603781.

25. Martinez, F. J., M. M. de Oca, R. I. Whyte, J. Stetz, S. E. Gay and B. R. Celli. "Lung-volume reduction improves dyspnea, dynamic hyperinflation, and respiratory muscle function." *Am J Respir Crit Care Med* 155 (1997): 1984–90. 10.1164/ajrccm.155.6.9196106. https://www.ncbi.nlm.nih.gov/pubmed/9196106.

26. O'Donnell, D. E., S. M. Revill and K. A. Webb. "Dynamic hyperinflation and exercise intolerance in chronic obstructive pulmonary disease." *Am J Respir Crit Care Med* 164 (2001): 770–7. 10.1164/ajrccm.164.5.2012122. https://www.ncbi.nlm.nih.gov/pubmed/11549531.

27. Vassaux, C., L. Torre-Bouscoulet, S. Zeineldine, F. Cortopassi, H. Paz-Diaz, B. R. Celli and V. M. Pinto-Plata. "Effects of hyperinflation on the oxygen pulse as a marker of cardiac performance in copd." *Eur Respir J* 32 (2008): 1275–82. 10.1183/09031936.00151707. https://www.ncbi.nlm.nih.gov/pubmed/18550609.

28. Heussel, C. P., F. J. Herth, J. Kappes, R. Hantusch, S. Hartlieb, O. Weinheimer, H. U. Kauczor and R. Eberhardt. "Fully automatic quantitative assessment of emphysema in computed tomography: Comparison with pulmonary function testing and normal values." *Eur Radiol* 19 (2009): 2391–402. 10.1007/s00330-009-1437-z. https://www.ncbi.nlm.nih.gov/pubmed/19458953.

29. Shah, P. L. and F. J. Herth. "Current status of bronchoscopic lung volume reduction with endobronchial valves." *Thorax* 69 (2014): 280–6. 10.1136/thoraxjnl-2013-203743. https://www.ncbi.nlm.nih.gov/pubmed/24008689.

30. Reymond, E., A. Jankowski, C. Pison, J. L. Bosson, M. Prieur, W. Aniwidyaningsih and G. R. Ferretti. "Prediction of lobar collateral ventilation in 25 patients with severe emphysema by fissure analysis with ct." *AJR Am J Roentgenol* 201 (2013): W571–5. 10.2214/AJR.12.9843. https://www.ncbi.nlm.nih.gov/pubmed/24059394.

31. de Oliveira, H. G., S. M. de Oliveira, R. R. Rambo and A. V. de Macedo Neto. "Fissure integrity and volume reduction in emphysema: A retrospective study." *Respiration* 91 (2016): 471–9. 10.1159/000446288. https://www.ncbi.nlm.nih.gov/pubmed/27241515.

32. Gompelmann, D., R. Eberhardt, D. J. Slebos, M. S. Brown, F. Abtin, H. J. Kim, D. Holmes-Higgin, S. Radhakrishnan, F. J. Herth and J. Goldin. "Diagnostic performance comparison of the chartis system and high-resolution computerized tomography fissure analysis for planning endoscopic lung volume reduction." *Respirology* 19 (2014): 524–30. 10.1111/resp.12253. https://www.ncbi.nlm.nih.gov/pubmed/24612306.

33. Goldin, J. G. and F. Abtin. "Update on radiology of emphysema and therapeutic implications." *Thorac Surg Clin* 19 (2009): 159–67, vii. 10.1016/j.thorsurg.2009.04.006. https://www.ncbi.nlm.nih.gov/pubmed/19662958.

34. Klooster, K., T. D. Koster, C. Ruwwe-Glosenkamp, D. Theilig, F. Doellinger, J. Saccomanno, H. A. M. Kerstjens, D. J. Slebos and R. H. Hubner. "An integrative approach of the fissure completeness score and chartis assessment in endobronchial valve treatment for emphysema." *Int J Chron Obstruct Pulmon Dis* 15 (2020): 1325–34. 10.2147/COPD.S242210. https://www.ncbi.nlm.nih.gov/pubmed/32606642.

35. Gompelmann, D., R. Eberhardt and F. J. Herth. "Collateral ventilation." *Respiration* 85 (2013): 515–20. 10.1159/000348269. https://www.ncbi.nlm.nih.gov/pubmed/23485627.

36. Shah, P. L. and F. J. Herth. "Dynamic expiratory airway collapse and evaluation of collateral ventilation with chartis." *Thorax* 69 (2014): 290–1. 10.1136/thoraxjnl-2013-204875. https://www.ncbi.nlm.nih.gov/pubmed/24355826.

37. Lee, S. W., S. Y. Shin, T. S. Park, Y. Y. Choi, J. C. Park, J. Park, S. Y. Oh, N. Kim, S. H. Lee, J. S. Lee, *et al.* "Clinical utility of quantitative ct analysis for fissure completeness in bronchoscopic lung volume reduction: Comparison between ct and chartis." *Korean J Radiol* 20 (2019): 1216–25. 10.3348/kjr.2018.0724. https://www.ncbi.nlm.nih.gov/pubmed/31270985.

38. Chandra, D., D. A. Lipson, E. A. Hoffman, J. Hansen-Flaschen, F. C. Sciurba, M. M. Decamp, J. J. Reilly, G. R. Washko and G. National Emphysema Treatment Trial Research. "Perfusion scintigraphy and patient selection for lung volume reduction surgery." *Am J Respir Crit Care Med* 182 (2010): 937–46. 10.1164/rccm.201001-0043OC. https://www.ncbi.nlm.nih.gov/pubmed/20538961.

39. Argula, R. G., C. Strange, V. Ramakrishnan and J. Goldin. "Baseline regional perfusion impacts exercise response to endobronchial valve therapy in advanced pulmonary emphysema." *Chest* 144 (2013): 1578–86. 10.1378/chest.12-2826. https://www.ncbi.nlm.nih.gov/pubmed/23828481.

40. Kristiansen, J. F., M. Perch, M. Iversen, M. Krakauer and J. Mortensen. "Lobar quantification by ventilation/perfusion spect/ct in patients with severe emphysema undergoing lung volume reduction with endobronchial valves." *Respiration* 98 (2019): 230–38. 10.1159/000500407. https://www.ncbi.nlm.nih.gov/pubmed/31167210.

41. Thomsen, C., D. Theilig, D. Herzog, A. Poellinger, F. Doellinger, N. Schreiter, V. Schreiter, D. Schurmann, B. Temmesfeld-Wollbrueck, S. Hippenstiel, *et al.* "Lung perfusion and emphysema distribution affect the outcome of endobronchial valve therapy." *Int J Chron Obstruct Pulmon Dis* 11 (2016): 1245–59. 10.2147/COPD.S101003. https://www.ncbi.nlm.nih.gov/pubmed/27354783.

The Concept of Lung Volume Reduction and the Best Evidence

3

Nathaniel Marchetti and Gerard J. Criner

INTRODUCTION

Chronic obstructive pulmonary disease (COPD) remains a common and morbid disease characterized by progressive airflow obstruction related to smoking or inhalation of other noxious gases such as air pollution or biomass fuels (1). Airflow obstruction occurs primarily in the small airways. Medical therapy is the mainstay of COPD therapy and improves the quality of life, reduces acute exacerbations, and improves symptoms. However, the effectiveness of medical therapy is limited in advanced disease, resulting in a poor quality of life despite aggressive therapy. Dyspnea is ubiquitous in patients with COPD and both static and dynamic hyperinflation are a major physiologic derangement contributing to dyspnea and exercise limitation (1, 2). Efforts to reduce hyperinflation medically, surgically, or with bronchoscopic approaches are available for those with hyperinflation. This chapter will briefly review how hyperinflation results in dyspnea and exercise limitation and review the evidence to support the concept of lung volume reduction as a major goal in treating advanced COPD.

PATHOPHYSIOLOGY OF HYPERINFLATION

The underlying physiologic derangement in COPD is expiratory airflow limitation, which is due to both emphysema and airway disease in the distal small airways. Small airways are narrowed due to smooth muscle hypertrophy, peri-bronchial fibrosis, airway inflammation, and mucus plugging. Emphysema results in the destruction of alveolar walls, leading to a loss of the tethering of the distal airways, predisposing the airway to expiratory collapse (1, 3). Lung emptying is determined by the expiratory time constant, which is the product of airway resistance and lung compliance. Because those with emphysema

DOI: 10.1201/9781003251439-3

have increased lung compliance and airways resistance, they are predisposed to developing hyperinflation (4). As the disease progresses, hyperinflation and gas trapping worsen due to increasing lung compliance and unopposed chest wall recoil, thus worsening static hyperinflation. The residual volume (RV) increases due to early airway closure and large volumes of air that are trapped in lung cysts and bullae (5, 6). Inspiratory muscles are incapable of expanding the lung much above RV, and while the total lung capacity (TLC) does increase, it will not increase to the same degree that the RV does. Thus, the difference between RV and TLC, vital capacity (VC), decreases as lung volumes increase in COPD. As the RV/TLC ratio increases, the VC continues to fall, and because FEV_1 depends on VC and can never exceed VC, FEV_1 decreases. Fessler and Permut proposed that FEV_1 can be explained with the following equation:

$$FEV_1 = (FEV_1/VC) \times (1\text{-}RV/TLC) \times (TLC)$$

Where 1-RV/TLC represents the fraction of TLC that can leave the lungs and FEV_1/VC represents the fraction of the volume that leaves in the first second to the total volume that can leave: 1-RV/TLC had strong correlation with FEV_1 (r = 0.88, p < 0.001), but the TLC and FEV_1VC did not correlate with FEV_1 in a group of ten patients with homogenous alpha-1 anti-trypsin deficiency (5). This suggests that hyperinflation and specifically RV contribute to a decline in FEV_1.

During exertion, the respiratory rate will increase, thereby reducing time spent during exhalation, and the end-expiratory lung volume (EELV) will increase even further, leading to dynamic hyperinflation (2) (Figure 3.1). As the EELV increases, the tidal volume cannot be increased as much as in individuals with normal lungs. To increase their minute ventilation, these individuals will increase breathing frequency, which will only result in more dynamic hyperinflation. Because TLC does not increase during exercise (7) as the EELV increases, the end-inspiratory lung volume begins to approach the inspiratory

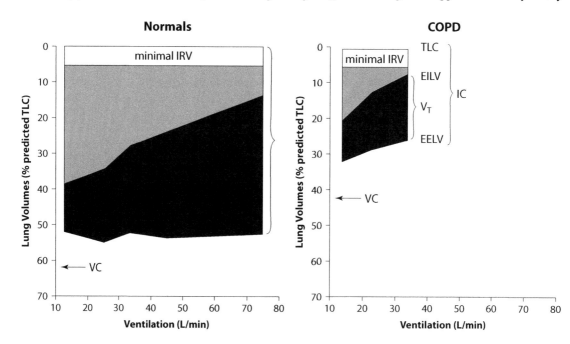

FIGURE 3.1 Lung volumes during exercise. The left panel is a normal individual who is able to expand tidal volume during exercise without having end-expiratory lung volumes rise. The right panel demonstrates operational lung volumes during exercise in a COPD patient. The end-expiratory lung volume rises and the inspiratory capacity falls, limiting expansion of tidal volume. Once the end-inspiratory lung volume approaches the inspiratory reserve volume, refractory dyspnea develops and exercise stops. Adapted with permission from O'Donnell et al. (2). Abbreviations: TLC, total lung capacity; VC, vital capacity; IRV, inspiratory reserve volume; EELV, end-expiratory lung volume; EILV, end-inspiratory lung volume; V_T, tidal volume.

reserve volume. O'Donnell demonstrated that once an inspiratory reserve volume of about 500 mL is reached during exercise, patients with COPD demonstrate an abrupt increase in dyspnea and exercise ceases (8). Patients with COPD often describe a sensation of not being able to "inhale deeply" during exercise. Using esophageal balloons, O'Donnell measured the effort-displacement ratio during exercise. The effort-displacement ratio is defined as the ratio between tidal swings of esophageal pressure (P_{es}) expressed relative to the maximum inspiratory pressure (PI_{max}) and the tidal volume (V_t) expressed relative to predicted vital capacity (P_{es}/PI_{max}:V_t/VC predicted). They found that this ratio increased dramatically compared with normal individuals during exercise. The authors concluded that the sensation COPD patients experience during exercise (inability to inhale deeply) is related to the increased respiratory effort for only a minimal increase in tidal volume (8, 9). This is known as neuromechanical dissociation, and it is a major factor in the sensation of exertional dyspnea in patients with advanced COPD who develop dynamic hyperinflation.

OTHER CONSEQUENCES OF HYPERINFLATION

Clearly, hyperinflation leads to dyspnea and exercise limitation, but there are other deleterious effects of hyperinflation. Jorgensen measured cardiac index (CI) and used transesophageal echocardiography to measure the left ventricular end-diastolic area index (EADI) pre- and post-operatively in ten patients undergoing lung volume reduction surgery (LVRS) (FEV_1 28 ± 2% predicted) and ten patients without COPD who had a lobectomy (FEV_1 82 ± 7% predicted). Measurements were taken just after induction with anesthesia and then following surgery once the chest was closed. Patients who underwent LVRS had lower CI and left ventricular EDAI compared with those who had a lobectomy. Immediately following LVRS, CI (1.86 ± 0.16 vs. 2.60 ± 0.18 L/min/m², p = 0.002) and left ventricular EADI (5.62 ± 0.55 vs. 6.61 ± 0.52 cm²/m², p = 0.009) improved significantly, while there was no change in either parameter following lobectomy (10). The same investigators subsequently performed cardiac magnetic resonance imaging (MRI) in 13 hyperinflated and gas-trapped (TLC 139 ± 24% predicted and RV 273 ± 64 %predicted) patients with emphysema and in ten healthy controls matched for age and body surface area. Compared with the healthy control group, those with emphysema had a significantly lower left ventricular end-diastolic volume index (84 ± 15 vs. 66 ± 12 mL/m², p = 0.002) as well as a lower right ventricular end-diastolic volume index (91 ± 15 vs. 73 ± 12 mL/m², p = 0.004). Patients with emphysema also had lower CI (2.5 ± 0.6 vs. 3.2 ± 0.7 mL/m², p = 0.02) as well as a lower intrathoracic blood volume index (0.29 ± 0.07 vs. 0.39 ± 0.05 L/m², p = 0.001) (11). Taken together, the authors suggest hyperinflation leads to decreased right and left ventricular filling, thereby affecting cardiac function. Watz et al. measured cardiac chamber sizes using echocardiography in 138 patients across all GOLD stages and demonstrated that with advancing GOLD stage, cardiac chamber size decreased. The inspiratory capacity to total lung capacity ratio (IC/TLC) correlated best with LV end-diastolic size (r = 0.56, p < 0.001), while RV (r = −0.45, p < 0.001) and functional residual capacity (FRC) (r = −0.50, p < 0.001) also had significant correlations with LV end-diastolic size (12). As part of a population-based study, the multi-ethnic study of atherosclerosis (MESA) study, 2,816 subjects had cardiac computed tomography (CT) scans, cardiac MRI, and spirometry. The amount of emphysema was measured in the visible lung (about 70% of lung volume) on the cardiac CT scan using mask density analysis. The investigators found that a ten-point increase in %-emphysema was linearly related to reductions in left ventricular end-diastolic volume (−4.1mL, −3.3 to −4.9, p < 0.001) and left ventricular stroke volume (−2.7mL, −2.2 to −3.3, p < 0.001), as well as a decreased cardiac output (−0.16 L/min, −0.14 to −0.23, p < 0.001). These effects were greatest among current smokers compared with former or non-smokers (13).

It has been postulated that static and dynamic hyperinflation could contribute to pulmonary hypertension in COPD due to widened intrathoracic pressure swings, cardiac effects of hyperinflation, direct compression of pulmonary vasculature due to hyperinflation, altered gas exchange, and pulmonary vascular remodeling. Despite the mechanistic possibilities, there are data to directly support the notion that static or dynamic hyperinflation leads to pulmonary hypertension (14).

Casanova et al. demonstrated that hyperinflation is related to increased mortality in COPD. They studied a cohort of 689 COPD patients recruited from multiple centers and followed them for an average of 34 months. They found that a decrease of 1% in the IC/TLC ratio was an independent predictor of all-cause mortality (RR 1.052, 1.022–1.083). Furthermore, an IC/TLC ratio of <25% was an important cut point with a sensitivity of 0.71, specificity of 0.69, and a negative predictive value of 0.87 for death during the study. Figure 3.2 shows the Kaplan–Meier curve for all-cause mortality in those with an IC/TLC ratio <25% compared with those with IC/TLC >25% (15). Additional evidence of hyperinflation being an independent predictor of mortality was demonstrated in a cohort of 310 COPD patients enrolled in the Korean

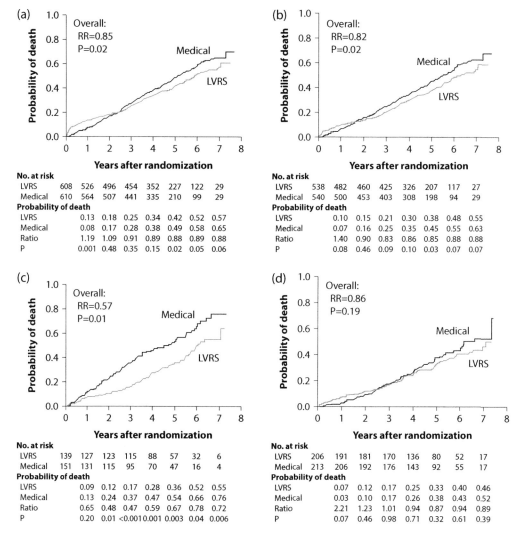

FIGURE 3.2   Kaplan–Meier survival curves as a function of years post-randomization to LVRS. The overall relative risk (RR) and p-value represent the 4.3 years median follow-up. Shown below each plot are the number of subjects at risk in each arm, the probability of death in each arm, the RR (LVRS:Medical) for each year, and the p-value for the difference in the probability. (a) All patients (n = 1,218). (b) Non-high-risk patients (n = 1,078). (c) Upper lobe predominant and low baseline exercise performance (n = 290). (d) Upper lobe predominant and high exercise capacity (n = 419). Adapted with permission from Naunheim et al. (32).

Obstructive Lung Disease (KOLD) study where patients were prospectively enrolled and followed over an average of five years. The investigators demonstrated that a higher RV/TLC ratio was an independent predictor of mortality (HR = 2.45, 1.16–5.17), and those with a higher RV/TLC and >10% emphysema on mask density analysis of CT imaging had an even greater risk of mortality (HR = 3.75, 1.81–7.73) (16).

Static and dynamic hyperinflation are major contributors to dyspnea, reduced exercise tolerance, decreased cardiac function, and increased risk of mortality in patients with COPD, thus making it an attractive target for therapy.

MEDICAL THERAPY

Fortunately, medical therapy for COPD has never been better and many options exist to reduce lung volumes medically, thereby improving symptoms related to hyperinflation. Prior to any invasive procedure, medical therapy should be maximized. Aggressive bronchodilator therapy is the mainstay, and combined long-acting muscarinic antagonist (LAMA) and long-acting beta agonist (LABA) have been shown to reduce static and dynamic hyperinflation (17–20) and even improve cardiac function by reducing hyperinflation (21). Supplemental oxygen (22) and pulmonary rehabilitation (23) reduce dynamic hyperinflation by altering respiratory mechanics primarily through a reduction in respiratory rate, thus allowing for longer expiratory time.

HISTORY OF LUNG VOLUME REDUCTION SURGERY

Brantigan first reported a case series of 33 hyperinflated COPD patients who had LVRS in 1959 (24). These initial cases were done unilaterally in two sequential procedures and combined with surgical lung denervation to help with mucus hypersecretion and bronchodilation. Although pulmonary function was not systematically measured, some patients reported improvements, but the procedure was not widely performed due to a reported mortality rate of 18%. Years later in 1995, Cooper reported a case series of 20 hyperinflated emphysema patients that had undergone LVRS without lung denervation (25). The same group had a follow-up case series detailing the outcomes of LVRS in 150 consecutive patients. They reported a 90-day mortality rate of 4% with dramatic improvements in FEV$_1$ (0.70 L, 25% predicted to 1.0 L 38% predicted) and in RV 6.0 L (288% predicted to 4.3 L 205% predicted) pre- and post-LVRS (26). Criner et al. published the first randomized trial demonstrating the effectiveness of LVRS (27) in 37 patients with advanced emphysema. Those undergoing LVRS had significant improvements in FEV$_1$ (26 ± 6.9 vs. 36 ± 13% predicted, p < 0.005), TLC (146 ± 26 vs. 125 ± 21% predicted, p < 0.005), RV (258 ± 58 vs. 192 ± 61% predicted, p = 0.001), and six-minute walk distance (6MWD) (282 ± 100 vs. 337 ± 99 m, p = 0.001) at three months compared with maximal medical therapy. A second single-center study randomized 48 patients to either medical therapy or LVRS and demonstrated improved FEV$_1$, shuttle walk distance, TLC, and RV at six months post-LVRS compared with medical therapy (28). The number of LVRS procedures increased dramatically during this time, but there were highly variable results among centers with mortality rates as high as 26%. Based on these data, the Agency for Healthcare Research and Quality (AHRQ) and Centers for Medicaid and Medicare (CMS) realized that a prospective randomized controlled clinical trial was needed to determine which patients with advanced emphysema would benefit from LVRS. The National Emphysema Treatment Trial (NETT) was designed to address these issues.

NATIONAL EMPHYSEMA TREATMENT TRIAL

There were 17 centers in NETT that enrolled patients with severe emphysema. They compared maximal medical therapy with LVRS along with maximal medical therapy (29). The main inclusion and exclusion criteria for the study are listed in Table 3.1. The primary endpoints of the study included 90-day survival and exercise performance on cardiopulmonary exercise testing, while secondary endpoints included lung function, patient symptoms, and quality of life. The study steering committee determined a priori that a 10 watt change in exercise performance and an eight-point change in St. George's Respiratory Questionnaire (SGRQ) were clinically meaningful changes since LVRS had significant morbidity and mortality. One of the goals of NETT was to define who would benefit from LVRS, so the investigators identified a priori the following prognostic factors: age, FEV_1 %-predicted, P_aCO_2, RV %-predicted, distribution of perfusion ion radionuclide lung scanning, homogeneity or heterogeneity of emphysema distribution on CT imaging, and the presence of hyperinflation on CXR (30). During the trial, but well before completion, the data safety monitoring board (DSMB) identified other important prognostic factors: diffusion capacity of carbon monoxide (DL_{CO}), maximal exercise capacity, RV/TLC ratio, ratio of expired ventilation in one

TABLE 3.1 Main inclusion and exclusion criteria from NETT

INCLUSION CRITERIA	EXCLUSION CRITERIA
BMI $\leq$31.1 kg/m² for men or $\leq$32.2 kg/m² for women	Previous lung transplant, LVRS, lobectomy, or median sternotomy
Stable on $\leq$20 mg prednisone	Bradycardia (HR <50 BPM), multifocal PVC, complex ventricular arrhythmia, or sustained SVT
CT imaging with bilateral emphysema	History of exercise-related syncope
FEV_1 $\leq$45% predicted	MI within six months and LVEF <45%
TLC $\geq$100% predicted	CHF within six months and LVEF <45%
RV $\geq$150% predicted	Uncontrolled hypertension (SBP >200 mm Hg or DBP >110 mm Hg)
P_aCO_2 $\leq$45 mm Hg	History of recurrent infections with clinically significant sputum production
6MWD $\geq$140 m	Significant pleural or interstitial lung disease
Ability to perform three minutes of unloaded cycling	Clinically significant bronchiectasis
Non-smoker for at least four months prior to screening	Pulmonary nodule requiring surgery
	Peak systolic pulmonary pressure >45 mm Hg or mean >30 mm Hg
	Oxygen requirement >6 LPM to keep saturation, $\geq$90% during exercise
	Unplanned weight loss >10% of usual body weight within 90 days
	Presence of systemic disease or cancer impacting survival in five years
	Inability to complete screening of baseline or follow-up data collection procedures

Abbreviations: BMI, body mass index; CT, computed tomography; LVEF, left ventricular function; PVC, premature ventricular contraction; SVT, supraventricular tachycardia; SBP, systolic blood pressure; DBP, diastolic blood pressure; 6MWD, six-minute walk distance.

minute to carbon dioxide excretion in one minute, presence or absence of upper lobe predominant emphysema, degree of dyspnea, quality of life, race or ethnic group, and sex.

By design, the surgical approach to LVRS was not uniform, as eight centers utilized only a median sternotomy approach, three centers used video-assisted thoracoscopic surgery (VATS), and the remaining six randomized to either approach: 25% to 30% of lung tissue was removed from each lung targeting the most emphysematous regions. Those with median sternotomy all had epidural catheters placed to help with pain control, and patients were expected to be extubated within two hours of the procedure when possible (30).

Primary outcomes of NETT

NETT investigators screened 3,777 patients to enroll 610 in maximal medical therapy arm and 608 to LVRS. Of those assigned to LVRS, 580 out of 608 (95.4%) underwent LVRS with 21 patients declining surgery and another seven who were deemed not operative candidates by the surgeon (29). The 90-day mortality was significantly higher in the LVRS group (7.9%, 5.9–10.3% vs. 1.3%, 0.6–2.6%, $p < 0.001$) compared with medical therapy. During follow-up (mean time of 29.2 months), the mortality was not different between LVRS and medical therapy despite the higher 90-day mortality in surgical arm (RR 1.01, $p = 0.90$). Patients that had LVRS were more likely to have improvements in FEV_1, 6MWD, dyspnea, and quality of life. Exercise performance at six, 12, and 24 months improved by 10 watts in 28%, 22%, and 15% of patients undergoing LVRS, respectively, compared with only 4%, 5%, and 3% at the same time points in the medical therapy group ($p < 0.001$) (29).

The NETT steering committee and the DSMB considered a 30-day mortality rate above 8% would justify stopping the trial. The investigators identified a subgroup of patients that had LVRS with an FEV_1 <20% predicted and either a DL_{CO} <20% predicted or homogeneous emphysema on CT imaging that had a 30-day mortality of 16% compared with 0% in the medical therapy arm. Additionally, the patients in the high-risk group that survived LVRS were far less likely to achieve clinically meaningful improvements in exercise performance and quality of life. Based on these data, those with an FEV_1 <20% predicted and either a DL_{CO} <20% predicted or homogeneous emphysema on CT imaging were excluded from enrolling in NETT and should not undergo LVRS (31). When the high-risk group was excluded from mortality analysis (1,078 patients remained), the 30-day mortality in the LVRS group was 2.2% vs. 0.2% in the medical group and the 90-day mortality in LVRS was 5.2% vs. 1.5% in the medical group (29).

The only baseline factors that discriminated mortality differences were craniocaudal distribution of emphysema on CT imaging and post rehabilitation pre-randomization exercise performance. No baseline factor was predictive of improvement in quality of life (29). The investigators divided patients into four subgroups based on exercise performance (high vs. low) and emphysema distribution (upper lobe predominant vs. non-upper lobe predominant). High exercise was defined a priori as achieving >40 watts for men and >25 watts for women on cardiopulmonary exercise testing. Those with upper lobe predominant emphysema and low exercise performance undergoing LVRS had a survival advantage compared with maximal medical therapy (risk ratio 0.47, $p = 0.005$) and were more likely to have clinically meaningful improvement in exercise performance and quality of life. Those with upper lobe predominant emphysema and high exercise capacity had no difference in mortality, but exercise performance and quality of life were meaningfully improved.

Among those with non-upper lobe predominant emphysema and low exercise performance, there was no statistical difference in mortality or exercise improvement, but quality of life improved among those that underwent LVRS. Among those with non-upper lobe predominant emphysema and high exercise performance, there was an increased risk of mortality in the LVRS group (risk ratio 2.06, $p = 0.02$), while LVRS had no effect on exercise or quality of life improvement. Table 3.2 summarizes the four groups and outcomes following LVRS compared with the medical group.

In summary, the first report of NETT demonstrated that LVRS did not improve mortality compared with medical therapy even when the high-risk group was excluded. However, there was an improvement

TABLE 3.2   Summary of NETT results: Subjects by emphysema distribution and exercise capacity

	MORTALITY	EXERCISE PERFORMANCE	QUALITY OF LIFE
Upper lobe predominant emphysema, low exercise	Improved	Improved	Improved
Upper lobe predominant emphysema, high exercise	No change	Improved	Improved
Non-upper lobe predominant emphysema, low exercise	No change	No change	Improved
Non-upper lobe predominant emphysema, high exercise	Worsened	No change	No change

in exercise performance, reduced dyspnea, and improved quality of life with LVRS. Based on a priori subgroups, LVRS improved survival, exercise performance, and quality of life in those with upper lobe predominant disease and low exercise capacity. Although the group with non-upper lobe predominant emphysema and low exercise had an improvement in quality of life following LVRS, it is felt that this is not worth the risk of surgery. The group with non-upper lobe predominant emphysema and high exercise had increased mortality with LVRS and should not undergo the procedure. The NETT investigators sought to learn about the long-term effects of LVRS on survival and exercise performance; therefore, they decided to continue following NETT patients.

NETT patients continued to have annual follow-up visits and long-term survival data were obtained via the Social Security Death Index (mean duration of 4.3 years). In all 1,218 patients, including the high-risk group, there was a survival advantage for those that underwent LVRS compared with medical therapy alone (RR = 0.85, p = 0.02) (Figure 3.2a). When the high-risk group was excluded, there was a similar survival advantage (RR = 0.82, p = 0.02) (Figure 3.2b). LVRS improved exercise capacity >10 watts in 23%, 15%, and 9% at years one, two, and three respectively compared with 5%, 3%, and 1% in the medical group (p < 0.001 at each time point). Additionally, there was meaningful improvement in quality of life (≥8-point improvement in SGRQ) in the LVRS group as far as four years from surgery. Those with upper lobe predominant emphysema and low exercise not surprisingly had the greatest survival advantage (Figure 3.2c) (RR = 0.57, p = 0.01), while those with upper lobe predominant emphysema and high exercise did not have a survival advantage (Figure 3.2d) (32).

Those with non-upper lobe predominant emphysema and low exercise did not have a survival advantage with LVRS. Although those in this group did have a better quality of life, the effect dissipated by year three and there was no improvement in exercise performance. Those with non-upper lobe predominant emphysema and high exercise that had LVRS did not have improved survival, exercise capacity, or quality of life with LVRS (32).

NETT demonstrated that the effect was durable in LVRS benefits patients with advanced upper lobe predominant emphysema. The benefits were meaningful to patients and included improved dyspnea, quality of life, exercise performance, and in those with low exercise at baseline improved survival. Most would agree that LVRS in non-upper lobe predominant disease does not have a favorable risk/benefit ratio.

As expected, there were complications other than mortality related to LVRS given that these patients all had advanced emphysema. In the first 90 days, 58.7% of LVRS patients had at least one complication. The most common complication was cardiac arrhythmia (23.5%), but others included reintubation (21.8%), pneumonia (18.2%), ICU readmission (11.7%), and requirement of tracheostomy (8.2%). Pulmonary morbidity was higher with advanced age, lower FEV_1, and lower DL_{CO}, while cardiac comorbidity was greater with age, preoperative steroid use, and non-upper lobe predominant emphysema (33). As expected, 90% of patients undergoing LVRS had an air leak within the first 30 days, and the median duration of the air leak was seven days. The rate of prolonged air leak (≥30 days) was 12% (34). Upper lobe predominant emphysema, lower diffusion capacity, and presence of adhesions were associated with greater risk of having an air leak. Patients that had air leaks were more likely to have complications (57% vs. 30%, p = 0.004) and longer hospital stay (11.8 ± 6.5 vs. 7.6 ± 4.4 days, p = 0.005). Despite air leak being common, only 4.4% of patients with an air leak required reoperation (34).

BRONCHOSCOPIC APPROACH TO LUNG VOLUME REDUCTION

Although LVRS is beneficial in carefully selected patients with advanced emphysema, many are reluctant to undergo the procedure due to concerns about morbidity and mortality associated with the procedure. Over the last 15 years, there has been extensive research into less invasive approaches to lung volume reduction. As a result of this work, there are now two different endobronchial valves (EBVs) approved for use in the United States. EBVs are placed in the airway at the lobar or segmental level with the goal of inducing lobar atelectasis, leading to a reduction in lung volume. The Spiration Valve System (SVS) (Spiration, Olympus, Tokyo, Japan) has an umbrella shape, where an occlusive cover is stretched over a titanium wire frame, allowing air and secretions to leave around the edges of the device (Figure 3.3). The Zephyr valve (Pulmonx, Inc., Neuchatel Switzerland) is a cylindrical device with a one-way duckbill valve placed in a nitinol wire cage (Figure 3.4). Expired air and secretions travel through the center of the device.

The Endobronchial Valve for Emphysema Palliation Trial (VENT) was a prospective randomized trial that utilized the Zephyr valve to achieve lung volume reduction (35). The investigators randomized 220 patients to EBV placement compared with 101 patients treated with maximal medical therapy. At six months, the FEV_1 improved to 4.3% in the EBV group while the FEV_1 declined to 2.5% in the medical therapy group. The 6MWD improved to 2.5% (9.3 m) in the EBV group and declined to 3.2% (10.7 m) in the medical therapy group. Although these changes were statistically significant, they were not clinically meaningful. Heterogeneity of emphysema (differences of 15%) between lobes in treated lungs and the presence of complete fissures were the only factors predictive of improvements in primary endpoints. EBV patients with intact fissures had a 16.2% improvement in FEV_1 at six months and 17.9% at 12 months, while those with incomplete fissures had FEV_1 changes of 2.0% and 2.8%, respectively (35).

The EUROVENT study, with 111 patients treated with EBV compared with 60 patients with medical therapy, demonstrated similar results. There were only modest gains in FEV_1, 6MWD, and quality of life,

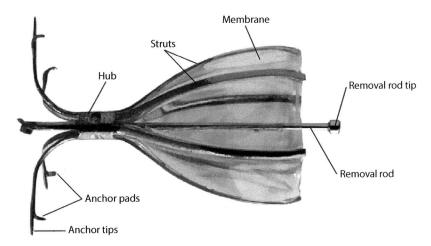

FIGURE 3.3 Spiration intrabronchial valve (Spiration, Olympus, Tokyo, Japan). Note the umbrella design with an occlusive cover over the titanium wire frame. The removal rod (the "umbrella handle") can be grasped by forceps to remove the valve while the anchors help keep the valve in place.

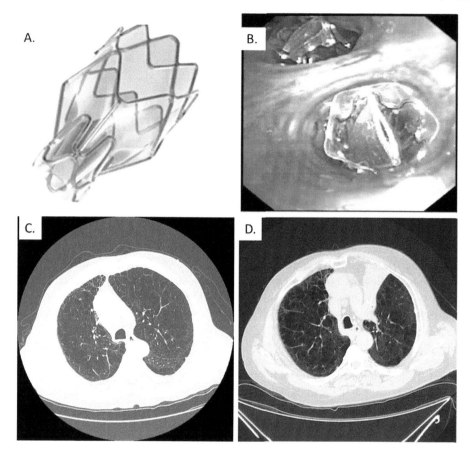

FIGURE 3.4   Zephyr valve (Pulmonx Inc., Neuchatel, Switzerland). (a) Valve ex vivo. (b) Endobronchial view of valves demonstrating the opening of the duckbill to permit deflation of the target lobe. (c) Representative HRCT image of severe left upper lobe emphysema. (d) HRCT image demonstrating complete left upper lobe atelectasis following endobronchial valve placement.

but those with intact fissures had better improvement in FEV_1 (16% vs. 2%) when treated with EBV (36). Additionally, those with intact fissures had greater target lobe volume reduction relative to baseline target lobe volume reduction. These two studies suggested that if collateral ventilation is absent, EBV placement could improve lung function and quality of life.

Initially, there was some debate on whether bilateral sub lobar placement with incomplete lobar atelectasis would be as good or better than unilateral lobar placement and total lobar atelectasis. Eberhardt compared unilateral treatment with the goal of total lobar atelectasis to bilateral subtotal atelectasis. They found that unilateral treatment resulted in much greater improvement in FEV_1 (+21.4% ± 10.7% vs. −0.03% ± 13.9%, p = 0.002), quality of life as measured by SGRQ (−11.8 ± 10.6 vs. −2.1 ± 8.5, p = 0.007), and improved 6MWD (48.9 ± 53.0 vs. −52.3 ± 81.2, p 0.02) compared with bilateral subtotal treatment (37). Based on these data, future designs of clinical trials for EBV should be focused on unilateral treatment with the goal of total lobar atelectasis.

From these early studies, it was also clear that treatment outcomes depended on fissure integrity (FI). Determining whether a patient has complete fissures can be determined by quantitative high-resolution computed tomography (HRCT) or balloon occlusion of the airway and monitoring flow with the Chartis system (Pulmonx) (38, 39). During bronchoscopy, a balloon-tipped catheter is inserted into the targeted bronchus and inflated to completely occlude the airway. The catheter measures flow at the distal tip and is used as a surrogate of FI if there is cessation of flow a few minutes after balloon inflation. Figure 3.5a is an

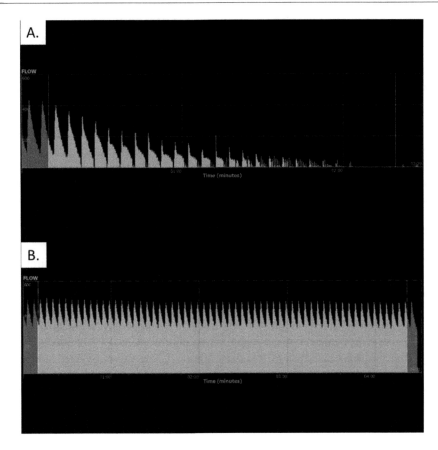

FIGURE 3.5   Chartis (Pulmonx Inc., Neuchatel, Switzerland) assessment demonstrating (a) a collateral ventilation negative patient and (b) a collateral ventilation positive patient.

example of collateral ventilation negative (intact fissure) clearly demonstrating cessation of flow. Figure 3.5b is an example of positive collateral ventilation indicating that the fissure is not intact. FI can also be measured by quantitative HRCT analysis, and it has been suggested that an FI of ≥90% complete indicates an acceptable parameter to proceed with EBV placement (40). Sensitivity and specificity for FI have been reported to be 77.8% and 73.3% for Chartis (Pulmonx) and 83.3% and 66.7% for HRCT analysis, respectively (39). While it is necessary to determine whether a fissure is intact prior to EBV placement, it is unclear if one method is better or whether both should be utilized.

Based on VENT trial results, all subsequent studies with EBV enrolled only patients with intact fissures and lack of collateral ventilation. The TRANSFORM study compared 65 patients treated with Zephyr valve (Pulmonx) to 32 patients in the control arm. Patients were only enrolled if Chartis assessment demonstrated a lack of collateral ventilation. Patients had to have FEV_1 between 15% and 45% predicted, TLC > 100% predicted and RV >180% predicted, a heterogeneity score of >10% between targeted lobe and ipsilateral lobe, and a 6MWD between 140 m and 450 m (41): 55% of patients treated with EBVs had an improvement in FEV_1 of at least 12% compared with the control group. Also, there was significant improvement in quality of life, 6MWD, and reduction in RV in those treated with EBV.

The LIBERATE trial randomized patients to EBV placement (n = 128) with Zephyr valve (Pulmonx, Inc.) or maximal medical therapy (n = 92). In addition to patients being severely obstructed and hyperinflated, the investigators only enrolled patients with ≥15% emphysema heterogeneity between lobes with >50% destruction in the targeted lobe (42). At 12 months, more patients had ≥15% improvement in FEV_1 in the EBV group compared with the maximal medical therapy (47.7% vs. 16.8%). The between-group difference (EBV − standard of care) for FEV_1 was 0.106 L ([0.047 to 0.165], p < 0.001), quality of life measured by SGRQ −7.05 ([−11.84 to −2.27], p < 0.001), and 6MWD 39.31 m ([14.64 to 63.98], p < 0.001). Responder analysis revealed that 56.4% had ≥12% improvement in FEV_1, 56.2% had improvement in SGRQ score of at least four points, and 84.2% had a decline in targeted lobe volume of at least 350 mL at one year. These data demonstrated that EBV placement in severely hyperinflated gas-trapped patients with heterogeneous emphysema and intact fissures had meaningful clinically important improvements in lung function, quality of life, and exercise performance that was durable to at least one year.

The SVS (Spiration, Olympus) valve was studied in the REACH trial, which enrolled 101 patients. FI was determined by quantitative HRCT analysis, and patients had to have FI of at least 90% to be enrolled. Only those with >15% heterogeneous emphysema were enrolled, and like other trials, inclusion criteria included an FEV_1 <45% predicted, TLC >100% predicted, and RV >150% predicted. At three months, the FEV_1 improved by 0.104 ± 0.178 L in the SVS group compared with 0.003 ± 0.147 in the control group. Responder analysis revealed that FEV_1 improvement of ≥15% occurred in 49%, 48%, and 41% of SVS patients at one, three, and six months, respectively, compared with 22%, 13%, and 21% in controls. There was also a significant improvement in quality of life at six months in the SVS group compared with controls (43).

The EMPROVE study was a randomized controlled trial utilizing the SVS valve (Spiration, Olympus) in 113 patients compared with 59 in the control arm (40). The inclusion criteria were like that of the REACH trial and the primary outcome for the study was change in FEV_1 at six months compared with baseline, but data were reported to 12 months. At six months, the SVS group improved by 0.099 L (0.069–0.128), whereas the control group changed by −0.002 L (−0.030–0.026) for a between-group difference of 0.101 L. The effect was durable to 12 months with a between-group improvement in FEV_1 of 0.099 L. There were significant improvements at six months for the between-group differences of targeted lung volume reduction (−0.947 L), SGRQ (−13.0), and dyspnea as measured by the Modified Medical Research Council score (−0.6) but not in 6MWD. Taken together, the REACH and EMPROVE studies demonstrated that the SVS valve (Spiration, Olympus) improved lung function, dyspnea, and quality of life in patients with heterogenous emphysema with intact fissures that have hyperinflation (TLC >100% predicted) and gas trapping (RV >150% predicted).

ENDOBRONCHIAL VALVES FOR HOMOGENEOUS EMPHYSEMA

Patients with advanced homogeneous emphysema who fail medical therapy have limited options as LVRS is contraindicated and lung transplantation is not always an option due to strict selection criteria, high morbidity and mortality, and limited organ availability. The IMPACT trial is a randomized controlled trial in patients with severe homogeneous emphysema utilizing the Zephyr (Pulmonx, Inc.) valve to achieve lung volume reduction. Inclusion criteria included FEV_1 15% to 45% predicted, TLC >100% predicted, and RV ≥200% predicted to either EBV placement (43 patients) or standard of care (50 patients) (44). Homogeneous emphysema was defined as a heterogeneity score of <15% between the target lobe and the ipsilateral non-target lobe. Patients also had to have <20% difference in perfusion between right and left lungs as measured by perfusion scintigraphy. All patients had intact fissures without evidence of collateral ventilation. The mean difference in FEV_1 between groups at three months was 17.0%, favoring the EBV group. There were significant improvements in quality of life measured by SGRQ score (−9.6 points), 6MWD (+40 m), and RV (−480 mL) in the EBV group compared with the control. A subsequent publication reported data for six months and demonstrated that there was a between-group improvement in FEV_1 of 120 ± 150 mL in the EBV group compared with controls. The improvements in quality of life measured by SGRQ (−7.51 points), 6MWD (+28.3 m), and RV (−430 mL) all persisted at six months. At 12 months, there were still improvements with EBV insertion compared with baseline in FEV_1 (50 mL),

SGRQ score (−4.01 points), and RV (−460mL) but not 6MWD (+3.7 m). These data suggest that carefully selected patients with severe homogenous can benefit from EBV treatment (45).

Endobronchial valve complication

Although EBV placement is associated with less morbidity and mortality than LVRS, there are significant complications associated with this procedure. The mortality rate in LIBERATE at 45 days was 3.1% (four patients) in the EBV group, and no deaths were reported in the control group. Three of the four deaths were related to pneumothorax (42). In the EMPROVE trial, the mortality rate was 5.3% in the first six months with one death attributed to possible pneumothorax compared with 1.7% in the control group (40). The two most common adverse events reported in clinical trials were pneumothoraces and exacerbations of COPD. Table 3.3 lists the rates for these complications among different studies where patients with intact fissures were enrolled. Most studies report a pneumothorax rate of around 30%. Not every patient who experiences a pneumothorax will require chest tube placement but many will. There are published expert opinions/guidelines on the management of pneumothorax post-EBV placement (46). The majority of pneumothoraces occur within the first few days following valve placement, and most experts recommend patients be observed in hospital for three or four days to allow for the timely treatment of pneumothorax. Other reported complications include hemoptysis, valve migration/expectoration, pneumonia, and the formation of granulation tissue.

LVRS versus endobronchial valve placement

Some patients with advanced emphysema could potentially be candidates for either LVRS or EBV placement. Most patients eligible for both therapies would prefer to proceed with EBV placement, but for those that have evidence of collateral ventilation or FI <90%, most experts would suggest they undergo LVRS (1). One recent randomized controlled trial randomly assigned patients to either unilateral LVRS (n = 41) or EBV placement (n = 47). Inclusion criteria included FEV_1 <60% predicted, TLC >100% predicted, and RV >170% predicted, and had heterogeneous emphysema based on CT imaging and lung perfusion. All patients had an absence of collateral ventilation as determined by both Chartis (Pulmonx, Inc.) assessment and quantitative analysis of FI >90% on CT imaging. The primary outcome was the i-BODE score at 12 months, which used an incremental shuttle walk test rather than 6MWD to calculate BODE score. At 12 months, there was improvement in i-BODE score in both groups, but the improvement was not different between the groups (LVRS −1.10 ± 1.44 vs. EBV −0.82 ± 1.61, p = 0.54) (47). The reduction in RV %-predicted was also similar between LVRS and EBV (−36.1% [−54.6 to −10%] vs. −30.1% [−53.7 to −9%], p = 0.81), respectively. There was a greater improvement in quality of life as measured by the COPD assessment test (CAT) in the LVRS group compared with EBV (−7 [−11 to −1] vs. −1 [−3 to 3], p = 0.005). The initial length of stay was longer in the LVRS group, but the EBV group was more likely to require further interventions. The authors concluded that unilateral LVRS was not statistically superior to EBV in patients eligible for either therapy. Most experts would suggest that those eligible for both procedures should undergo EBV first, and if treatment goals are not reached, LVRS would still be an option.

CONCLUSION

Static and dynamic hyperinflation in advanced emphysema is associated with increased dyspnea, poor exercise performance, cardiac dysfunction, poor quality of life, and increased mortality. This makes hyperinflation an attractive target for treatment in these patients. The first line of therapy should always be

TABLE 3.3 Summary of pneumothorax and acute exacerbation of COPD events in EBV trial with intact fissure

	LIBERATE (42) (N = 128)	TRANSFORM (41) (N = 65)	IMPACT (44) (N = 43)	BELIEVER HIFI (48) (N = 25)	STELVIO (49) (N = 34)	REACH (43) (N = 72)	EMPROVE (40) (N = 113)	TOTAL (N = 480)
Pneumothorax events	46	20	12	2	6	5	31	122
Patients with pneumothorax	44 (34.4%)	16 (29.2%)	12 (25.6%)	2 (8%)	6 (18%)	5 (7.5%)	32 (28.3%)	116 (24.2%)
Patients with AECOPD	10 (7.8%)	3 (4.65%)	10 (16.3%)	16 (64%)	4 (12%)	5 (7.6%)	19 (16.8%)	67 (14.0%)

AECOPD, acute exacerbation of COPD.

maximizing less morbid treatments such as bronchodilators, pulmonary rehabilitation, and oxygen when indicated, but if patients fail this therapy, they should be evaluated for invasive techniques for lung volume reduction. Those with homogeneous disease or non-upper lobe predominant emphysema that are gas trapped and hyperinflated should proceed with EBV placement if eligible. Patients with heterogeneous emphysema and evidence of collateral ventilation could be candidates for LVRS. Patients with heterogeneous emphysema could be eligible for either EBV placement or LVRS, and most would first pursue EBV placement due to less morbidity. Further work is needed in developing bronchoscopic procedures for those not eligible for LVRS that have evidence of collateral ventilation.

REFERENCES

1. Agusti A, Celli B, Criner G, Halpin D, Varla MVL, de Oca MM, et al. Global strategy for the diagnosis, management, and prevention of chronic obstructive pulmonary disease (2024 Report) 2023. Available from: https://goldcopd.org/2024-gold-report.
2. O'Donnell DE, Revill SM, Webb KA. Dynamic hyperinflation and exercise intolerance in chronic obstructive pulmonary disease. *Am J Respir Crit Care Med*. 2001;164(5):770–7.
3. Butler J, Caro CG, Alcala R, Dubois AB. Physiological factors affecting airway resistance in normal subjects and in patients with obstructive respiratory disease. *J Clin Invest*. 1960;39(4):584–91.
4. Hogg JC, Chu F, Utokaparch S, Woods R, Elliott WM, Buzatu L, et al. The nature of small-airway obstruction in chronic obstructive pulmonary disease. *N Engl J Med*. 2004;350(26):2645–53.
5. Fessler HE, Permutt S. Lung volume reduction surgery and airflow limitation. *Am J Respir Crit Care Med*. 1998;157(3 Pt 1):715–22.
6. Fessler HE, Scharf SM, Ingenito EP, McKenna RJ, Sharafkhaneh A. Physiologic basis for improved pulmonary function after lung volume reduction. *Proc Am Thorac Soc*. 2008;5(4):416–20.
7. Stubbing DG, Pengelly LD, Morse JL, Jones NL. Pulmonary mechanics during exercise in normal males. *J Appl Physiol Respir Environ Exerc Physiol*. 1980;49(3):506–10.
8. O'Donnell DE, Hamilton AL, Webb KA. Sensory-mechanical relationships during high-intensity, constant-work-rate exercise in COPD. *J Appl Physiol*. (1985).2006;101(4):1025–35.
9. O'Donnell DE, Bertley JC, Chau LK, Webb KA. Qualitative aspects of exertional breathlessness in chronic airflow limitation: pathophysiologic mechanisms. *Am J Respir Crit Care Med*. 1997;155(1):109–15.
10. Jörgensen K, Houltz E, Westfelt U, Nilsson F, Scherstén H, Ricksten SE. Effects of lung volume reduction surgery on left ventricular diastolic filling and dimensions in patients with severe emphysema. *Chest*. 2003;124(5):1863–70.
11. Jörgensen K, Müller MF, Nel J, Upton RN, Houltz E, Ricksten SE. Reduced intrathoracic blood volume and left and right ventricular dimensions in patients with severe emphysema: an MRI study. *Chest*. 2007;131(4):1050–7.
12. Watz H, Waschki B, Meyer T, Kretschmar G, Kirsten A, Claussen M, et al. Decreasing cardiac chamber sizes and associated heart dysfunction in COPD: role of hyperinflation. *Chest*. 2010;138(1):32–8.
13. Barr RG, Bluemke DA, Ahmed FS, Carr JJ, Enright PL, Hoffman EA, et al. Percent emphysema, airflow obstruction, and impaired left ventricular filling. *N Engl J Med*. 2010;362(3):217–27.
14. Wrobel JP, Thompson BR, Williams TJ. Mechanisms of pulmonary hypertension in chronic obstructive pulmonary disease: a pathophysiologic review. *J Heart Lung Transplant*. 2012;31(6):557–64.
15. Casanova C, Cote C, de Torres JP, Aguirre-Jaime A, Marin JM, Pinto-Plata V, et al. Inspiratory-to-total lung capacity ratio predicts mortality in patients with chronic obstructive pulmonary disease. *Am J Respir Crit Care Med*. 2005;171(6):591–7.
16. Kim YW, Lee CH, Hwang HG, Kim YI, Kim DK, Oh YM, et al. Resting hyperinflation and emphysema on the clinical course of COPD. *Sci Rep*. 2019;9(1):3764.
17. Calzetta L, Ora J, Cavalli F, Rogliani P, O'Donnell DE, Cazzola M. Impact of LABA/LAMA combination on exercise endurance and lung hyperinflation in COPD: A pair-wise and network meta-analysis. *Respir Med*. 2017;129:189–98.
18. Oba Y, Keeney E, Ghatehorde N, Dias S. Dual combination therapy versus long-acting bronchodilators alone for chronic obstructive pulmonary disease (COPD): a systematic review and network meta-analysis. *Cochrane Database Syst Rev*. 2018;12(12):CD012620.

19. O'Donnell DE, Voduc N, Fitzpatrick M, Webb KA. Effect of salmeterol on the ventilatory response to exercise in chronic obstructive pulmonary disease. *Eur Respir J.* 2004;24(1):86–94.
20. O'Donnell DE, Sciurba F, Celli B, Mahler DA, Webb KA, Kalberg CJ, et al. Effect of fluticasone propionate/salmeterol on lung hyperinflation and exercise endurance in COPD. *Chest.* 2006;130(3):647–56.
21. Herth F, Hohlfeld JM, Haas J, de la Hoz A, Jin X, Kreitner KF, et al. The effect of tiotropium/olodaterol versus fluticasone propionate/salmeterol on left ventricular filling and lung hyperinflation in patients with COPD. *BMJ Open Respir Res.* 2020;7(1).
22. O'Donnell DE, D'Arsigny C, Webb KA. Effects of hyperoxia on ventilatory limitation during exercise in advanced chronic obstructive pulmonary disease. *Am J Respir Crit Care Med.* 2001;163(4):892–8.
23. O'Donnell DE, McGuire M, Samis L, Webb KA. General exercise training improves ventilatory and peripheral muscle strength and endurance in chronic airflow limitation. *Am J Respir Crit Care Med.* 1998;157(5 Pt 1):1489–97.
24. Brantigan OC, Mueller E, Kress MB. A surgical approach to pulmonary emphysema. *Am Rev Respir Dis.* 1959;80(1, Part 2):194–206.
25. Cooper JD, Trulock EP, Triantafillou AN, Patterson GA, Pohl MS, Deloney PA, et al. Bilateral pneumectomy (volume reduction) for chronic obstructive pulmonary disease. *J Thorac Cardiovasc Surg.* 1995;109(1):106–16; discussion 16-9.
26. Cooper JD, Patterson GA, Sundaresan RS, Trulock EP, Yusen RD, Pohl MS, et al. Results of 150 consecutive bilateral lung volume reduction procedures in patients with severe emphysema. *J Thorac Cardiovasc Surg.* 1996;112(5):1319–29; discussion 29-30.
27. Criner GJ, Cordova FC, Furukawa S, Kuzma AM, Travaline JM, Leyenson V, et al. Prospective randomized trial comparing bilateral lung volume reduction surgery to pulmonary rehabilitation in severe chronic obstructive pulmonary disease. *Am J Respir Crit Care Med.* 1999;160(6):2018–27.
28. Geddes D, Davies M, Koyama H, Hansell D, Pastorino U, Pepper J, et al. Effect of lung-volume-reduction surgery in patients with severe emphysema. *N Engl J Med.* 2000;343(4):239–45.
29. Fishman A, Martinez F, Naunheim K, Piantadosi S, Wise R, Ries A, et al. A randomized trial comparing lung-volume-reduction surgery with medical therapy for severe emphysema. *N Engl J Med.* 2003;348(21):2059–73.
30. Rationale and design of The National Emphysema Treatment Trial: a prospective randomized trial of lung volume reduction surgery. The National Emphysema Treatment Trial Research Group. *Chest.* 1999;116(6):1750–61.
31. Fishman A, Fessler H, Martinez F, McKenna RJ, Naunheim K, Piantadosi S, et al. Patients at high risk of death after lung-volume-reduction surgery. *N Engl J Med.* 2001;345(15):1075–83.
32. Naunheim KS, Wood DE, Mohsenifar Z, Sternberg AL, Criner GJ, DeCamp MM, et al. Long-term follow-up of patients receiving lung-volume-reduction surgery versus medical therapy for severe emphysema by the National Emphysema Treatment Trial Research Group. *Ann Thorac Surg.* 2006;82(2):431–43.
33. Naunheim KS, Wood DE, Krasna MJ, DeCamp MM, Ginsburg ME, McKenna RJ, et al. Predictors of operative mortality and cardiopulmonary morbidity in the National Emphysema Treatment Trial. *J Thorac Cardiovasc Surg.* 2006;131(1):43–53.
34. DeCamp MM, Blackstone EH, Naunheim KS, Krasna MJ, Wood DE, Meli YM, et al. Patient and surgical factors influencing air leak after lung volume reduction surgery: lessons learned from the National Emphysema Treatment Trial. *Ann Thorac Surg.* 2006;82(1):197–206; discussion -7.
35. Sciurba FC, Ernst A, Herth FJ, Strange C, Criner GJ, Marquette CH, et al. A randomized study of endobronchial valves for advanced emphysema. *N Engl J Med.* 2010;363(13):1233–44.
36. Herth FJ, Noppen M, Valipour A, Leroy S, Vergnon JM, Ficker JH, et al. Efficacy predictors of lung volume reduction with Zephyr valves in a European cohort. *Eur Respir J.* 2012;39(6):1334–42.
37. Eberhardt R, Gompelmann D, Schuhmann M, Reinhardt H, Ernst A, Heussel CP, et al. Complete unilateral vs partial bilateral endoscopic lung volume reduction in patients with bilateral lung emphysema. *Chest.* 2012;142(4):900–8.
38. Herth FJ, Eberhardt R, Gompelmann D, Ficker JH, Wagner M, Ek L, et al. Radiological and clinical outcomes of using Chartis™ to plan endobronchial valve treatment. *Eur Respir J.* 2013;41(2):302–8.
39. Schuhmann M, Raffy P, Yin Y, Gompelmann D, Oguz I, Eberhardt R, et al. Computed tomography predictors of response to endobronchial valve lung reduction treatment. Comparison with Chartis. *Am J Respir Crit Care Med.* 2015;191(7):767–74.
40. Criner GJ, Delage A, Voelker K, Hogarth DK, Majid A, Zgoda M, et al. Improving lung function in severe heterogenous Emphysema with the Spiration Valve System (EMPROVE). A Multicenter, Open-Label Randomized Controlled Clinical Trial. *Am J Respir Crit Care Med.* 2019;200(11):1354–62.
41. Kemp SV, Slebos DJ, Kirk A, Kornaszewska M, Carron K, Ek L, et al. A multicenter randomized controlled trial of zephyr endobronchial valve treatment in heterogeneous emphysema (TRANSFORM). *Am J Respir Crit Care Med.* 2017;196(12):1535–43.

42. Criner GJ, Sue R, Wright S, Dransfield M, Rivas-Perez H, Wiese T, et al. A multicenter randomized controlled trial of zephyr endobronchial valve treatment in heterogeneous emphysema (LIBERATE). *Am J Respir Crit Care Med.* 2018;198(9):1151–64.
43. Li S, Wang G, Wang C, Gao X, Jin F, Yang H, et al. The REACH trial: A randomized controlled trial assessing the safety and effectiveness of the Spiration® Valve System in the treatment of severe emphysema. *Respiration.* 2019;97(5):416–27.
44. Valipour A, Slebos DJ, Herth F, Darwiche K, Wagner M, Ficker JH, et al. Endobronchial valve therapy in patients with homogeneous emphysema. Results from the IMPACT Study. *Am J Respir Crit Care Med.* 2016;194(9):1073–82.
45. Eberhardt R, Slebos DJ, Herth FJF, Darwiche K, Wagner M, Ficker JH, et al. Endobronchial valve (Zephyr) treatment in homogeneous emphysema: One-year results from the IMPACT randomized clinical trial. *Respiration.* 2021;100(12):1174–85.
46. van Dijk M, Sue R, Criner GJ, Gompelmann D, Herth FJF, Hogarth DK, et al. Expert statement: Pneumothorax associated with one-way valve therapy for emphysema: 2020 update. *Respiration.* 2021;100(10):969–78.
47. Buttery SC, Banya W, Bilancia R, Boyd E, Buckley J, Greening NJ, et al. Lung volume reduction surgery. *Eur Respir J.* 2023;61(4).
48. Davey C, Zoumot Z, Jordan S, McNulty WH, Carr DH, Hind MD, et al. Bronchoscopic lung volume reduction with endobronchial valves for patients with heterogeneous emphysema and intact interlobar fissures (the BeLieVeR-HIFi study): a randomised controlled trial. *Lancet.* 2015;386(9998):1066–73.
49. Klooster K, ten Hacken NH, Hartman JE, Kerstjens HA, van Rikxoort EM, Slebos DJ. Endobronchial valves for emphysema without interlobar collateral ventilation. *N Engl J Med.* 2015;373(24):2325–35.

Surgical Concepts and the Techniques of Lung Volume Reduction Surgery

4

Laurens J. Ceulemans, Christelle M. Vandervelde, Claudio Caviezel and Walter Weder

INTRODUCTION

Chronic obstructive pulmonary disease (COPD) is one of the most disabling lung conditions and is the third leading cause of death worldwide (1). It is the result of a complex inflammatory reaction and affects both (small) airways and lung parenchyma.

The destructive process of the lung alveoli is called emphysema and results in a loss of elastic recoil and a limited area available for gas exchange. As a result, the small airways collapse (2), causing chronic irreversible airflow limitation, air entrapment, and lung hyperinflation.

This constant state of hyperinflation causes disabling symptoms like increased dyspnea, increased work of breathing, restricted exercise tolerance, frequent exacerbations, and poor quality of life, resulting in early death (3). Medical treatment may delay progression and temporarily alleviate the symptoms but cannot reverse the underlying pathophysiology of the disease, or the damage to the parenchyma, so that many patients remain severely symptomatic and evolve toward end-stage emphysema.

Lung transplantation may be the ultimate treatment for end-stage emphysema patients. Unfortunately, the prevalence of severe emphysema is far beyond the availability of suitable donor lungs, and many patients are not eligible for this life-saving, but invasive, procedure due to their advanced age or comorbidities. Therefore, less invasive interventions that may improve lung function and symptoms in patients with severe emphysema have been investigated.

Lung volume reduction surgery (LVRS) is one of the few therapies directly targeting hyperinflation in emphysema patients by addressing the excess residual volume (RV) (4). However, due to initial poor selection criteria at the turn of the millennium, it has been one of the most underutilized and controversial

DOI: 10.1201/9781003251439-4

topics in thoracic surgery. Nevertheless, over the last few years, with the wider integration of multidisciplinary patient selection, minimal invasive surgical techniques (thoracoscopy and robotic-assisted surgery), and enhanced recovery programs, outcomes have drastically improved, resulting in increasing case numbers in specialized centers.

In this chapter, we focus on the surgical treatment of end-stage emphysema. Both a historical overview and the current LVRS strategy (candidate selection; pre-, peri-, and post-operative patient care; surgical technique; and enhanced recovery program) are addressed.

THE HISTORY OF LUNG VOLUME REDUCTION SURGERY

Early surgical approaches to treat lung emphysema were focused on altering the chest wall or diaphragm (5–7). The first introduction of LVRS was made in 1959 by Otto Brantigan (8), who described it as a reduction pneumoplasty with the main objectives to improve respiratory mechanics and the lung's outward traction to maintain the small airways. It consisted of a staged bilateral thoracotomy followed by resection of the most emphysematous parts of the lung and lung denervation by radical hilar stripping. The most affected side was operated first, followed by the contralateral side three months later. Due to the high peri-operative mortality rate of 16% and the lack of data demonstrating subjective improvement in survivors, his work was not widely accepted.

During the following four decades, various groups experimented with versions of Brantigan's method. Bullae excisions, plications of the air sac, segmentectomies, lobectomies, and pneumonectomies were attempted, resulting in very sporadic success (9).

In the early 1990s, Joel Cooper (1995) (10) introduced the dawn of a new era on LVRS after modifying Brantigan's technique to a bilateral LVRS via median sternotomy. In 20 patients with heterogeneous non-bullous emphysema, he reported no peri-operative mortality and forced expiratory volume in one second (FEV_1)-improvement of 82% at six months, associated with marked relief of dyspnea and improvement in quality of life (QoL) (11). Re-evaluation of Cooper's technique in 150 consecutive patients demonstrated an increase in FEV_1 of 51%, peri-operative mortality in six patients (4%), and continuing improvement in QoL (12).

In Zurich (Switzerland), Walter Weder started a bilateral LVRS VATS program in 1993 and reported from 1994 to 1995 the initial results of 20 patients with no peri-operative mortality, improvement of FEV_1 of 41%, increase in walking distance (12 min: 495 m to 688 m, p < 0.001), and a substantial relief of dyspnea at three months (13). The same technique was reported in 1996 by Keenan et al. (14) from Pittsburgh (USA) who performed a unilateral LVRS by VATS in 57 patients, resulting in one peri-operative death and significant improvements in forced vital capacity (2.69 L after vs. 2.26 L before) and FEV_1 (1.04 L after vs. 0.82 L before), with 63% of patients showing an improvement of more than 20%.

These promising results provided an impetus for several new LVRS programs to implement their own LVRS program and called for a randomized National Emphysema Treatment Trial (NETT), performed in North America, evaluating the efficacy of LVRS on QoL and survival benefit in comparison with medical treatment (15). Out of the 1,218 patients included in the NETT, VATS was only used in 30% of cases.

The results were published in 2003 and the trial confirmed a significant improvement in survival, exercise capacity, and QoL in non-high-risk emphysema patients. Unfortunately, patients with FEV_1 <20%, DLCO <20%, and homogenous morphology on a computed tomography (CT) scan were also included and, not surprisingly, were identified as a high-risk cohort and experienced a mortality of 16% (16). Based on the latter group, the report led to several misconceptions in medical society, concluding that LVRS was an invasive and risky procedure.

Further analysis of the data showed that for LVRS patients with heterogeneous emphysema (predominantly upper lobe) and low baseline exercise capacity, a significant improvement was attained in survival (up to five years), exercise capacity (up to three years), and QoL (up to five years) (17). Although several other studies (11, 18–22) have confirmed the efficacy and safety of LVRS, a supposed high surgical morbidity and mortality, the high cost of the procedure, and poorly defined patient selection criteria seem to have influenced both the medical community and patients, as the number of LVRS procedures remained low (12, 23). Additionally, the continuing hope for less invasive endoscopic alternatives undoubtedly delayed the integration of a surgical procedure in the multidisciplinary treatment armamentarium.

In the last two decades, with further development of the VATS approach and increased experience at high-volume centers, surgical mortality has steadily improved (22, 24–27) (ranging from 0% at six months to 4% in-hospital), with a significant and maximal functional improvement (spirometry, dyspnea scores, and QoL) from three months up to five years after LVRS. These data, together with appropriate multidisciplinary patient selection, further bolster the general acceptance of LVRS in the field of thoracic surgery.

These solid results inspired expert centers to investigate expanding indications in patients with severe hyperinflation and other morphology than heterogeneous upper lobe disease. In a retrospective analysis of prospectively collected, single-center data from Zurich, 138 out of 250 patients had a homogenous morphology of emphysema with no or very limited target zones for resection. In this subgroup, similar to heterogeneous patients, significant improvements in FEV_1 (+35%) and six-minute walk distance (+79 m) at three months were shown, with no differences in peri-operative and one-year mortality (18). Additionally, in experienced centers, LVRS can cautiously be considered in a subgroup of highly selected patients with severely impaired diffusion capacity (DLCO <20%) and the presence of major hyperinflation and heterogeneous emphysema. In a retrospective analysis of 33 patients, good results have been achieved for these patients at three months with a significant increment of FEV_1 (23% to 29%) and DLCO (15% to 20%) and no mortality at three months (28). Subgroups of patients presenting with mild to moderate pulmonary hypertension (sPAP >35 mmHg, median sPAP: 41 mmHg), with heterogenous emphysema and clear target zones, also have the potential to benefit from LVRS with the ability to no longer be considered as absolute contraindication (29). Since endothelial function and blood pressure have been found to improve three months after LVRS, the procedure may have a positive impact on cardiovascular outcomes as well (30).

"VOLUME IS THE ISSUE, NOT THE TISSUE"

The chest wall, lungs, and diaphragm normally coordinate mechanically with each other to optimize elastic recoil. In emphysema, lung hyperinflation is pressing the diaphragm down, inhibiting its full function. The increased distensibility of the emphysematous lung parenchyma results in a lung that is easily inflated but tends to remain pathologically inflated throughout the breathing cycle, especially during effort. Dynamic hyperinflation during exercise is difficult to assess but can be identified from specific questions to the patient. An important consequence of the defect is that portions of severely emphysematous lung act as non-functional, volume-occupying areas impairing diaphragmatic and chest wall function.

Emphysema is a generalized pulmonary disease, but all areas of the lungs are not equally involved. The areas that are more involved are probably completely or at least heavily useless as respiratory tissue. Volume reduction aims to reshape the normal lung volume by removal/shaving severely damaged, poorly ventilated, and expanded lung tissue. It restores the lung to its original form and may cause the diaphragm to return to its former, dome-like shape. This results in increased expiratory flow rates, improved alveolar gas exchange, and improved mechanical function of the diaphragm and thoracic cage, leading to decreased work while breathing.

Surgery provides a unique volume-oriented approach as surgical resection has the inherent benefit of personalized reshaping of the lungs. One or several target zones for resection are identified on CT scans or ventilation/perfusion scintigraphy, leaving the better-preserved lung parenchyma intact.

PATIENT SELECTION

Patient selection is crucial to the success of the procedure and should be performed at an experienced center with a multidisciplinary team approach to emphysema treatment, including the option (or at least in close collaboration with a center) of lung transplantation. Referrals are based on advanced emphysema that is not adequately responsive to standard medical therapy. Chest CT, ventilation/perfusion scintigraphy, spirometry, plethysmography, six-minute walking distance, and echocardiography are conducted to identify eligible LVRS candidates. Cardiac assessment is recommended to evaluate coronary disease, pulmonary artery pressure, and right ventricular function. Patients must be highly motivated to undergo surgical treatment and be willing to participate in a pulmonary and physical rehabilitation program.

Indications

In general, eligible ambulatory emphysema patients are good candidates for LVRS if there is a suitable morphology identified by CT scan (Figures 4.1 and 4.2); FEV_1 ranges between 15% and 45% predicted (pred); with a residual volume (RV) >150% pred; modified Medical Research Council dyspnea score ≥ 2; smoking cessation (confirmed by urinary cotinine test) for ≥ 6 months; and mean pulmonary artery pressure <45 mmHg (invasively confirmed if cardiac ultrasound is considered unreliable). However, among all the parameters, most important is severe hyperinflation of the lungs and morphology on CT scans (31).

Contraindications

Patients with a very low functional reserve (FEV_1 <20% and DLCO <20%) should be carefully assessed and only considered if a markedly heterogeneous or bullous-like morphology can be identified and have a marked hyperinflation (RV >250%). Patients with important bronchiectasis, more than two exacerbations in the past year, and any comorbid disease rendering them unfit for surgery are considered ineligible.

Surgery is also considered a higher risk in patients with a BODE index of seven or above (BODE: body mass index (BMI), airflow obstruction, dyspnea, and exercise capability). Extreme cachexia or obesity (BMI 32 kg/m^2 for women, 31 for men kg/m^2) and patients older than 75 years – they were formerly

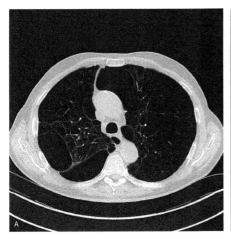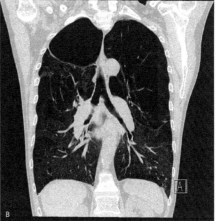

FIGURE 4.1 Transverse and coronal CT sections from a patient with severe heterogenous emphysema, selected for LVRS surgery. Both apexes show severe emphysematous destruction with some prominent bullae.

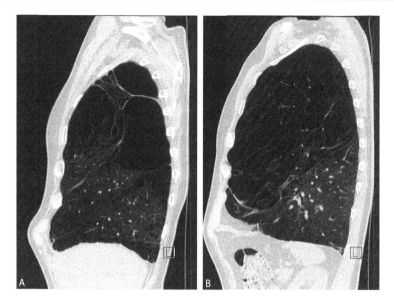

FIGURE 4.2 Both sagittal CT sections from a patient with severe heterogenous emphysema, selected for LVRS. Target areas are clearly identified in both upper lobes with still well-preserved tissue in the middle and lower lobes.

listed as absolute contraindications. However, in general, patients should be fit enough to undergo surgery, and therefore, advanced calendar age, BMI, or previous thoracic surgery should be considered as relative contraindications and assessed on an individual basis to strike a balance between anticipated benefits and risk of the procedure.

Multidisciplinary emphysema expert team

A multidisciplinary team should consist of pulmonologists experienced in COPD and lung transplantation, thoracic surgeons, chest radiologists, and an interventional pulmonologist.

A visual assessment of the type and distribution of emphysema (morphology of hyperinflation), any unexpected findings, and an estimation of fissure integrity by a dedicated chest radiologist is needed. Software is used to support the quantification of emphysema destruction, target lobe selection, and fissure integrity measurement (StratX®, Corelinesoft®). The decision-making of this multidisciplinary emphysema expert team (MEET) finally addresses the target area for volume reduction in the context of individual morbidity risk and benefit.

SURGICAL CONCEPT: PERSONALIZED REMODELING OF THE LUNGS

Surgery offers a unique volume-oriented strategy since resection has the intrinsic advantage of resecting several target zones while leaving the better-preserved lung parenchyma unaltered and the shape of the lung intact. The resection of an entire lobe comparable to valve treatment resulting in total atelectasis is almost never indicated.

The history of LVRS has clearly shown that selected emphysematous patients can benefit from a remodeling intervention that aims to restore chest geometry, by reshaping the overinflated lungs, to its normal size (26, 32, 33). Identifying the target zones for resection is crucial in preparing an LVRS procedure. Every morphology is unique and can generally be categorized in three types: marked heterogeneous, intermediate heterogeneous, and homogeneous (34).

The standard of surgical care nowadays is a bilateral minimal invasive VATS approach to tackle all target areas; however, intra-operative evaluation of the patient's safety is crucial, sometimes showing a unilateral or staged bilateral approach to be more suitable. The question of whether a bilateral staged approach is better or worse is scientifically not finally solved and has to be decided on an individual level. In general, in patients with bilateral target zones, the bilateral approach is preferred over unilateral LVRS, since the functional benefits achieved are of greater dimension compared with the unilateral procedure (35). On the other hand, a staged bilateral procedure can lower post-operative morbidity and improve functional results up to six years (36–38).

Implementation of an enhanced recovery program (ERP), a clinical pathway to accelerate recovery based on a multimodal program with optimal pain relief, stress reduction with regional anesthesia, early extubation, early enteral nutrition, and early mobilization has been shown to improve patient outcomes. At our institution (UZ Leuven), we recently demonstrated that ERP for LVRS results in fewer complications and a reduced length of stay related to decreased incidence and duration of air leaks.

Pre-operative phase

All patients have to be evaluated in the outpatient clinic. Alongside careful assessment, they have to be informed of the pathophysiology of emphysema, so that they understand the purpose of the reduction surgery as well as the expected alteration in breathing pattern post-operatively. They receive pre-operative counselling by a social worker, dietitian, and physiotherapist. Patients are encouraged to participate in a pre-operative pulmonary rehabilitation program.

Operative phase

Anesthesia and positioning

To provide adequate pain control, a patient-controlled epidural analgesia (PCEA) is positioned before induction. Alternatively, intercostal block analgesia using long-acting anesthetic can be considered. Prophylactic antibiotics (amoxycillin-clavulanic acid) are administered at induction if no allergies are reported. Patients receive an arterial catheter, a peripheral venous catheter, and a urinary catheter. A deep venous catheter should be avoided to prevent catheter-related infection post-operatively.

Following induction, a double-lumen tube is placed and the patient is positioned in a lateral decubitus position, which allows for safer adhesiolysis and improved angle for stapling compared with a supine positioning. In case of a bilateral procedure, the patient is turned to the other side when the first side is completed without any difficulties and when no or only a minor air leak is present. If no adhesions are expected and the patient has a markedly heterogeneous upper lobe morphology, supine positioning can be considered. The table is folded at the level of the xiphoid to extend the thorax laterally, widening the intercostal spaces. Protection of the brachial plexus with a plexus cushion and support of the ipsilateral arm on a leg holder are customary.

Low-tidal volume ventilation, longer expiration times to avoid hyperinflation during LVRS, and early extubation in the operating room are critical in helping to avoid air leaks caused by the disruption of the suture line or surrounding lung tissue. The use of short-acting anesthetics, appropriate post-operative pain management, and preservation of the patient's euvolemic and normothermic condition are all necessary to achieve early extubation (39).

Surgical technique

Several techniques have been described for LVRS, and currently it is still dependent on the experience of the institution and the surgeon. Nowadays, it is preferably performed by minimally invasive VATS and consists of unilateral or bilateral LVRS by stapling.

Preferentially, a 10 mm 30-degree camera is used. The number of ports depends on the location of the target areas, ranging from uniportal up to four ports (upper and lower lobe targets), with the camera in the sixth intercostal space on the midaxillary line. This first port is placed under vision to avoid damage to the lung. The second port is normally placed just anterior to, but one intercostal space higher than, the first incision on the inframammary line and the third port inferior to the tip of the scapula in the same intercostal space as the first incision. All ports are minimally 10 mm wide – a mini-Alexis can be used as well if lubricated.

Lung manipulation should be performed with care using minimally invasive forceps or a 10 mm cherry dissector (Ethicon Endo-Surgery, Cincinnati, OH). A no-touch policy of the lung parenchyma that remains has to be followed. Ipsilateral lung ventilation is stopped only at the moment of incision, thereby allowing the most diseased parts to remain inflated (39). Complete and careful adhesiolysis if necessary is the first step (Figure 4.3, step 1), allowing full re-expansion of the lung after the procedure. The phrenic nerve must be protected. Dissection of the pulmonary ligament is recommended in most cases.

A volume-based parenchymal resection/shaving of the more peripheral target areas is performed, according to a pre-operative defined plan based on detailed CT analysis. By minimal touch reshaping (Figure 4.3, step 2) of the voluminous lung, the most severely destroyed tissues are confirmed and their volume can be assessed. The lack of resorption atelectasis is helpful in identifying target areas for resection. Deflation by cautery should be avoided since the purpose is to resect actual volume. When these target zones are identified, pre-stapling compression of the lung can be performed gently with endoscopic forceps (Figure 4.3, step 3).

Volume reduction is then realized by performing a series of (reinforced) staplings (Tri-Staple™ 2.0, Signia), starting with 45 mm, since the first stapling will be closest to the thoracic wall. We aim at reducing the additional lung volume as calculated from the estimated total lung capacity (TLC) subtracted from the measured TLC.

To avoid tearing of the fragile lung tissue, it is advised not to force the stapler over the lung, but slide the lung gently between the stapler, which can be lubricated with paraffin (Figure 4.3, step 4).

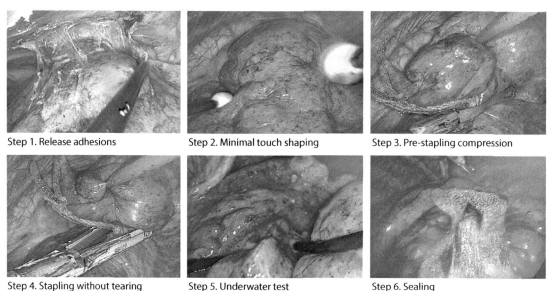

Step 1. Release adhesions   Step 2. Minimal touch shaping   Step 3. Pre-stapling compression

Step 4. Stapling without tearing   Step 5. Underwater test   Step 6. Sealing

FIGURE 4.3 Surgical technique.

In case of heterogeneous upper lobe predominant emphysema, the lateral one-third of lung parenchyma and the apical part (lung parenchyma superior to the arch of the azygos vein or aorta) are stapled, with avoidance of the fissures, so that the resulting line of resection follows an inverted J-shape (hockey-stick resection). Each consecutive stapler line begins at the last centimeter of the previous stapler line to prevent an air leak at the junction.

In there are doubts about an air leak, the lung can be submerged in water while restarting ventilation to exclude an air leak (Figure 4.3, step 5). When the lung appears fragile, a polyglycolic acid (PGA) sheet (Neoveil®; Gunze; Kyoto, Japan) along the staple line can be applied to reinforce the tissue, which is most prone to post-operative tearing during re-expansion (40), or covered with Progel™ Pleural Air Leak Sealant (Becton Dickinson and Company, Franklin Lakes, NJ) (41, 42) (Figure 4.3, step 6). Talc-pleurodesis is rarely performed and only in patients who are not eligible for lung transplant. One curved chest drain (20–28 G) is placed in the chest-cavity, pointed with the curve in the posterior sinus and the tip pointed apically. In case of very fragile tissue or minimal air leak, a second straight drain can be positioned. Mechanical ventilation is gradually resumed under visual control to assure the remaining lung is expanding completely. Aggressive recruitment should be avoided (43). No or minor suction (−3–5 cm) is required. In case of a major air leak, the suction can temporarily be increased up to −10 cm H_2O. The resected lung tissue is sent for pathological investigation.

Post-operative phase

To prevent coughing or Valsalva and to limit the time that the delicate, surgically repaired lungs are exposed to positive pressure ventilation, early extubation is important. This should be realized slowly so that the build-up of pCO2 during the operation can be decreased as well as preventing bronchospasm or coughing, which can pose major risk factors for air leaks. Switching from a double-lumen tube to a laryngeal mask can prevent coughing. Because a high PaO2 may be harmful in a patient with pre-operative CO2 retention, the PaO2 is kept close to baseline (44). The use of non-invasive ventilatory support is considered if progressive hypercapnia occurs, with no more than two liters of oxygen per minute to avoid the risk of additional CO_2 retention. No standard admission to the intensive care unit is planned unless medically required. Adequate use of non-narcotic analgesics, prophylactic use of antibiotics, chest physiotherapy to manage secretions, and early, pain-free mobilization (day of surgery) are vital in the prevention of respiratory failure or infection.

PCEA is removed at post-operative day (POD) two to three. Ranitidine (unless a proton-pump inhibitor is part of the patient's maintenance therapy), beta-2 adrenergic agonist aerosol, acetylcysteine, prophylactic dose of low-molecular-weight heparin, and an oral osmotic laxative are administered according to the protocol.

Vigilant and limited intravenous fluid administration is maintained until PCEA removal. Weight should be monitored daily and in case of volume overload, diuretics should be administered to prevent heart decompensation or pulmonary overload. Daily respiratory and general physiotherapy is mandatory and starts two to three hours post-operatively when patients are still in the recovery room. Patients receive protein-enriched meals from POD1. The urinary catheter is removed on POD1. Chest drains are removed early in the absence of an air leak and drainage of less than 200 cc. Air leak is daily evaluated in function of breathing, talking, Valsalva, or coughing.

When prolonged air leak (more than seven days) occurs, or in case of a major air leak early on, a re-intervention should be considered to prevent prolonged hospitalization. It is advised that all patients are included in a three-month respiratory rehabilitation program.

Complications

An air leak (lasting more than seven days after surgery) is the most common event, occurring in around 20–25% patients (21) and can usually be managed with continued pleural drainage until resolution. The presence and duration are associated with patient characteristics and pre-existing disease (use of inhaled steroids, low forced expiratory volume in one second, homogenous emphysema, and the degree of pleural adhesions) (45). The use of buttressed staplers (46) and the staple line coverage with sealants could potentially reduce the incidence of prolonged air leak (47). Failure for early extubation in the operating room resulting in prolonged ventilation and pneumonia are extremely rare.

Out of the potential cardiac complications, arrhythmias are most frequent. Approximately 22% of patients in the NETT experienced post-operative arrhythmia that required additional medical treatment (15). Infrequently, gastro-intestinal complications may occur (48). However, in our experience, this is much less commonly seen.

Other surgical options

While resectional LVRS is still the gold standard, non-resectional LVR is also described. This technique is performed by plicating the most emphysematous lung regions and using non-cutting stapling (27, 49). The main hypothesis is to minimize air leaks by avoiding discontinuation of the pleura and buttressing the staple line, leaving the non-resected tissue as coverage over the manipulated area.

Surgery can be carried out through either general or epidural anesthesia (awake surgery). In a single-center, randomized trial, non-resectional (awake) LVRS was compared with resectional (non-awake) LVRS (32 vs. 31 patients, respectively) and resulted in a shorter hospital stay in the awake, non-resectional patients (6 days vs. 7.5 days) with similar lung functional improvements at six months (50). However, the bias of comparing two different techniques in different settings (awake/non-awake) must be considered. Additionally, when lung tissue is not resected, the risk of infection and resultant malignancies must be considered. Other prospectively multi-center collected data are needed to confirm the potential benefits of non-resectional and awake surgery.

Experience with awake thoracic surgery is increasing worldwide with the primary objective to improve outcomes by avoiding side-effects associated with general anesthesia and one-lung ventilation (pneumonia, bronchospasm, lung injury related to ventilation) (51). However, non-awake LVRS can only be performed after thorough patient selection. Patients with radiologic evidence of extensive pleural adhesions, contraindications for epidural anesthesia, and uncomfortable with the idea of being awake during surgery are contraindicated for awake surgery. Technically demanding cases are preferably performed under general anesthesia since maintaining diaphragmatic motion and cough reflexes can hinder surgical manipulation.

According to the general evolution in oncologic surgery, robotic LVRS could become more prominent due to its minimal invasive approach, maximal exposure, and potential future software applications. One example is the potential implementation of 3D visualization, as the goal of LVRS is to target the most destroyed areas identified on pre-operative imaging (52).

REFERENCES

1. WHO. The top 10 causes of death fact sheet 2019 [Internet]. Available from: https://www.who.int/news-room/fact-sheets/detail/the-top-10-causes-of-death
2. Decramer M, Janssens W, Miravitlles M. Chronic obstructive pulmonary disease. *Lancet.* 2012;379(9823):1341–51.
3. Mannino DM, Buist AS. Global burden of COPD: risk factors, prevalence, and future trends. *Lancet* [Internet]. 2007;370(9589):765–73. Available from: http://dx.doi.org/10.1016/S0140-6736(07)61380-4
4. Shah PL, Herth FJ, van Geffen WH, Deslee G, Slebos DJ. Lung volume reduction for emphysema. *Lancet Respir Med [Internet].* 2017;5(2):147–56. Available from: http://dx.doi.org/10.1016/S2213-2600(16)30221-1
5. Freund WA. Zur operativen Behandlung gewisser Lungenkrankheiten, insbesondere des auf starrer Thoraxidlatation beruhenden alveolären Emphysems (mit einem Operationsfalle). *Zeitschrift für Exp Pathol und Ther* [Internet]. 1906 Nov;3(3):479–98. Available from: http://link.springer.com/10.1007/BF02622074

6. Abbott OA, Hopkins WA, Van Fleit WE, Robinson JS. A new approach to pulmonary emphysema. *Thorax* [Internet]. 1953 Jun 1;8(2):116–32. Available from: https://thorax.bmj.com/lookup/doi/10.1136/thx.8.2.116

7. Allison PR. Giant bullous cysts of the lung. *Thorax* [Internet]. 1947 Dec 1;2(4):169–75. Available from: https://thorax.bmj.com/lookup/doi/10.1136/thx.2.4.169

8. Brantigan OC, Mueller E, Kress MB. A surgical approach to pulmonary emphysema. *Am Rev Respir Dis.* 1959;80(1, Part 2):194–206.

9. Knudson RJ, Gaensler EA. Surgery for emphysema. *Ann Thorac Surg* [Internet]. 1965 May;1(3):332–62. Available from: http://dx.doi.org/10.1016/S0003-4975(10)66764-1

10. Cooper JD, Trulock EP, Triantafillou AN, Patterson GA, Pohl MS, Deloney PA, et al. Bilateral pneumectomy (volume reduction) for chronic obstructive pulmonary disease. *J Thorac Cardiovasc Surg* [Internet]. 1995 Jan;109(1):106–19. Available from: https://linkinghub.elsevier.com/retrieve/pii/S0022522395704264

11. Stanifer PB, Ginsburg ME. Lung volume reduction surgery in the post-National Emphysema Treatment Trial era. *J Thorac Dis.* 2018;10(7):S2744–7.

12. Whittaker HR, Connell O, Campbell J, Elbehairy AF, Hopkinson NS, Quint JK. Eligibility for lung volume reduction surgery in patients with COPD identified in a UK primary care setting. *Chest* [Internet]. 2020 Feb;157(2):276–85. Available from: https://doi.org/10.1016/j.chest.2019.07.016

13. Bingisser R, Zollinger A, Hauser M, Bloch KE, Russi EW, Weder W. Bilateral volume reduction surgery for diffuse pulmonary emphysema by video-assisted thoracoscopy. *J Thorac Cardiovasc Surg* [Internet]. 1996 Oct;112(4):875–82. Available from: https://linkinghub.elsevier.com/retrieve/pii/S0022522396700867

14. Keenan RJ, Landreneau RJ, Sciurba FC, Ferson PF, Holbert JM, Brown ML, et al. Unilateral thoracoscopic surgical approach for diffuse emphysema. *J Thorac Cardiovasc Surg* [Internet]. 1996 Feb;111(2):308–16. Available from: https://linkinghub.elsevier.com/retrieve/pii/S0022522396704397

15. Fishman A, Martinez F, Naunheim K, Piantadosi S, Wise R, Ries A, et al. A randomized trial comparing lung-volume–reduction surgery with medical therapy for severe emphysema. *N Engl J Med* [Internet]. 2003 May 22;348(21):2059–73. Available from: http://www.nejm.org/doi/abs/10.1056/NEJMoa030287

16. Fishman A, Fessler H, Martinez F, McKenna Jr RJ, Naunheim K, Piantadosi S, Weinmann G, Wise R. Patients at high risk of death after lung-volume–reduction surgery. *N Engl J Med* [Internet]. 2001 Oct 11;345(15):1075–83. Available from: http://www.nejm.org/doi/abs/10.1056/NEJMoa11798

17. Naunheim KS, Wood DE, Mohsenifar Z, Sternberg AL, Criner GJ, DeCamp MM, et al. Long-term follow-up of patients receiving lung-volume-reduction surgery versus medical therapy for severe emphysema by the National Emphysema Treatment Trial Research Group. *Ann Thorac Surg* [Internet]. 2006 Aug;82(2):431–43. e19. Available from: https://linkinghub.elsevier.com/retrieve/pii/S0003497506010563

18. Weder W, Tutic M, Lardinois D, Jungraithmayr W, Hillinger S, Russi EW, et al. Persistent benefit from lung volume reduction surgery in patients with homogeneous emphysema. *Ann Thorac Surg* [Internet]. 2009 Jan;87(1):229–37. Available from: https://linkinghub.elsevier.com/retrieve/pii/S0003497508022236

19. Ginsburg ME, Thomashow BM, Yip CK, DiMango AM, Maxfield RA, Bartels MN, et al. Lung volume reduction surgery using the NETT selection criteria. *Ann Thorac Surg* [Internet]. 2011 May;91(5):1556–61. Available from: http://dx.doi.org/10.1016/j.athoracsur.2011.01.054

20. van Agteren JE, Carson KV, Tiong LU, Smith BJ. Lung volume reduction surgery for diffuse emphysema. *Cochrane Database Syst Rev* [Internet]. 2016 Oct 14;2016(10). Available from: http://doi.wiley.com/10.1002/14651858.CD001001.pub3

21. Seadler B, Thuppal S, Rizvi N, Markwell S, Sawyer J, McCullough K, et al. Clinical and quality of life outcomes after lung volume reduction surgery. *Ann Thorac Surg* [Internet]. 2019 Sep;108(3):866–72. Available from: https://doi.org/10.1016/j.athoracsur.2019.03.089

22. Ginsburg ME, Thomashow BM, Bulman WA, Jellen PA, Whippo BA, Chiuzan C, et al. The safety, efficacy, and durability of lung-volume-reduction surgery: a 10-year experience. *J Thorac Cardiovasc Surg* [Internet]. 2016;151(3):717–24.e1. Available from: http://dx.doi.org/10.1016/j.jtcvs.2015.10.095

23. Criner GJ, Cordova F, Sternberg AL, Martinez FJ. The National Emphysema Treatment Trial (NETT) part II: lessons learned about lung volume reduction surgery. *Am J Respir Crit Care Med* [Internet]. 2011 Oct 15;184(8):881–93. Available from: https://www.atsjournals.org/doi/10.1164/rccm.201103-0455CI

24. Ciccone AM, Meyers BF, Guthrie TJ, Davis GE, Yusen RD, Lefrak SS, et al. Long-term outcome of bilateral lung volume reduction in 250 consecutive patients with emphysema. *J Thorac Cardiovasc Surg.* 2003;125(3):513–25.

25. Tutic M, Lardinois D, Imfeld S, Korom S, Boehler A, Speich R, et al. Lung-volume reduction surgery as an alternative or bridging procedure to lung transplantation. *Ann Thorac Surg.* 2006;82(1):208–13.

26. Cassart M, Hamacher J, Verbandt Y, Wildermuth S, Ritscher D, Russi EW, et al. Effects of lung volume reduction surgery for emphysema on diaphragm dimensions and configuration. *Am J Respir Crit Care Med* [Internet]. 2001 Apr 1;163(5):1171–5. Available from: http://www.ncbi.nlm.nih.gov/pubmed/18347203

27. Pompeo E, Rogliani P, Cristino B, Fabbi E, Dauri M, Scrgiacomi G. Staged unilateral lung volume reduction surgery: from mini-invasive to minimalist treatment strategies. *J Thorac Dis*. 2018;10(Suppl 23):S2754–62.

28. Caviezel C, Schaffter N, Schneiter D, Franzen D, Inci I, Opitz I, et al. Outcome after lung volume reduction surgery in patients with severely impaired diffusion capacity. *Ann Thorac Surg* [Internet]. 2018;105(2):379–85. Available from: https://doi.org/10.1016/j.athoracsur.2017.09.006

29. Caviezel C, Aruldas C, Franzen D, Ulrich S, Inci I, Schneiter Di, et al. Lung volume reduction surgery in selected patients with emphysema and pulmonary hypertension. *Eur J Cardio-thoracic Surg*. 2018;54(3):565–71.

30. Clarenbach CF, Sievi NA, Brock M, Schneiter D, Weder W, Kohler M. Lung volume reduction surgery and improvement of endothelial function and blood pressure in patients with chronic obstructive pulmonary disease: a randomized controlled trial. *Am J Respir Crit Care Med*. 2015;192(3):307–14.

31. Barbarossa A, Van Raemdonck D, Weder W, Ceulemans LJ. Urgent lung volume reduction surgery is effective for secondary pneumothorax in emphysema patients. *Interdiscip Cardiovasc Thorac Surg* [Internet]. 2023 Jun 1;36(6):0–2. Available from: https://academic.oup.com/icvts/article/doi/10.1093/icvts/ivad099/7192179

32. Sciurba FC, Rogers RM, Keenan RJ, Slivka WA, Gorcsan J, Ferson PF, et al. Improvement in pulmonary function and elastic recoil after lung-reduction surgery for diffuse emphysema. *N Engl J Med* [Internet]. 1996 Apr 25;334(17):1095–9. Available from: http://journals.lww.com/00008483-199705000-00009

33. Weder W, Ceulemans LJ, Opitz I, Schneiter D, Caviezel C. Lung volume reduction surgery in patients with homogeneous emphysema. *Thorac Surg Clin* [Internet]. 2021;31(2):203–9. Available from: https://doi.org/10.1016/j.thorsurg.2021.02.007

34. Weder W, Thurnheer R, Stammberger U, Bürge M, Russi EW, Bloch KE. Radiologic emphysema morphology is associated with outcome after surgical lung volume reduction. *Ann Thorac Surg*. 1997;64(2):313–20.

35. Meyers BF, Sultan PK, Guthrie TJ, Lefrak SS, Davis GE, Patterson GA, et al. Persistent benefit from lung volume reduction surgery in patients with homogeneous emphysema. *Ann Thorac Surg* [Internet]. 2009 Jan;87(1):229–37. Available from: https://linkinghub.elsevier.com/retrieve/pii/S0003497508022236

36. Oey I, Steiner M, Morgan M, Waller D. Patient-directed volume reduction for emphysema: sequential surgical and endobronchial techniques. *Ann Thorac Surg* [Internet]. 2021;112(1):295–301. Available from: https://doi.org/10.1016/j.athoracsur.2020.08.015

37. Oey IF, Morgan MDL, Spyt TJ, Waller DA. Staged bilateral lung volume reduction surgery — the benefits of a patient-led strategy. *Eur J Cardio-Thoracic Surg* [Internet]. 2010 Apr;37(4):846–52. Available from: https://academic.oup.com/ejcts/article-lookup/doi/10.1016/j.ejcts.2009.10.025

38. Pompeo E, Mineo T. Long-term outcome of staged versus one-stage bilateral thoracoscopic reduction pneumoplasty. *Eur J Cardio-Thoracic Surg* [Internet]. 2002 Apr;21(4):627–33. Available from: https://academic.oup.com/ejcts/article-lookup/doi/10.1016/S1010-7940(02)00038-6

39. Brister NW, Barnette RE, Kim V, Keresztury M. Anesthetic considerations in candidates for lung volume reduction surgery. *Proc Am Thorac Soc* [Internet]. 2008 May 1;5(4):432–7. Available from: http://pats.atsjournals.org/cgi/doi/10.1513/pats.200709-149ET

40. Kawai N, Kawaguchi T, Suzuki S, Yasukawa M, Tojo T, Taniguchi S. Low-voltage coagulation, polyglycolic acid sheets, and fibrin glue to control air leaks in lung surgery. *Gen Thorac Cardiovasc Surg* [Internet]. 2017 Dec 30;65(12):705–9. Available from: http://link.springer.com/10.1007/s11748-017-0829-2

41. Klijian A. A novel approach to control air leaks in complex lung surgery: a retrospective review. *J Cardiothorac Surg*. 2012;7(1):3–8.

42. Allen MS, Wood DE, Hawkinson RW, Harpole DH, McKenna RJ, Walsh GL, et al. Prospective randomized study evaluating a biodegradable polymeric sealant for sealing intraoperative air leaks that occur during pulmonary resection. *Ann Thorac Surg*. 2004;77(5):1792–801.

43. Boasquevisque CHR, Yildirim E, Waddel TK, Keshavjee S. Surgical techniques: lung transplant and lung volume reduction. *Proc Am Thorac Soc*. 2009;6(1):66–78.

44. Sharafkhaneh A, Falk JA, Minai OA, Lipson DA. Overview of the perioperative management of lung volume reduction surgery patients. *Proc Am Thorac Soc*. 2008;5(4):438–41.

45. DeCamp MM, Blackstone EH, Naunheim KS, Krasna MJ, Wood DE, Meli YM, et al. Patient and surgical factors influencing air leak after lung volume reduction surgery: lessons learned from the National Emphysema Treatment Trial. *Ann Thorac Surg* [Internet]. 2006 Jul;82(1):197–207. Available from: https://linkinghub.elsevier.com/retrieve/pii/S0003497506003924

46. Stammberger U, Klepetko W, Stamatis G, Hamacher J, Schmid RA, Wisser W, et al. Buttressing the staple line in lung volume reduction surgery: a randomized three-center study. *Ann Thorac Surg*. 2000;70(6):1820–5.

47. Moser C, Opitz I, Zhai W, Rousson V, Russi EW, Weder W, et al. Autologous fibrin sealant reduces the incidence of prolonged air leak and duration of chest tube drainage after lung volume reduction surgery: a prospective randomized blinded study. *J Thorac Cardiovasc Surg* [Internet]. 2008;136(4):843–9. Available from: http://dx.doi.org/10.1016/j.jtcvs.2008.02.079

48. Cetindag IB, Boley TM, Magee MJ, Hazelrigg SR. Postoperative gastrointestinal complications after lung volume reduction operations. *Ann Thorac Surg* [Internet]. 1999 Sep;68(3):1029–33. Available from: https://linkinghub.elsevier.com/retrieve/pii/S0012369215463044
49. Mineo TC, Pompeo E, Mineo D, Tacconi F, Marino M, Sabato AF. Awake nonresectional lung volume reduction surgery. *Ann Surg*. 2006;243(1):131–6.
50. Pompeo E, Rogliani P, Tacconi F, Dauri M, Saltini C, Novelli G, et al. Randomized comparison of awake nonresectional versus nonawake resectional lung volume reduction surgery. *J Thorac Cardiovasc Surg* [Internet]. 2012 Jan;143(1):47–54.e1. Available from: https://linkinghub.elsevier.com/retrieve/pii/S0022522311010683
51. Tacconi F, Pompeo E. Non-intubated video-assisted thoracic surgery: where does evidence stand? *J Thorac Dis* [Internet]. 2016 Apr;8(S4):S364–75. Available from: http://jtd.amegroups.com/article/view/7440/6849
52. Caviezel C, Schneiter D, Lauk O, Opitz I. Firefly robotic lung volume reduction surgery: case report. *J Vis Surg*. 2021;7:19–19.

Image Analysis to Identify Target Areas for Lung Volume Reduction

5

Maruti Kumaran, Yogesh Gupta and Chandra Dass

INTRODUCTION

Chronic obstructive pulmonary disease (COPD) is the third leading cause of death worldwide, causing 3.23 million deaths in 2019, and is the seventh leading cause of poor health worldwide [1]. Conventional medical management for COPD primarily involves the use of short or long-acting bronchodilators, corticosteroids, supplemental oxygen, and pulmonary rehabilitation. These medical interventions, however, primarily target patient airway inflammation and are unable to address the irreversible destruction of lung parenchyma and hyperinflation of airspaces associated with emphysema, and thus offer limited clinical benefit to those with advanced disease [2]. Lung volume reduction (LVR) procedures such as lung volume reduction surgery (LVRS) and bronchoscopic lung volume reduction (BLVR) using endobronchial valves (EBV) have been increasingly employed in recent years as alternative options for those patients who are symptomatic despite optimal medical management. The clinical benefits of LVR procedures result mainly from improvements in the mechanical function of the respiratory muscles by decreasing the functional residual capacity and reducing dynamic hyperinflation during exercise [3, 4]. Additionally, redistribution of blood perfusion into the untreated lung improves VQ quotient [5]. Improved right ventricle hemodynamics from decreased intrathoracic pressure also contributes to the overall clinical benefits [6]. With more medical centers currently adapting LVRS and BLVR, the radiology community will be expected to make meaningful contributions to maximize the clinical outcome of these procedures. With this goal in mind, this chapter focuses on the current role of imaging in appropriate patient selection and target lobe selection, as well as identifying post-procedural adverse events for their timely management.

DOI: 10.1201/9781003251439-5

LUNG VOLUME REDUCTION SURGERY

LVRS is a promising palliative treatment option for select patients and involves reducing the volume of each lung by between 20% and 30% by wedge excising the least functional part of the lungs. The National Emphysema Treatment Trial (NETT) demonstrated that LVRS improves pulmonary function, exercise capacity, and quality of life in select subgroups – especially in patients with predominantly upper lobe disease and low-exercise capacity [7, 8]. The role of imaging in LVRS is twofold, namely, appropriate selection of surgical candidates and the management of post-surgical adverse events.

Pre-procedural imaging assessment

The primary role of HRCT imaging is to identify the optimal candidate by assessing the severity and anatomic distribution of emphysema and identifying other conditions that may preclude LVRS [7, 8]. The major imaging finding generally thought to be favorable for LVRS is upper lobe predominant severe emphysema coexisting with a higher percentage of less emphysematous and near normal remaining lung (Figure 5.1). Several factors that are considered relative contraindications to LVRS are homogeneous distribution of emphysema, absence of preserved lung tissue, severe airway disease, significant pleural disease, interstitial lung disease, giant bulla, lung mass or concerning nodules, severe pulmonary hypertension, previous intervention (pleurodesis, thoracotomy), and profound chest wall deformities. [9]. Planar perfusion lung scintigraphy may have a complementary role in confirming upper zone predominant emphysema phenotype for LVRS by quantifying the upper lung zonal hypoperfusion [10].

Post-procedural imaging assessment

Primary pulmonary complications in the immediate post-operative period include air leak and pneumonia. Air leak is the most common complication after LVRS, and prolonged air leak is defined as an air leak lasting more than five to seven days after surgery [11]. Due to the high proportion of patients with air leaks, careful attention to the proper function of the chest tubes is key to prevent development of a pneumothorax. A chest radiograph is obtained daily to confirm full lung re-expansion. Pneumonia is considered the second most common pulmonary complication after LVRS. The role of imaging in terms

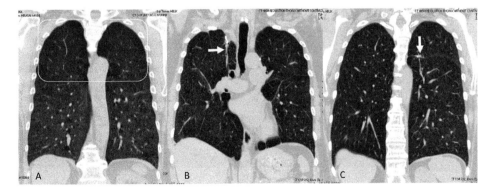

FIGURE 5.1 Ideal LVRS candidate. (A) Upper lobe predominant severe emphysema (white rectangle) coexisting with a higher percentage of less emphysematous remaining lung. (B, C) Status post-bilateral LVRS with biapical surgical sutures and scarring (white arrow).

of other less common post-operative complications (thrombo-embolic disease, bleeding, surgical wound complications, etc.) is no different than any other thoracotomy surgical procedure.

BRONCHOSCOPIC LUNG VOLUME REDUCTION

LVRS is under-utilized due to concerns about the invasiveness of the procedure, associated patient comorbidities, and narrow patient eligibility criteria [12]. Fortunately, BLVR using two FDA-approved EBV (Zephyr® Valve System Pulmonx®, Palo Alto, CA, USA; Spiration® Valve System SVS – Olympus Respiratory America®, Redmond, WA, USA) is currently increasingly available as an alternative option for those patients who are symptomatic despite optimal medical management but are poor candidates for LVRS [13, 14] (Figure 5.2). Given the results of multiple randomized clinical trials, it has been established that the clinical outcomes of BLVR using EBV can be maximized when clinical- and blood chemistry-based criteria are applied to specific image-based COPD phenotypes. The rest of this chapter highlights the role of imaging before the procedure, in the early post-procedure, and in long-term surveillance of these patients.

Pre-procedural imaging assessment

HRCT acquisition. After spirometric confirmation of COPD, potential candidates for EBV therapy are initially screened according to the clinical eligibility criteria as per the expert panel recommendations [13–15] based on multiple randomized clinical trials [16–25]. Obtaining a non-contrast volumetric chest HRCT scan (typical protocol: kVp 120; mAs 120; spiral mode with a pitch factor 1; slice thickness 0.5–1.5 mm; gantry speed 0.5 s; breath hold at total lung capacity; coronal and sagittal reconstruction; mediastinal

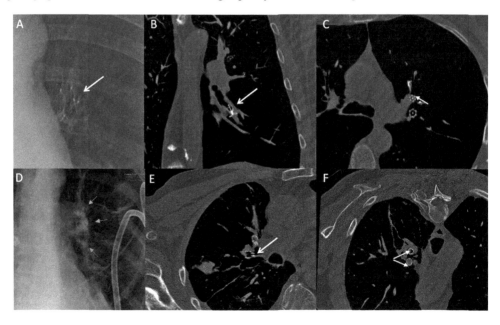

FIGURE 5.2 CXR and HRCT imaging appearance of endobronchial valves. (A–C) Expected appearance of Spiration valves (arrows) on frontal chest radiograph (A) and on multiplanar CT images of the chest in profile (B) and end on (C). (D–F) The expected appearance of Zephyr valves (arrows) on frontal chest radiograph (D) and on multiplanar CT images of the chest in profile (E) and end on (F).

and lung window display) is the next step in the patient selection algorithm. HRCT is quality controlled by a chest radiologist for adequate coverage, signal-to-noise ratio, and to identify any motion artifact (the latter is detrimental to the subsequent computer-based quantification process).

HRCT analysis. HRCT analysis serves three important purposes:

1. Confirmation of emphysema and hyperinflation. The multiplanar HRCT images are first visually evaluated for the type and severity of emphysema, their lobar distribution (heterogenous vs. homogenous), areas of hyperinflation, parenchymal destruction, and interlobar fissure integrity.
2. Exclusion criteria. The images are then carefully screened for any HRCT exclusion criteria, some of which are absolute contraindications for BLVR and others are relative (Table 5.1 and Figure 5.3).
3. Target lobe selection. This pivotal step is based on certain quantitative CT (QCT) parameters, derived commonly using some commercially available software, as per the recently updated recommendation of the expert panel, as described below [13].
   A) Emphysema score. This software-generated score quantifies the extent and lobar distribution of emphysema in a more reproducible way than visual qualitative evaluation [26]. The score is expressed as a percentage of voxels in each lobe below certain attenuation (HU) threshold (aka. low attenuation area [LAA]), typically <-910 HU (Figure 5.4). It has been found that EBV treatment is useful when at least 50% of the lobe is emphysematous applying these criteria. The lobe with the highest emphysema score is the preferred target lobe for valve placement.
   B) The heterogeneity index is the relative percentage difference in the emphysema scores between the ipsilateral lobes [13]. Although no clear definition of interlobar heterogeneity exists, a 10–15% heterogeneity index has been used in most clinical trials [13, 26]. Although earlier clinical trials focused on heterogeneous emphysema distribution, STELVIO 2015 [20] and IMPACT 2016 [21] trials included patients with homogeneous emphysema, suggesting the possible effectiveness of EBV therapy in this subgroup as well [15, 21–27]. Moreover, in contrast to NETT results, EBV therapy appears to be equally effective in both upper and lower lobe predominant emphysema [28].
   C) Inspiratory lobar volume. As these valves work primarily by reversing lung hyperinflation, it is imperative to select the most hyperinflated lobe as the target lobe for treatment (Figure 5.4). A higher emphysema score generally means greater hyperinflation and is

TABLE 5.1   HRCT-based exclusion criteria

HRCT FINDING	COMMENTS
Defective major fissure (>20%)	Higher likelihood of significant CV
Large bulla >30% ipsilateral lung volume	Bronchial communication cannot be assured
Predominant paraseptal emphysema	Bronchial communication cannot be assured
Suspicious lung nodules	Needs further evaluation
Severe bronchiectasis	Valve migration
Active infection	Treated before valve deployment
Associated fibrotic ILD (CPFE)	Poor lung compliance
Severe pulmonary hypertension	Potential worsening
Severe pleural thickening/subpleural scarring	Increased risk of pneumothorax
Prior ipsilateral intervention	Lung transplant, LVRS, pleurodesis
Any incidental findings that need further assessment	Large aneurysm, mediastinal mass, significant lymphadenopathy, diaphragm paralysis, etc.

Note: Exclusion criteria are based on peer-reviewed updated expert panel recommendations and multiple randomized controlled trials [13–25].

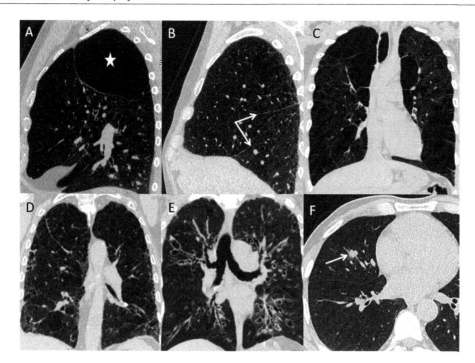

FIGURE 5.3   HRCT-based exclusion criteria for EBV treatment. Unenhanced HRCT images of the chest demonstrate various exclusion criteria for BLVR. (A) A sagittal image shows giant apical bullae (star). (B) A sagittal image demonstrates an incomplete major fissure (arrows). (C) A coronal image demonstrates predominant paraseptal emphysema. (D) A coronal image demonstrates combined pulmonary fibrosis and emphysema. (E) A coronal image shows bronchiectasis with bronchitis. (F) Axial image demonstrates a suspicious RML nodule (arrow).

expected to result in a better post-procedure outcome. For consistency and reproducibility, computer software-generated inspiratory lobar volume is used as an index of severity of hyperinflation.

D) Fissure integrity and collateral ventilation. Collateral ventilation (CV) is airflow between adjacent lobes through channels that bypass the normal bronchial tree. CV mitigates the intended deflation of the treated lobe and only lobes with minimal or no collateral ventilation are eligible for valve implantation. Since the morphologic fissure integrity (fissure completeness) is highly correlated with CV, visual or computer analysis of HRCT images for completeness of the interlobar fissures is performed in all three orthogonal planes. Automated computer software analysis for this purpose is currently encouraged over visual analysis due to higher interobserver variability with the latter [29, 30]. The fissure completeness score thus obtained helps to choose the target lobe (Figure 5.4).

The results are generally interpreted as follows:

Fissure completeness <80%: Suggests higher likelihood of significant CV, not considered eligible for EBV treatment.

Fissure completeness >90%: Suggests lower likelihood of CV and high success rate (additional invasive evaluation is optional).

Fissure completeness 80–90%: Suggests intermediate likelihood of CV, and an additional confirmation testing is currently recommended [31].

In practice, additional real-time assessment of CV is done immediately before the BLVR procedure using a proprietary system (e.g., Chartis® pulmonX, Redwood City, CA, USA). In a direct comparison of HRCT automated computer software-based fissure analysis and the Chartis® system, both were found to be equally effective for predicting the response to EBV therapy [32–34]. Both methods were concordant

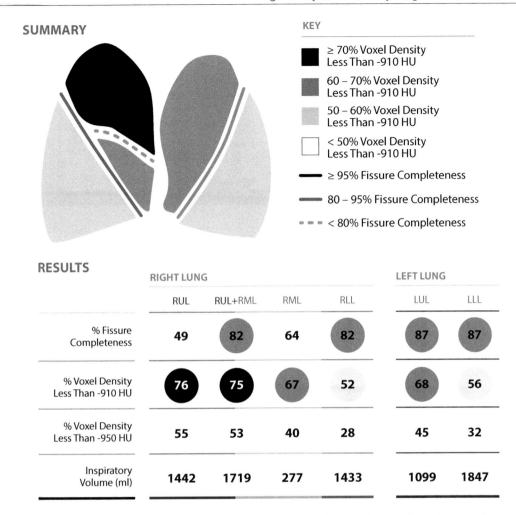

SUMMARY

KEY

- ≥ 70% Voxel Density Less Than -910 HU
- 60 – 70% Voxel Density Less Than -910 HU
- 50 – 60% Voxel Density Less Than -910 HU
- < 50% Voxel Density Less Than -910 HU
- ≥ 95% Fissure Completeness
- 80 – 95% Fissure Completeness
- < 80% Fissure Completeness

RESULTS

	RIGHT LUNG				LEFT LUNG	
	RUL	RUL+RML	RML	RLL	LUL	LLL
% Fissure Completeness	49	82	64	82	87	87
% Voxel Density Less Than -910 HU	76	75	67	52	68	56
% Voxel Density Less Than -950 HU	55	53	40	28	45	32
Inspiratory Volume (ml)	1442	1719	277	1433	1099	1847

FIGURE 5.4 StratX Report Card displaying percentage fissure completeness (top row), emphysema destruction score (middle two rows, <–910 and <–950 HU), and inspiratory lobar volume (bottom row). Highly incomplete fissures are noted by a dashed line (right minor fissure). Partially incomplete fissures are denoted by a solid gray line (both major fissures). Highly complete fissures are denoted by a solid black line. Chartis evaluation is recommended in this patient to assess the physiological significance of the major fissures. A lighter lobar color tone denotes lesser emphysema, while a darker lobar color tone represents more emphysema. The right upper lobe has the highest emphysema destruction score (76%) and is the target lobe. Given that the right minor fissure is highly incomplete, both the right upper and middle lobes must be considered as a single unit for EBV deployment.

in two-thirds of the patients, thus a certain proportion of patients may require assessment with both techniques to predict the optimal treatment response with a higher likelihood [32–35].

Lung perfusion imaging (SPECT-CT). In patients with more than one eligible lobe, especially in those with homogeneous or mildly heterogeneous emphysema, perfusion scintigraphy may be helpful to identify a single target lobe [21]. While planar lung scintigraphic imaging (as usually done for LVRS) is able to provide zonal perfusion, lung perfusion SPECT- CT is the preferred modality to map the relative lobar perfusion for BLVR (Figure 5.5). The lobe with a lower perfusion is targeted for therapy. It has been shown that higher perfusion in the untreated ipsilateral lobe is a strong predictor of exercise capacity improvement after valve therapy [36]. Alternatively, dual energy CT iodine distribution mapping can provide similar relative lobar perfusion information.

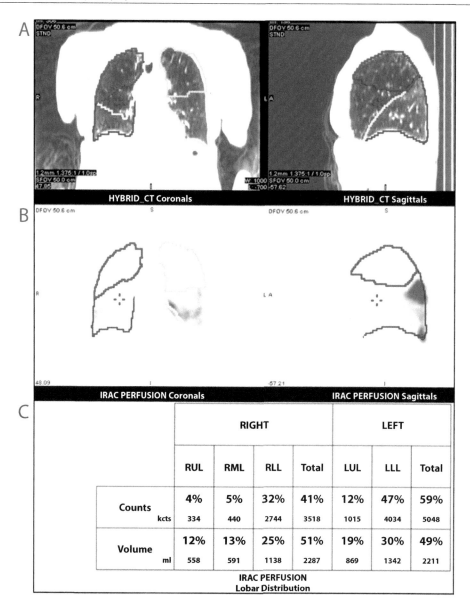

FIGURE 5.5 Quantification of relative lobar perfusion using SPECT-CT. (A) Images from the CT portion of the study show the fissures delineated semiautomatically. (B) Images from the perfusion portion of the study with superimposed fissures obtained from the CT. (C) The table shows relative lobar perfusion based on radionuclide counts (upper row) and absolute lobar volume based on CT densitometry (lower row). In this patient, both upper lobes were considered equally good target candidates on the basis of quantitative CT analysis (not shown). The fractional lobar perfusion from SPECT-CT was 4% in the RUL and 12% in the LUL. The RUL with lower perfusion was chosen as the target lobe, saving the LUL with better perfusion. LLL, left lower lobe; LUL, left upper lobe; RLL, right lower lobe; RUL, right upper lobe.

The ideal target lobe for BLVR is the one with (a) a higher emphysema destruction score, (b) bordered by intact fissure(s), (c) larger inspiratory volume, and (d) lower perfusion (Table 5.2). For the purpose of target lobe analysis, the right middle lobe (RML) is not considered an "independent lobe"; it is evaluated either with the right upper lobe (RUL+RML) or with the right lower lobe (RLL+RML). Both valve manufacturers provide a cloud-based quantitative CT (QCT) analysis service by generating a "Report Card"-type printout of the results (StratX® Report by PulmonX®; VIDA SeleCT® by SVS®) on emphysema

TABLE 5.2   Ideal target lobe selection criteria

IMAGING CRITERIA	PREFERRED FINDING
1. Severity of emphysema	Lobe with higher emphysematous score (<−950 HU)
2. Collateral ventilation	Lobe with intact fissure(s)
3. Lobar volume	Most hyperinflated lobe
4. Lobar perfusion	Least perfused lobe

destruction score, fissure integrity score, and the lobar inspiratory volume for choosing the correct target lobe (Figure 5.4). However, it is important to acknowledge that there is substantial inter-software variability in the results, and it is recommended to use the same scanning protocol and QCT software for longitudinal monitoring of these patients [6]. This type of report generation can also be used to objectively evaluate lung volume changes after EBV deployment.

Early post-procedural imaging assessment

Following EBV procedures, the primary role of imaging is monitoring for immediate post-procedural complications such as pneumothorax (PTX), pneumonia, COPD exacerbations, and valve migration [15, 37], apart from the expected gradual collapse of the treated lobe (Figure 5.6). PTX is by far the most common complication, occurring in about 20% to 30% of the cases following EBV placement [20] (Figure 5.7). Suspected risk factors include rapid deflation of the target lobe or the presence of pleural adhesions [24, 38]. Since roughly 75% of PTXs occur within the first three days following the procedure, the current practice for many institutions is to admit the patient for three to five days for observation with daily chest radiographs. While small asymptomatic PTX may be managed with observation and repeat radiographs as necessary, moderate to large PTX or symptomatic PTX may require chest tube placement, with further management determined by the patient's clinical progression and imaging findings from chest radiography, bedside sonography, or even low-dose CT (Figure 5.8). If imaging shows re-expansion of the collapsed nontarget lobe with no more air leak, the chest tube can be removed. Evidence of continued air leaks would necessitate the removal of one or more valves, surgical intervention, or pleurodesis [13].

Other early post-procedural complications such as COPD exacerbations and pneumonia occur in up to 20% of patients and are easily identifiable with chest radiographs (Figure 5.9). Valve migration occurs much less commonly, roughly in about 6% of patients [15]. It is usually a consequence of inappropriate valve sizing or inappropriate valve deployment and leads to incomplete lobar deflation or re-expansion of the previously collapsed lobe. In terms of surveillance, misplaced valves may be difficult to visualize on

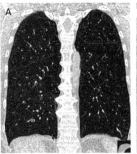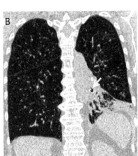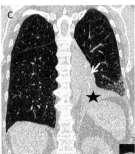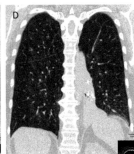

FIGURE 5.6   Normal post-EBV placement changes. (A) CT images of the chest in coronal plane demonstrate emphysematous lungs before EBV treatment. (B–D) HRCT scan obtained after placement of multiple endobronchial valves (arrow) in the left lower lobe shows progressive volume loss (star) at four hours (B), four days (C), and one year (D).

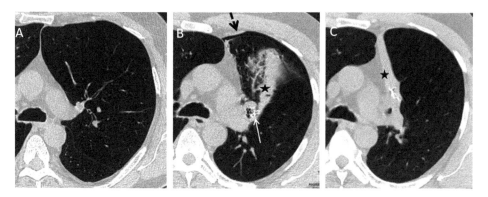

FIGURE 5.7   Post-EBV placement pneumothorax. CT of the thorax in axial plane. (A) Emphysematous lung before treatment. (B) Following placement on endobronchial valves in the left upper lobe segmental bronchi (white arrow), there is partial atelectasis (star) and a small ex-vacuo pneumothorax (black arrows). (C) Progressive atelectasis (star) and resolution of pneumothorax with no active intervention.

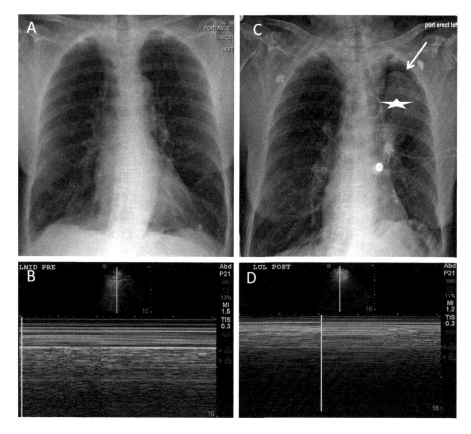

FIGURE 5.8   Bedside M-mode lung sonogram in post-EBV placement pneumothorax. (A, B) Pre-EBV placement images. (A) Baseline chest radiograph demonstrates hyperinflated lungs. (B) The corresponding M-mode ultrasound tracing shows a normal "seashore" pattern. (C, D) Post-EBV placement images. (C) Chest radiograph demonstrating left upper lobe atelectasis (star) and a small pneumothorax (arrow). (D) The corresponding M-mode ultrasound tracing shows an abnormal "barcode" pattern.

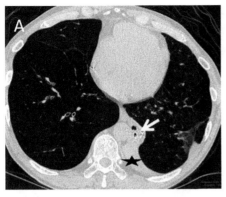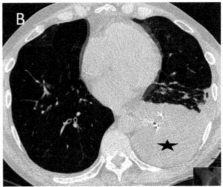

FIGURE 5.9   Post-EBV placement infection. (A, B) Axial CT images of the chest demonstrate complete left lower lobe atelectasis (star) after EBV placement (arrow) (A). Subsequent consolidation (star) within the collapsed left lower lobe with new pleural effusion (B), representing target lobe post-obstructive pneumonia.

chest radiographs, so often an HRCT may be required. Airway kinking or folding is an extremely rare complication that can be identified on CT [28].

Long-term post-procedural imaging surveillance

Significant volume reduction of the treated lobe may be observed within the first few days, although, in some patients, it may take up to a month (Figure 5.6). Criteria for premature re-evaluation of these patients have been established, and imaging plays an important role in their identification and management [13–15]. It is recommended to obtain a low-dose CT scan around 30 to 45 days after the procedure to assess valve placement, particularly if there is no perceived clinical improvement or breathing deterioration. The CT is evaluated by mainly focusing on the valve count, valve location (migration/malpositioning), and target lobe(s) volume reduction (TLVR), among others.

Valve position. EBV position in the airway is best evaluated by CT using the multiplanar reconstruction technique (MPR) (Figure 5.10). The ideal position of the valve is for the long axis of the EBV to be coaxial with the long axis of the airway lumen while having the widest segment of the valve be circumferentially in direct contact with the airway wall. With proper placement, the main body of the valve must be distal to the ostium, and the valve extractor extends proximal to the ostium, rendering it accessible for removal with grasping forceps. In addition to confirming the position of the valves, radiologists should also confirm the number of valves present; any missing valve needs to be accounted for either by identifying it in an unintended location or with a history of "coughing the valve out." Further bronchoscopic evaluation and valve replacement are recommended depending on the CT findings.

Target lobe(s) volume reduction. TLVR is one of the predictors of successful clinical treatment, as higher the TLVR achieved, the greater the improvement in lung functional parameters. Although the minimal clinically important difference for TLVR (and consequent reduction in residual volume) was originally defined as 350 mL, more recent experience suggests that a higher TLVR is necessary to achieve a clinically relevant benefit [24].

Diaphragmatic contour. Following significant lung volume reduction, the hemidiaphragms are expected to move cephalad, regaining upward convex contour, resulting in improved amplitude of their excursion [39]. These morphological changes are visually assessed using erect chest radiographs or coronal reformatted CT images obtained at full inspiration. A diaphragm sonogram can be used for dynamic evaluation pre- and post-procedure.

Malignancy surveillance. Atelectasis following a BLVR procedure can make the detection of new cancers within the collapsed lung extremely difficult from routine imaging. With a higher incidence of

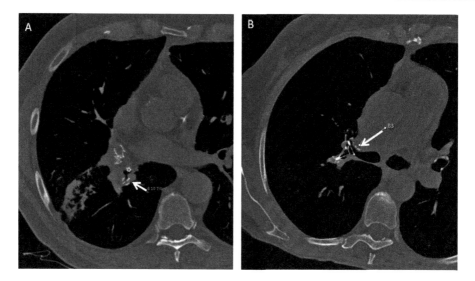

FIGURE 5.10 Target lobe failure to collapse due to a malpositioned EBV. Multiplanar HRCT images demonstrate multiple right lower lobe segmental EBV placement. (A) The EBV in the right lower lobe posterior basal segmental bronchus (arrow) is tilted about 45 degrees compared with the long axis of the lumen of the bronchus. (B) Different patient with EBV in the right upper lobe anterior segmental bronchus (arrow) that is proximally migrated into the lobar bronchus.

lung cancer in emphysematous patients, the radiologist may need to scrutinize the collapsed lobe with a high index of suspicion for any occult mass. Removal of the valves may be necessary and PET-CT scans may be useful for further evaluation [40].

CONCLUSION

With the increasing rate of COPD-related mortalities worldwide and the availability of LVRS and BLVR as effective palliative treatment methods for COPD patients with advanced emphysema, it is important that chest radiologists understand their roles in the clinical team taking care of these patients. The clinical benefits of the LVR procedure are maximized in certain imaging-based COPD phenotypes, and imaging plays a pivotal role in identifying this subgroup and guiding the management of post-procedural adverse events.

REFERENCES

1. WHO.   https://www.who.int/news-room/fact-sheets/detail/chronic-obstructive-pulmonary-disease-(copd). (Last accessed on Aug 09, 2023).
2. Hartman JE, Welling JBA, Klooster K, et al. Survival in COPD patients treated with bronchoscopic lung volume reduction. *Respir Med.* 2022 May;196:106825.
3. Hopkinson NS, Toma TP, Hansell DM, et al. Effect of bronchoscopic lung volume reduction on dynamic hyperinflation and exercise in emphysema. *Am J Respir Crit Care Med.* 2005;171:453–460.
4. Coxson HO, Nasute Fauerbach PV, Storness-Bliss C, et al. Computed tomography assessment of lung volume changes after bronchial valve treatment. *Eur Respir J.* 2008;32:1443–1450.

5. Pizarro C, Ahmadzadehfar H, Essler M, et al. Effect of endobronchial valve therapy on pulmonary perfusion and ventilation distribution. *PLoS One*. 2015;10:e0118976.

6. Pizarro C, Schueler R, Hammerstingl C, et al. Impact of endoscopic lung volume reduction on right ventricular myocardial function. *PLoS One*. 2015;10:e012137.

7. Fishman A, Martinez F, Naunheim K, et al. National Emphysema Treatment Trial Research Group: a randomized trial comparing lung-volume-reduction surgery with medical therapy for severe emphysema. *N Engl J Med*. 2003;348:2059–2073.

8. Criner GJ, Cordova F, Sternberg AL, et al. The National Emphysema Treatment Trial (NETT) part II: lessons learned about lung volume reduction surgery. *Am J Respir Crit Care Med*. 2011;184:881–893.

9. Washko GR, Hoffman E, Reilly JJ. Radiographic evaluation of the potential lung volume reduction surgery candidate. *Proc Am Thorac Soc*. 2008;5(4):421–426.

10. Chandra D, Lipson DA, Hoffman EA, et al; National Emphysema Treatment Trial Research Group. Perfusion scintigraphy and patient selection for lung volume reduction surgery. *Am J Respir Crit Care Med*. 2010 Oct 1;182(7):937–946.

11. Lacour M, Caviezel C, Weder W, et al. Postoperative complications and management after lung volume reduction surgery. *J Thorac Dis*. 2018 Aug;10(Suppl 23):S2775–S2779.

12. Naunheim KS, Wood DE, Krasna MJ, et al. Predictors of operative mortality and cardiopulmonary morbidity in the National Emphysema Treatment Trial Research Group: predictors of operative mortality and cardiopulmonary morbidity in the National Emphysema Treatment Trial. *J Thorac Cardiovasc Surg*. 2006;131:43–53.

13. Herth FJ, Slebos DJ, Criner GJ, et al. Endoscopic lung volume reduction: an expert panel recommendation–Update 2019. *Respiration*. 2019;97:548–557.

14. Valipour A. Valve therapy in patients with emphysematous type of chronic obstructive pulmonary disease (COPD): from randomized trials to patient selection in clinical practice. *J Thorac Dis*. 2018;10:S2780.

15. Ramaswamy A, Puchalski J. Bronchoscopic lung volume reduction: recent updates. *J Thorac Dis*. 2018;10:2519–2527.

16. Ninane V, Geltner C, Bezzi M, et al. Multicentre European study for the treatment of advanced emphysema with bronchial valves. *Eur Respir J*. 2012;39:1319–1325.

17. Wood DE, Nader DA, Springmeyer SC, et al. The IBV Valve trial: a multicenter, randomized, double-blind trial of endobronchial therapy for severe emphysema. *J Bronchology Interv Pulmonol*. 2014;21:288–297.

18. Sciurba FC, Ernst A, Herth FJ, et al. A randomized study of endobronchial valves for advanced emphysema (VENT study). *N Engl J Med*. 2010;363:1233–1244.

19. Davey C, Zoumot Z, Jordan S, et al. Bronchoscopic lung volume reduction with endobronchial valves for patients with heterogeneous emphysema and intact interlobar fissures: a randomised controlled trial (BeLieVeR-HIFi study). *Lancet*. 2015;386:1066–1073.

20. Klooster K, ten Hacken NH, Hartman JE, et al. Endobronchial valves for emphysema without interlobar collateral ventilation (STELVIO study). *N Engl J Med*. 2015;373:2325–2335.

21. Valipour A, Slebos DJ, Herth F, et al. Endobronchial valve therapy in patients with homogeneous emphysema: results from the IMPACT study. *Am J Respir Crit Care Med*. 2016;194:1073–1082.

22. Kemp SV, Slebos DJ, Kirk A, et al. A multicenter randomized controlled trial of zephyr endobronchial valve treatment in heterogeneous emphysema (TRANSFORM). *Am J Respir Crit Care Med*. 2017;196:1535–1543.

23. Criner GJ, Sue R, Wright S, et al. A multicenter RCT of Zephyr® endobronchial valve treatment in heterogeneous emphysema (LIBERATE). *Am J Respir Crit Care Med*. 2018;198:1151–1164.

24. Li S, Wang G, Wang C, et al. The REACH trial: a randomized controlled trial assessing the safety and effectiveness of the Spiration® Valve System in the treatment of severe emphysema. *Respiration*. 2018;14:1–2.

25. Criner GJ, Delage A, Voelker K, et al. Improving lung function in severe heterogenous emphysema with the Spiration® Valve System (EMPROVE). A multicenter, open-label randomized controlled clinical trial. *Am J Respir Crit Care Med*. 2019;200:1354–1362.

26. Lynch DA, Newell JD. Quantitative imaging of COPD. *J Thorac Imaging*. 2009;24:89–194.

27. Gompelmann D, Sarmand N, Herth FJ. Interventional pulmonology in chronic obstructive pulmonary disease. *Curr Opin Pulm Med*. 2017;23:261–268.

28. Eberhardt R, Herth FJ, Radhakrishnan S, et al. Comparing clinical outcomes in upper versus lower lobe endobronchial valve treatment in severe emphysema. *Respiration*. 2015;90:314–320.

29. Koenigkam-Santos M, de Paula WD, Owsijewitsch M, et al. Incomplete pulmonary fissures evaluated by volumetric thinsection CT: semi-quantitative evaluation for small fissure gaps identification, description of prevalence and severity of fissural defects. *Eur J Radiol*. 2013;82:2365–2370.

30. Van Rikxoort EM, Goldin JG, Galperin-Aizenberg M, et al. A method for the automatic quantification of the completeness of pulmonary fissures: evaluation in a database of subjects with severe emphysema. *Eur Radiol*. 2012;22:302–309.

31. Fiorelli A, Santini M, Shah P. When can computed tomography-fissure analysis replace Chartis collateral ventilation assessment in the prediction of patients with emphysema who might benefit from endobronchial valve therapy? *Interact Cardiovasc Thorac Surg.* 2018;26:313–318.
32. Schuhmann M, Raffy P, Yin Y, et al. Computed tomography predictors of response endobronchial valve lung reduction treatment. Comparison with Chartis. *Am J Respir Crit Care Med.* 2015;191:767–774.
33. Reymond E, Jankowski A, Pison C, et al. Prediction of lobar collateral ventilation in 25 patients with severe emphysema by fissure analysis with CT. *Am J Roentgenol.* 2013;201:W571–W575.
34. Gompelmann D, Eberhardt R, Slebos DJ, et al. Diagnostic performance comparison of the Chartis System and high resolution computerized tomography fissure analysis for planning endoscopic lung volume reduction. *Respirology.* 2014;19:524–530.
35. Koster TD, van Rikxoort EM, Huebner RH, et al. Predicting lung volume reduction after endobronchial valve therapy is maximized using a combination of diagnostic tools. *Respiration.* 2016;92:150–157.
36. Thomsen C, Theilig D, Herzog D, et al. Lung perfusion and emphysema distribution affect the outcome of endobronchial valve therapy. *Int J Chron Obstruct Pulmon Dis.* 2016;11:1245–1259.
37. Low SW, Lee JZ, Desai H, et al. Endobronchial valves therapy for advanced emphysema: a meta-analysis of randomized trials. *J Bronchology Interv Pulmonol.* 2019;26:81–89.
38. Van Geffen WH, Klooster K, Hartman JE, et al. Pleural adhesion assessment as a predictor for pneumothorax after endobronchial valve treatment. *Respiration.* 2017;94:224–231.
39. Grabenhorst M, Schmidt B, Liebers U, et al. Radiologic manifestations of bronchoscopic lung volume reduction in severe chronic obstructive pulmonary disease. *AJR Am J Roentgenol.* 2015 Mar;204(3):475–486.
40. Tummino C, Maldonado F, Laroumagne S, et al. Lung cancer following bronchoscopic lung volume reduction for severe emphysema: a case and its management. *Respiration.* 2012;83(5):418–420.

Nuclear Medicine Techniques in Pre- and Post-Procedural Evaluation of Lung Volume Reduction Interventions and of Single Pulmonary Nodule

6

Sean Ide Bolet, Gerard Criner and Simin Dadparvar

INTRODUCTION

Severe COPD causes patients significant morbidity and mortality, has remained difficult to treat, and is without a cure in modern medicine. One of the physiological changes that impact the patient's breathing

DOI: 10.1201/9781003251439-6

is decreased pulmonary elastic recoil that results from hyperinflation of the lung tissue.[1] The hyperinflation of lung tissue is secondary to chronic alveolar destruction, leading to obstructed and air-filled regions of lung tissue that become physiologically non-contributory to overall lung function. Lung volume reduction surgery (LVRS) was initially developed to target the issue of lung hyperinflation in severe emphysema patients who have exhausted medical management. Later, the initial National Emphysema Treatment Trial (NETT) proved that LVRS was strongly impactful and beneficial in improving the survival of patients suffering from upper lobe heterogenous emphysema along with diminished baseline exercise capacity.[2] Beyond NETT, further single-center trials have further emphasized the strength of the indication for LVRS in patients suffering from severe upper lobe heterogenous COPD.[3–7]

LVRS provides improved respiratory function with the removal of significant amounts of diseased lung tissue. Improvement in respiratory function results from the overall decompression of the thoracic cavity. The increased thoracic cavity volume post-lung volume reduction allows for an increase in pulmonary elastic recoil associated with the re-expansion of the remaining healthy lung tissue.

After NETT, further investigation and intervention have been aimed at the less invasive option of bronchoscopic lung volume reduction (BLVR).[8] Nuclear medicine techniques have played a key role in delineating who can receive treatment, treatment planning, monitoring physiological changes after treatment, and determining the clinical efficacy of LVRS and BLVR. This chapter will explore and highlight the clinical significance of the utilization of nuclear medicine techniques, primarily single-photon emission computed tomography/computed tomography (SPECT/CT), in pre-procedural planning, patient selection, and monitoring patients' response to therapy. It will further explore current nuclear medicine methodology and additionally highlights the utility of SPECT/CT in pulmonary nodule/mass resection.

NUCLEAR MEDICINE TECHNIQUES IN LUNG VOLUME REDUCTION SURGERY

LVRS is a well-researched and time-tested means of targeting lung hyperinflation in patients who have severe emphysema and have exhausted medical management. Nuclear medicine has continually played a role in pre-procedural planning and monitoring patients' clinical outcomes post-operatively.

Pre-operative evaluation of regional lung function is an imperative aspect of predicting and planning surgery. In the past, methods of SPECT or planar perfusion and ventilation have served as a semiquantitative method of determining regional lung function through arbitrarily defined geometric zones that imprecisely determine lobar anatomy. As the methodology is imprecise, it can lead to concerning ambiguity in pre-operative assessment. This leads to the more recent approach that utilizes a combination of SPECT and CT, denoted SPECT/CT, which provides a fully quantitative analysis of perfusion at the lobar level. Early studies of pre-operative fused multidetector-row CT (MDCT) and SPECT scintigram, a type of SPECT/CT (GE DISCOVERY 670 DR, Milwaukee, WI, USA), demonstrated utility in determining the surgical approach for LVRS and concluded that the implementation of SPECT/CT improved surgical outcomes.[9] The following study further highlights the utility of SPECT/CT over planar with SPECT, and quantitative and qualitative assessed MDCT as the best predictor of post-operative clinical outcomes. Twenty-five consecutive patients pre-operatively underwent planar SPECT, MDCT, and SPECT/CT in the trial. The post-operative clinical outcomes were investigated following pre- and post-operative FEV1 and the six-minute walk test (6MWT). Upper versus lower lobe (U/L) ratios were established on SPECT/CT from calculations of regional uptakes between upper and lower lung fields in the operated lung field. For comparison of predicting clinical outcomes among imaging modalities, the U/Ls ratios were statistically correlated with the corresponding clinical outcome. The study resulted in the best correlation with clinical outcomes in LVRS candidates with pre-operative use of SPECT/CT over pure planar SPECT or MDCT.[10] As evidenced by prior studies, SPECT/CT is the superior modality in pre-operative assessment as it is the only true quantitative assessment of perfusion at the lobar level and it provides the most accurate pre-operative prediction of post-surgery lung function. SPECT/CT has become a standard of practice at Temple University Hospital (TUH) and in other institutions.[11]

NUCLEAR MEDICINE TECHNIQUES IN SINGLE PULMONARY NODULE AND PULMONARY MASS RESECTION

Lung cancer is responsible for more deaths annually than any other cancer and accounts for 25% of all cancer mortality in the United States.[12] The most significant risk factor for the development of lung cancer is a history of smoking.[13] Unfortunately, smoking is also a major risk factor for the development of COPD, which often leads to patients suffering from both conditions. The only curative treatment for malignant masses in the lungs is via wide-margin surgical resection. Previous literature has suggested evidence of SPECT/CT as a suitable candidate in pr-eoperative lung resection planning and as a reliable predictor of post-lung resection pulmonary function, especially FEV1.[14,15]

However, patients suffering from superimposed COPD may not be viable surgical candidates, especially when evaluating their pulmonary function tests (PFTs).[16] The utilization of SPECT/CT in planning the patient's treatment course becomes imperative in predicting surgical outcomes. SPECT/CT not only plays a role in imaging the tumor and its location but also allows for the determination of lung perfusion data, which allows physicians to determine which treatment intervention is possible.[16] In a single-center study at TUH, a cohort of 16 patients with emphysema was investigated, 14 of whom had a history of 50 pack-years of smoking, one who had a history of alpha-1 antitrypsin deficiency, and one who was a non-smoker. In each patient, a perfusion/ventilation scan was performed with an average dose of 5 mCi of Tc-99-mAA and 10 mCi of Xe-133-gas in which each lobe was individually analyzed for counts and volume. The pulmonary function test performed reported a mean pre-operative FEV1 of 2.0 L for each patient undergoing surgery and an FEV1 of 0.85 L for patients not undergoing surgery. Furthermore, SPECT/CT analysis was utilized to predict post-operative FEV1 changes. Overall, nine patients underwent surgery, and seven patients did not undergo surgery, secondary to three being poor surgical candidates, three having benign masses/nodules, and one deferred surgery for continued CT monitoring. Post-surgery, all patients reported doing subjectively well without the need for increased oxygen requirements in the post-operative period. Those undergoing resections were also found to maintain a higher average FEV1 after the operation. The study highlights the need and successful utilization of pre-procedural SPECT/CT in the post-surgical prediction of pulmonary function in patients needing surgical resection of a single pulmonary nodule or lung mass in the setting of superimposed severe emphysema. Quantitative perfusion SPECT/CT for pre-operative lobar assessment is the current recommendation rather than previously used traditional regional quantitative perfusion[17] (Figure 6.1).

LUNG PERFUSION STUDIES

The primary agent used in lung perfusion studies is Technetium-99m macroaggregated albumin (MAA). The agent highlights the lung vasculature by the mechanism of capillary blockade.[18] A typical dosage is between 2 and 5 mCi, which correlates to an effective dose of 200,000 to 500,000 particles. These

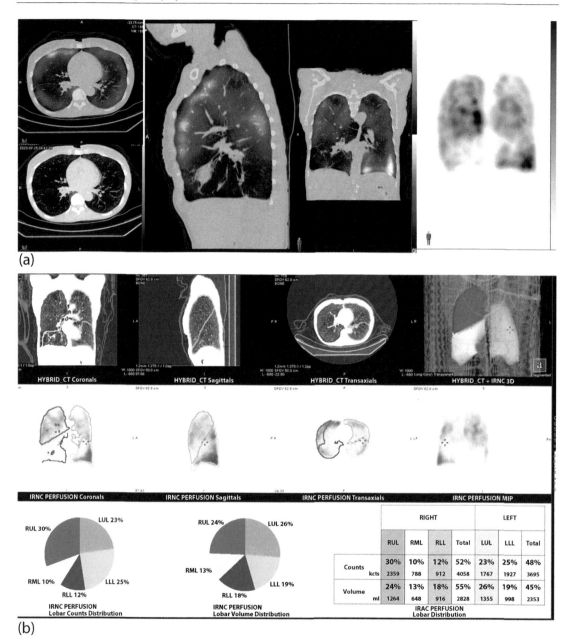

FIGURE 6.1   A 62-year-old female with biopsy proven small cell lung cancer in the right lower lobe, pre-op evaluation for resection. (A) Pre-operative lung scan with SPECT/CT showing lung perfusion. (B) Quantitative SPECT/CT for identifying perfusion (counts) in the right lower lobe containing the pulmonary mass.

particles are injected intravenously at a slow rate over several respiratory cycles. Blood must not be drawn back into the syringe during the injection, as it creates hot emboli affecting the final image. Once administered, imaging can begin immediately. Standard imaging protocol involves obtaining 500,000 to 700,000 counts per image. Several views can be obtained including posterior, anterior, right/left lateral, and right/left posterior oblique; however, oblique views are optional.

LUNG VENTILATION STUDIES

Lung ventilation studies are primarily for our purposes investigated using Xe^{133}. Xe^{133} offers several advantages such as its rapid washout and a short half-life of 30 seconds along with no central airway deposition. It furthermore offers superior sensitivity over Tc-99m DTPA in the identification of COPD. It also does not produce any artifact that interferes with the perfusion imaging agent, given the low photopeak of Xe^{133} at 81 keV. It does suffer from some disadvantages as the rapid washout also limits the number of views/projections available. Given that the photopeak of Xe^{133} is lower than that of Tc-99m MAA, it becomes imperative that you perform the ventilation scan sequentially before the perfusion scan. If the Tc-99m MAA were to be administered first, it would result in a down scatter that would degrade the quality of the ventilation scan.[19] Of note, lung ventilation studies have been limited in the setting of the COVID-19 pandemic, and thus further research and physiological monitoring of ventilation both pre- and post-BLVR have been limited.

NUCLEAR MEDICINE TECHNIQUES IN BRONCHOSCOPIC LUNG VOLUME REDUCTION

After NETT, investigation and intervention have been aimed at the less invasive and more cost-effective option of BLVR to target severe emphysema. Compared with LVRS, BLVR therapy overall provides significantly lower mortality and morbidity while being cheaper and reducing hospital length of stay.[20]

Nuclear medicine techniques have been prominent in the analysis of a multitude of criteria including patient selection, lung lobe targeting, and monitoring physiological changes in response to treatment. Unfortunately, some of the trials in 2020 and 2021 on the role of ventilation shifts post-BLVR procedures have been limited due to the COVID-19 pandemic, as ventilation studies were suspected to increase the mechanical spread of the SARS-CoV-2 virus.

SPECT/CT: CURRENT METHODOLOGY IN LOBE TARGET SELECTION

In the past, nuclear scintigraphy was the method for determining areas of low perfusion. However, more recently, a perfusion lung scan with SPECT/CT plays an imperative role in pre-procedural planning, especially in identifying which lobe to target with valve(s) placement. The quantification of relative lobar perfusion is performed with SPECT/CT. The CT portion of the study provides images that allow for lung fissures delineation. The integrity of the fissures is important for assessing collateral ventilation.[21] The perfusion aspect of the study is then superimposed on the fissures delineated on CT. Lobar perfusion identified via radionuclide counts and absolute volume determined from CT densitometry is then together formed into a table showing counts against volume in each of the lobes of the left and right lungs. The lobe with the lowest perfusion (counts) then usually becomes the target of the placed valve[22] (Figure 6.2).

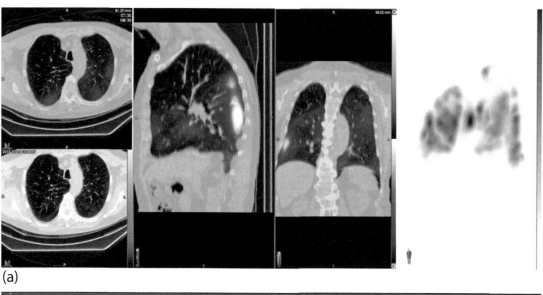

(a)

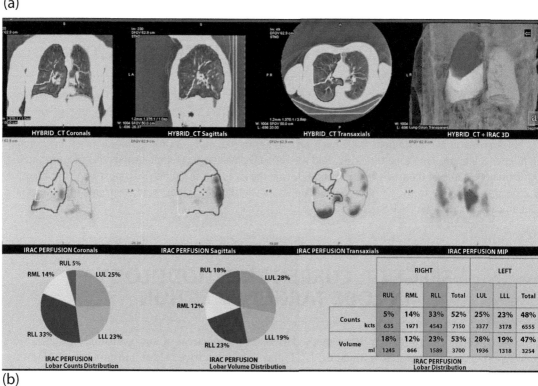

(b)

FIGURE 6.2   A 76-year-old male with severe emphysema referred for pre-BLVR (February 20, 2019) evaluation. (A) Lung scan with SPECT/CT with heterogenous perfusion. (B) Quantitative SPECT/CT for identifying the lobe with the lowest perfusion as target for BLVR shows right upper lobe with the lowest count.

SPECT/CT IN IDENTIFYING MULTIPLE TARGET LOBES

SPECT/CT has clearly shown to be impactful in the targeting of lobes with the lowest perfusion to obtain significant physiological and clinical improvements. However, there are instances in which pre-procedural planning may contraindicate targeting the lowest perfusion lobe. The following TUH study investigated SPECT/CT as a pre-operative assessment tool and asked how patients suffering from severe emphysema (RV >150%, TLC >100%) would be impacted if a lobe other than the lowest perfusion lobe was targeted. Target lobes were selected based on lobar counts and volumes, the integrity of the fissures, and the percent of emphysema destruction. Emphysema destruction utilized a <−950 Hounsfield unit (HU) cutoff, which was assessed by quantitative CT analysis programs. All patients were pre-operatively assessed with Tc-99m MAA perfusion and counts/volume were identified. At 45 days post-procedure, confirmation of volume reduction was determined by quantitative CT and FEV1. A total of 55 patients at TUH were evaluated consecutively in this group; 22 were excluded for a myriad of reasons. Of the 33 remaining patients, 24 were placed in the concordant group. The concordant group had the lobe with the lowest perfusion identified on SPECT/CT targeted for valve insertion. The remaining nine patients were in the discordant group in which an alternative lobe other than the lowest perfusion lobe was targeted for valve insertion. Between the concordant and discordant groups, there was no statistically significant difference in the improvement of FEV1 or target lobe volume reduction, post-operatively. The study concluded that SPECT/CT provides information on alternative targets for valve placement, which can still provide clinically meaningful benefits in the setting that other pre-procedural considerations prevent, such as the targeting of the lowest perfusion lobe. This study also showed the unique advantage of a Tc99m MAA perfusion lung scan with SPECT/CT over planar nuclear scintigraphy in that SPECT/CT provides highly precise lobar information that is not affected/altered by regional hyperinflation, whereas nuclear scintigraphy in the same situation would produce inaccurate zonal approximations in the setting of regional hyperinflation.[21]

SPECT/CT IN HETEROGENOUS EMPHYSEMA

One of the most important roles of SPECT/CT is in patients with diffuse homogeneous emphysema or patients who have more than one lobe that could be targeted. Having this tool is paramount in identifying the best possible target lobe. However, it is important to stress that this method of pre-procedural planning for BLVR works in both patients suffering from homogeneous and heterogeneous severe emphysema.[23] Currently, minimally invasive BLVR has shown to be most effective when the target lobe has a significantly greater degree of destruction compared with the ipsilateral non-targeted lobe.

SPECT/CT IN BLVR PRE-PROCEDURAL PLANNING

The niche role of SPECT/CT in pre-procedural BLVR planning has been investigated in a single-center study at TUH. Thirty-four patients were investigated who underwent high-resolution computerized tomography (HRCT) and SPECT/CT and who then subsequently underwent BLVR. In the following ventilation-perfusion analysis, Xe[133] was used to determine ventilation, and Tc-99-MAA was utilized to determine lung perfusion. It was determined that the overall correlation between emphysema score on HRCT and the counts/volume ratio determined via SPECT/CT had a moderate correlation, and the strongest of correlations was found in the RUL. The correlations in the RML, RLL, LLL, and LUL were overall weak for all lobes. Importantly, the correlation of emphysematous destruction and counts/volume ratio was also moderate in the lobe targeted by BLVR therapy. The concluding correlation is that emphysematous destruction found on HRCT does not correlate strongly with counts/volume. This conclusion emphasizes that SPECT/CT plays an independent, unique, and necessary role in pre-procedural BLVR planning.[24]

Nuclear medicine techniques have further been imperative in monitoring the patient's physiological response to treatment. Studies have investigated ventilation changes, perfusion changes, ventilation/perfusion mismatch changes, and DL_{CO} changes post-BLVR procedure.

SPECT/CT IN PREDICTING VENTILATION SHIFTS POST-BLVR

Early data regarding BLVR and SPECT/CT imaging have shown there were conflicting results regarding the shifts in ventilation post-valve placement; this is likely due to the nature of the overlap of these studies with the COVID-19 pandemic as limited data could be collected for ventilation studies. Furthermore, ventilation imaging was limited to posterior-anterior views in the few patients with ventilation data, providing suboptimal data for analysis. A trial from TUH highlighted ventilation shifts after BLVR. All patients in the analysis had undergone BLVR and had both pre- and post-procedural HRCT and perfusion scintigraphy with the average follow-up scans being nine months post-valve placement. BLVR is the most effective in patients suffering from a high degree of destruction in the targeted lobe and concurrent absence to a low degree of destruction in the ipsilateral non-targeted lobe. Pearson correlations were determined between lobar emphysema destruction, clinical outcomes, and between target zone and non-target zone ventilation changes. A total of seven consecutive patients were included. It was further demonstrated that the target lobes for valve placement had severe emphysematous destruction with advanced emphysema destruction scores. The study found no correlation between ventilation change to volume reduction in the target lobe and moderate clinical changes with changes in target lobe ventilation. In five of the seven patients, the largest shift/change in ventilation was observed in the hemithorax contralateral to the target lobe. It was primarily concluded that the most significant amplitude shifts in ventilation were to areas of the lowest emphysematous destruction after target lobe volume reduction was performed.[25]

SPECT/CT IN PREDICTING PERFUSION SHIFTS POST-BLVR

An advantage of BLVR over previously prominent LVRS is that the vasculature is left in place with valve placement. The following study investigated the hypothesis that post-valve placement, the physiological hypoxic vasoconstrictive response in the lungs will shunt blood to the lobes with better ventilation. The study analyzed the effects of BLVR on ventilation and perfusions and its impact on gas exchange. A single-center study was performed at TUH in which all patients underwent SPECT/CT perfusion/ventilation scans, arterial blood gas studies, and pulmonary function tests before BLVR. The study found a statistically significant volume reduction of the target lobe. Furthermore, patients also had a significant decrease in perfusion of the target lobe independent of the complete or partial collapse of the lobe. All patients were found to have improvements in arterial blood gases with increased PaO_2 and decreased $PaCO_2$. The study concluded that an important therapeutic benefit of BLVR over LVRS is the perfusion shift associated with the hypoxic vasoconstrictive response, allowed by the vasculature left in place, which shifts perfusion to

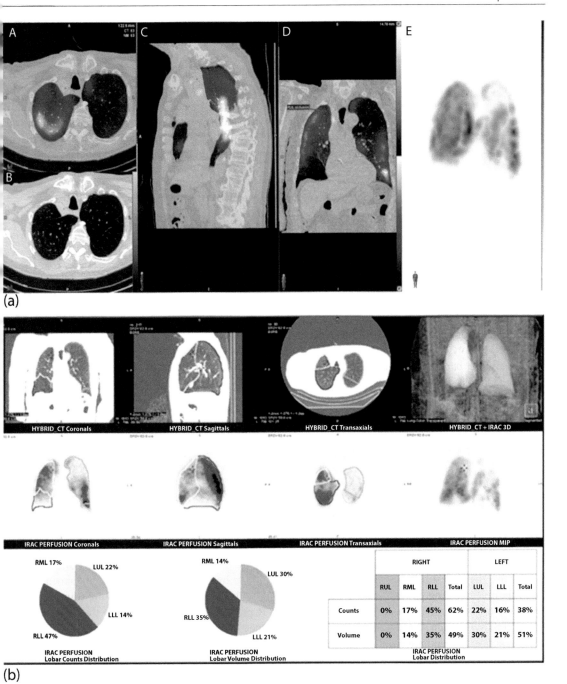

FIGURE 6.3 A 76-year-old male with severe emphysema referred for post-BLVR (6-month post-operative) evaluation. (A) Lung scan with SPECT/CT looking at lung perfusion post-valve placement(s) in the right upper lobe. (B) Quantitative SPECT/CT for identifying complete collapse of the right upper lobe confirmed occlusion of the right upper lobe bronchus. When comparing to Figure 6.2b, an increase in perfusion and volume of ipsilateral and contralateral lobes is noted.

more well-aerated lobes of the lung.[26] These findings are further supported by a case where a 70-year-old man underwent BLVR and received pre- and post-procedural SPECT/CT. His PFTs showed evidence of severe obstructive lung disease. After BLVR placement, six-month follow-up ventilation, and perfusion scans done through quantitative SPECT/CT, there was evidence of a significant reduction in both perfusion and ventilation in the target lobes with improved perfusion and ventilation to well-aerated regions of the lungs.[27] Furthermore, these findings are further corroborated by another separate TUH single study retrospective analysis of prospectively collected data of 47 patients who utilized SPECT/CT pre- and post-BLVR therapy to determine perfusion shifts. SPECT/CT data showed a significant decrease in perfusion of the target lobe with a significant increase in perfusion to the ipsilateral non-targeted lobe[28] (Figure 6.3).

SPECT IN PREDICTING CLINICAL AND PHYSIOLOGICAL RESPONSE POST-BLVR

A retrospective analysis done at TUH investigated 77 consecutive patients undergoing BLVR with pre- and post-SPECT/CT along with pre- and post-PFT and 6MWT. The study showed strong evidence that when the lobe targeted for collapse through BLVR was identified using the lowest counts on SPECT/CT, patients saw statistically significant improvements in PFT values, particularly FEV1, TLC, RV/TLC, and FVC. Furthermore, this study supported that when SPECT/CT is used in lobe selection, patients see significant clinical benefits with meaningful clinical improvements, specifically dyspnea ratings improved post-procedure.[29]

FUTURE AIMS: TC99M MAA LUNG SCAN WITH SPECT/CT IN PATIENT SELECTION

The treatment of emphysema with BLVR is a rapidly growing treatment modality. Nuclear medicine's impact, particularly SPECT/CT, is undeniable. Currently, studies support SPECT/CT's use in pre-procedural planning and predicting improvements in both clinical and physiological variables. Research is ongoing and includes using SPECT/CT to better define patient selection criteria and understand which patients can receive the largest benefit from BLVR. Furthermore, we hypothesize SPECT/CT will play a significant role in identifying patients who are poor surgical candidates or cannot obtain lung transplants and are likely to see significant improvement with a BLVR procedure. Unfortunately, in the United States, Krypton 81 ventilation scans are no longer available. Once the ventilation lung scan with Technegas™ is in our reach, lobar ventilation quantitation can be of value to assess the ventilation of each lobe in pre- and post-BLVR insertion.

REFERENCES

1. Papandrinopoulou D, Tzouda V, Tsoukalas G. *Pulm Med.* 2012;2012:542769. doi:10.1155/2012/542769
2. Fishman A, Martinez F, Naunheim K, et al. *N Engl J Med.* May 22 2003;348(21):2059–73. doi:10.1056/NEJMoa030287

3. Brenner M, McKenna RJ, Jr., Chen JC, et al. *Ann Thorac Surg.* Feb 2000;69(2):388–93. doi:10.1016/s0003-4975(99)01339-9

4. Flaherty KR, Kazerooni EA, Curtis JL, et al. *Chest.* May 2001;119(5):1337–46. doi:10.1378/chest.119.5.1337

5. Ciccone AM, Meyers BF, Guthrie TJ, et al. *J Thorac Cardiovasc Surg.* Mar 2003;125(3):513–25. doi:10.1067/mtc.2003.147

6. Tutic M, Lardinois D, Imfeld S, et al. *Ann Thorac Surg.* Jul 2006;82(1):208–13; discussion 213. doi:10.1016/j.athoracsur.2006.02.004

7. Ginsburg ME, Thomashow BM, Bulman WA, et al. *J Thorac Cardiovasc Surg.* Mar 2016;151(3):717–24.e1. doi:10.1016/j.jtcvs.2015.10.095

8. Criner GJ, Cordova F, Sternberg AL, Martinez FJ. *Am J Respir Crit Care Med.* Oct 15 2011;184(8):881–93. doi:10.1164/rccm.201103-0455CI

9. Okuda I, Maruno H, Kohno T, Yamase H, Mori K, Kokubo T. *Kyobu Geka.* Mar 2006;59(3):197–203. PMID: 16528991.

10. Takenaka D, Ohno Y, Koyama H, et al. *Eur J Radiol.* 2010/06/01/ 2010;74(3):465–72. doi:10.1016/j.ejrad.2009.03.008

11. Wechalekar K, Garner J, Gregg S. *Semin Nucl Med.* Jan 2019;49(1):22–30. doi:10.1053/j.semnuclmed.2018.10.011

12. Society AC. Key statistics for lung cancer. Accessed 2022. https://www.cancer.org/cancer/lung-cancer/about/key-statistics.html#:~:text=Lung%20cancer%20is%20by%20far,because%20people%20are%20quitting%20smoking.

13. Wheaton AG, Liu Y, Croft JB, et al. *MMWR Morb Mortal Wkly Rep.* Jun 21 2019;68(24):533–8. doi:10.15585/mmwr.mm6824a1

14. Krishnakumar R, Vijayalakshmi K, Rangarajan GK, Vinodkumar MC, Krishnamurthy A. *Pol J Radiol.* Jan 2011;76(1):80–4.

15. Suh HY, Park S, Ryoo HG, et al. *Nucl Med Mol Imaging.* Dec 2019;53(6):406–13. doi:10.1007/s13139-019-00617-7

16. Piai DB, Quagliatto R, Toro I, Cunha Neto C, Etchbehere E, Camargo E. *Eur Respir J.* 2004;24(2):258. doi:10.1183/09031936.04.00123503

17. Gibbons M, Dadparvar S. *J Nucl Med.* 2020;61(supplement 1):1485.

18. Mettler FA, Guiberteau MJ. *Essentials of nuclear medicine and molecular imaging.* 7th edition. ed. Elsevier; 2019:viii, 543 pages.

19. Chapter 10 - Pulmonary System. In: Ziessman HA, O'Malley JP, Thrall JH, eds. *Nuclear Medicine (Fourth Edition).* W.B. Saunders; 2014:204–26.

20. Zantah M, Gangemi AJ, Criner GJ. *Ann Transl Med.* Nov 2020;8(21):1469. doi:10.21037/atm-20-1551

21. Nijor S, Gangemi A, Patel R, et al. *J Nuclear Med.* 2020;61(supplement 1):1493.

22. Dass C, Goldbach A, Dako F, Kumaran M, Steiner R, Criner GJ. *J Thorac Imaging.* May 1 2021;36(3):131–41. doi:10.1097/rti.0000000000000549

23. Valipour A, Slebos DJ, Herth F, et al. *Am J Respir Crit Care Med.* Nov 1 2016;194(9):1073–82. doi:10.1164/rccm.201607-1383OC

24. Patel R, Gangemi AJ, Dadparvar S, et al. *Am J Respir Crit Care Med.* 2020;201. https://doi.org/10.1164/ajrccm-conference.2020.201.1_MeetingAbstracts.A5043

25. Gangemi AJ, Dadparvar S, Patel R, et al. *American Thoracic Society*; 2020:A6863–A6863. *American Thoracic Society International Conference Abstracts.* https://doi.org/10.1164/ajrccm-conference.2020.201.1_MeetingAbstracts.A6863

26. Zantah M, Patel R, Gangemi AJ, et al. *American Thoracic Society International Conference Abstracts.* https://doi.org/10.1164/ajrccm-conference.2020.201.1_MeetingAbstracts.A4310

27. Zantah M, Dominguez Castillo E, Patel R, et al. *American Thoracic Society*; 2020:A3190–A3190. *American Thoracic Society International Conference Abstracts.* https://doi.org/10.1164/ajrccm-conference.2020.201.1_MeetingAbstracts.A3190

28. Van Der Rijst N, ;Gayen S, ;Dadparvar S, ;et al ;May 1, 2022, ;A2133–A2133. https://doi.org/10.1164/ajrccm-conference.2022.205.1_MeetingAbstracts.A2133

29. Sisti J, Ross L, Ide Bolet S, et al. Society of Nuclear Medicine and Molecular Imaging. 2023. SNMMI 2023 Meeting Abstracts.

Precision Treatment for Severe Lung Emphysema and the Impact of a Multidisciplinary Lung Team

7

Luis C. Losso, Marina Dornfeld C. Castro,
Mario C. Ghefter and Marcel M. Sandrini

PRECISION MEDICINE, SEVERE LUNG EMPHYSEMA AND TREATABLE TRAITS

Chronic obstructive pulmonary disease (COPD) is a complex and heterogenous lung health condition characterized by chronic respiratory symptoms due to abnormalities of the airways and/or alveoli that cause persistent, progressive, airflow obstruction.

COPD is a frequent, preventable, and treatable health status, secondary to the inhalation of toxic particles, gases, air pollution, and mainly tobacco smoke; more rarely, it may still have a genetic origin in cases of alfa-1 antitrypsin deficency.[1,2] It results from the interaction between gene and environment in an individual over their lifetime. It can damage the lungs during development and aging, and it is one of the most prevalent diseases in the world. The condition has a high burden of personal, social, and public health impacts due to its influence in high morbimortality.[1-3] It is currently one of the top three causes of death in the world, and 90% of these deaths occur in low- and middle-income countries.

DOI: 10.1201/9781003251439-7

In essence, COPD is a "complex disease," as it has several components with nonlinear dynamic interactions, and it is also a "heterogenous disease," meaning that not all of these components are present in all patients or in a given patient throughout their lifetime.[3,4] COPD has a mix of distinct biological mechanisms that go beyond the traditional pathophysiological mechanisms of pulmonary disease and extrapulmonary comorbidities and psychosocial, behavioral, and environmental factors that significantly impact the health status and risk of morbidity and mortality of patients.[5]

COPD may share cellular and molecular mechanisms (also named "endotypes") and present observable similar clinical, functional, imaging, and/or biological features (also named "phenotypes"), the last produced by the interactions of the "genotype" and the environment.[3,6] The definition of a "phenotype" requires a unifying and consistent natural history, consistent clinical and physiological characteristics, underlying pathobiology with identifiable biomarkers and genetics, and predictable responses to general and specific therapies.[6]

Accordingly, the concept of clinical "phenotypes" evolved to that of "treatable traits" defined as therapeutic targets identified by a "phenotype" through validated biomarkers, constituting the fundamentals of the concept of "precision medicine."[7] A treatable trait is defined as the treatment targeted to the individual needs of each patient on the basis of genetic, biomarker, phenotypic, or psychosocial characteristics that distinguish a given patient from other patients with similar clinical presentations.[8] The final objective of "precision medicine" is to improve individual clinical outcomes for each patient while minimizing unnecessary side effects for those less likely to respond to a given treatment.[8]

Once new measurements have become available and systems approaches allow a new level of integration of clinical and biological knowledge, the physician's task to manage patients individually toward better outcomes has evolved.[3] Consequently, COPD patients require an individualized and precise approach, be it a medical or an interventional treatment, one ideally suited for "precision medicine" focusing on improving the assessment, treatment, and outcomes.[3]

A new paradigm to advance medical care, "precision medicine," is part of a transformation in patient care: a personalized medicine that goes beyond individualized medicine since it intends that, based on the individual's genome (personalized), predictions about future risks can be made and, accordingly, preventive strategies can be implemented.[9] This is why it is also known as "P4 medicine" for being predictive, preventive, personalized, and participatory.[9]

One example of "phenotype" in COPD is the heterogeneity and distribution of the emphysema versus airway wall thickness.[1,4] Computed tomography is the biomarker that identifies those specific and different "phenotypes." Lung hyperinflation is another important "phenotype" in COPD, particularly in severe pulmonary emphysema. Air trapping caused by damage to the lungs is identified by other specific biomarkers represented by pulmonary functional tests including body plethysmography and carbon monoxide diffusion measurements. They will be fundamental in the design of personalized medical or interventional treatment.

Progress in the development and validation of biomarkers (i.e., an objectively mensurable biological, functional, imaging, and/or clinical characteristic) that can facilitate the implementation of "precision medicine" in airway diseases and allow the clinician to build-up a clearer picture of the main drivers of morbidity enables provision of the right treatment, at the right time, to the right person.[3,5,7] They represent indicators of normal biological processes, pathogenic processes, or biological responses and should be able to predict the response to treatment (including adverse effects), monitor treatment effects, and/or predict clinically relevant outcomes (mortality, exacerbations, and lung function decline).[3,5,7]

Some "phenotypes," also known as "treatable traits," of the disease are explored in Box 7.1. They are being incorporated to evolve, improve, and refine the current scenario, but the list is not exhaustive and should be in constant debate.

BOX 7.1 CLINICALLY RELEVANT DOMAINS TO POTENTIALLY CONSIDER IN THE FUTURE MANAGEMENT OF CHRONIC OBSTRUCTIVE PULMONARY DISEASE

Frequent exacerbations
Bacterial colonization
Airway smooth muscle contraction
Eosinophilic inflammation
Target lung denervation
Pulmonary hyperinflation
Pulmonary hypertension
Chronic respiratory failure
Alfa-1 antitrypsin deficiency
Extrapulmonary treatable traits
Severe disability
Lung microbiome

In the context of chronic airways diseases, "precision medicine" can therefore be a promising strategy to improve their management.[5] In contrast to the limitations of standard evaluation and stepwise therapy, the "treatable traits" approach has emerged as a new individualized strategy, including the multilevel and dynamic heterogeneity of the disease.[1,7]

In COPD, this approach has the potential to deliver clinically relevant outcomes: the identification of genetic markers that facilitate the assessment of the risk of future events; biomarker validation and new therapeutic targets identification; and clinical decision support systems and other integrated care tools.[4]

"Precision medicine" in COPD does not need to be restricted to severe or refractory disease.[5] It is also adaptable to all levels of healthcare to make it simpler or more complex depending on local practical circumstances, including the primary focus of assessment at all levels of care, while some traits may be more appropriately assessed and dealt with in tertiary care, even by a specialized multidisciplinary lung team center.[3,4] As a result, it represents a cost-effective strategy related to an expected larger therapeutic response.[3,4]

If all these previous considerations about "precision medicine" are added to the impact of a multidisciplinary lung team, specialized in advanced pulmonary diseases, in the interventional treatment strategy of patients with severe emphysema, then personalized and individualized medicine will achieve its goal.

Lung volume reduction interventions for severe emphysema with the hyperinflation "phenotype" show strong evidence of survival benefit over medical treatment in patients with heterogeneous upper lobe predominant disease and poor exercise capacity.[10,11]

But despite the fact that such interventions – minimally invasive thoracoscopic surgery and/or bronchoscopy – are nowadays recommended as a "precision treatment" for the emphysema hyperinflation "phenotype," the number of procedures performed remains low.[5] This fact reflects a sense of nihilism among physicians and their reluctance to offer invasive interventions for those very limited patients with severe emphysema, depriving them of shortness of breath relief, improved quality of life, and survival. Probably, this attitude is due to the complex nature of chronic obstructive respiratory disease, its possibility of high burden of illness despite the pharmacotherapy, the frequent associated comorbidities, the systemic consequences, and the significant social and economic impact.

It has been much debated that the attitudes of healthcare professionals not offering lung volume reduction procedures to patients were because most respiratory physicians were unsure or did not know the advantages and low morbimortality risk of the interventions and clearly significantly overestimated the risk of the surgery. A survey also showed a significant proportion of respiratory physicians reported having limited access to advanced multidisciplinary lung team centers with expertise in lung volume reduction procedures to discuss their cases of severe disease.

This finding is supported by a patient-centered study that reported patients having to fight for specialist referral. They were disappointed by the poor knowledge of healthcare professionals on the issue. It is not uncommon for patients to have to search these treatments themselves, and there is a general lack of knowledge and understanding of outcomes and pathways across the healthcare system.[12]

Patient selection is key for the successful lung volume reduction therapeutic option, and with the advent of more surgical techniques, the selection has become more complex. The complexity of assessment and the variety of treatments will inevitably result in a difference of opinion between health professionals and patients, hence a meaningful discussion at a multidisciplinary team meeting is mandatory.[13]

Identifying the right patient who will benefit from one of the individualized targeted options available is crucial. Engaging a multidisciplinary lung team enables the management of the complexities that characterize this patient population and could be a useful platform in identifying precise treatable traits to implement a targeted and successful lung volume reduction program.[14]

The multidisciplinary lung team meetings should use the expertise of each member and ensure a team-based approach.[15,16] It should be coordinated by a pulmonary physician involved in advanced lung diseases and be composed of a thoracic radiologist, thoracic surgeon, interventional bronchoscopist, respiratory physiologist, transplant physician, specialist nurse, psychologist, and respiratory physiotherapist. The whole team should be involved in cases selection and meet on a regular basis.

The multidisciplinary lung team should provide an in-depth discussion of each patient with severe pulmonary emphysema. They can also provide a learning environment for training referral clinicians, leading to improved outcomes for the patient. Referrals should be invited and asked to participate.[16]

By developing a multidisciplinary lung team meeting format, patient cases can be presented to be discussed and the individual's identified treatable traits can be identified using a multidimensional assessment approach, followed by planning the treatment of the identified traits.[7] Then, a multidisciplinary lung team review should be held as part of each clinic to review an individual patient's progress and to plan the next phase of care or intervention.[12]

Patients should be referred to the multidisciplinary lung team by a respiratory physician, always after an initial medical assessment. Referral to a specialized lung center is appropriate when the symptoms persist despite maximal guideline-based medical therapy.[17]

Communication with the referring physician is essential for ongoing support of the program. A referral form should be generated and made readily available to the referrers, informing the results of the baseline and ongoing assessments, in addition to the outcomes of any additional therapies. Rerouting patient to the referring physicians may occur if a patient is deemed not suitable for an interventional procedure by the multidisciplinary lung team, declines to participate, or after optimized treatment.[18]

Written consent to participate in a multidisciplinary lung team center, be the target of multidisciplinary discussion, or receive certain therapies including invasive procedures may be requirements in some situations or healthcare systems.

The multidisciplinary lung team appraises the risk and benefits to individual patients, and they tailor the risk management pre- and post-procedure to reduce morbidity. The main discussion points include the analysis of chest computed tomography (CT) with a visual qualitative analysis platform to identify the presence and quantify the percentage of the emphysema-like lung (low-attenuation areas), the lobar and zonal distribution of the low-attenuation regions, the integrity of lung fissures, and changes in airway walls and luminal caliber, as well as the severity of gas trapping at expiratory CT of the pulmonary function tests, body plethysmography, lung diffusion capacity, arterial blood gas analysis, cardiopulmonary exercise test, lung perfusion scan, COPD assessment test (CAT), dyspnea scale (modified Medical Research Council scale), six-minute walk test (6MWT), body mass index, airway obstruction, dyspnea, and exercise capacity (BODE), performance score, and transthoracic echocardiogram.[19–21]

The potential benefits of an interventional procedure is considered to determine whether unilateral surgical or bronchoscopic intervention is appropriate: the predictable complications as well as establishing the risk that comorbidities pose in limiting the benefits or increasing the risk of procedure; the assessment of pulmonary reserve and overall risk especially vascular and cardiac; identifying target lobes, i.e., lobes with the highest emphysema destruction and poor function as determined by perfusion scan; and the optimization of fitness before bronchoscopy or surgery and perioperative management.[22]

Once the treatment/intervention has been decided, further coordination among multidisciplinary team members regarding pre-operative medical optimization and post-procedure care is orchestrated through standardized referral coordinated through the service specific administrator. Patients who may be suitable for staged bilateral lung volume reduction are identified from the initial multidisciplinary lung team outcome to be re-discussed in the multidisciplinary team meeting in due course.[18]

The two flowcharts (Flowchart 1 and Flowchart 2) show the path that patients take from the initial diagnosis of severe lung emphysema made by a respiratory medical center to reach the severe lung emphysema unit. At this unit, medical, laboratory, functional, and imaging evaluations define the presence of the emphysema hyperinflation phenotype – from that moment on, patients will be submitted to the evaluation of the multidisciplinary team, and their individual health situation will be evaluated and precision treatment will be proposed in each case.

Flowchart 1

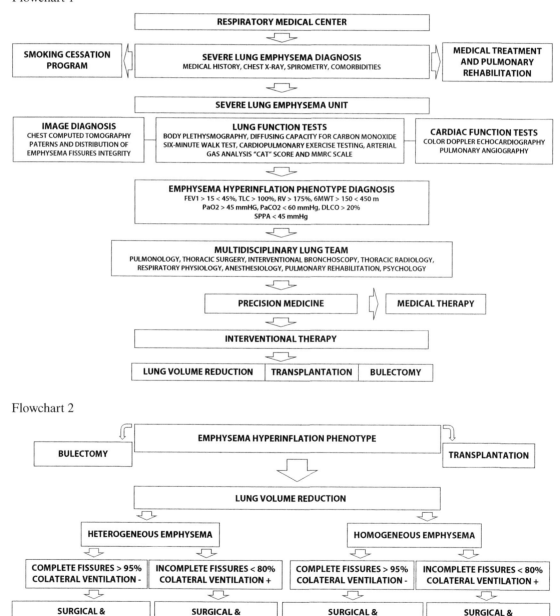

Flowchart 2

CONCLUSION

The outcomes of a successful lung volume reduction program are not only dependent on the quality of medical or interventional techniques and post-operative care. Precision case selection and work-up by a dedicated multidisciplinary lung team approach for severe emphysema patients plays an invaluable and integral part in the program.

The recognition of the precise treatable traits of severely sick patients, in view of multilevel, dynamic, and heterogeneous issues and, eventually, the discovery and validation of appropriate biomarkers can likely help in the endeavor in using precision medicine.

A lung team center provides a multidisciplinary approach to the management of emphysema that enables a multilevel assessment, the optimization of treatment management, and self-management skills, including interventional procedures where indicated.

REFERENCES

1. Faner R, Agustí A. Multilevel, dynamic chronic obstructive pulmonary disease heterogeneity. A challenge for personalized medicine. *Ann Am Thorac Soc.* 2016;13(5):S466–S70.
2. Global strategy for the diagnosis, management, and prevention of chronic obstructive pulmonary disease 2024. Accessed November 2024. https://goldcopd.org.
3. Agusti A, Bel E, Thomas M, et al. Treatable traits: toward precision medicine of chronic airway diseases. *Eur Respir J.* 2016;47(2):410–9.
4. Agusti A. The path to personalised medicine in COPD. *Thorax.* 2014;69(9):857–64.
5. Agustí A, Bafadhel M, Beasley R, et al. Precision medicine in airway diseases: moving to clinical practice. *Eur Respir J.* 2017;50(4):1701655.
6. Wenzel SE. Asthma phenotypes: the evolution from clinical to molecular approaches. *Nat Med.* 2012;2012;18(5):716–25.
7. McDonald VM, Fingleton J, Agusti A, et al. Treatable traits: a new paradigm for 21st century management of chronic airway diseases: treatable Traits Down Under International Workshop Report. *Eur Respir J.* 2019;53(5):1802058.
8. Jameson JL, Longo DL. Precision medicine-personalized, problematic, and promising. *N Engl J Med.* 2015;372(23):2229–34.
9. Galas DJ, Hood L. Systems biology and emerging technologies will catalyze the transition. *Interdisciplinary Bio Central.* 2009;1:1–4.
10. Lim E, Sousa I, Shah PL, et al. Lung volume reduction surgery reinterpreted with longitudinal data analysis methodology. *Ann Thorac Surg.* 2020;109:1496–502.
11. van Geffen WH, Slebos DJ, Herth FJ, et al. Surgical and endoscopic interventions that reduce lung volume for emphysema: a systemic review and meta-analysis. *Lancet.* 2019;7:313–24.
12. Buttery S, Lewis A, Oey I, et al. Patient experience of lung volume reduction procedures for emphysema: a qualitative service improvement project. *ERJ Open Res.* 2017;3:00031–02017.
13. Chew J, Mahadeva R. The role of a multidisciplinary severe chronic obstructive pulmonary disease hyperinflation service in patient selection for lung volume reduction. *J Thoracic Dis.* 2018;10(27):3335–43.
14. Kouritas V, Milton R, Kefaloyannis E, et al. The impact of a newly established multidisciplinary team on the interventional treatment of patients with emphysema. *Clin Med In Circ Resp Pul Med.* 2019;13:1–9.
15. Rea H, McAuley S, Stewart A, et al. A chronic disease management programme can reduce days in hospital for patients with chronic obstructive pulmonary disease. *Intern Med J.* 2004;34(11):608–14.
16. McDonald VM, Higgins I, Wood LG, et al. Multidimensional assessment and tailored interventions for COPD: respiratory utopia or common sense? *Thorax.* 2013;68(7):691–4.
17. Raskin J, Marks T, Miller A. Phenotypes and characterization of COPD: a pulmonary rehabilitation perspective. *J Cardiopulm Rehabil Prev.* 2018;38(1):43–8.

18. Oey I, Waller D. The role of the multidisciplinary emphysema team meeting in the provision of lung volume reduction. *J Thorac Dis.* 2018;10(23):2824–29.
19. Lynch DA, Austin JH, Hogg JC, et al. CT-definable subtypes of chronic obstructive pulmonary disease: a statement of the Fleischner Society. *Radiology.* 2015;277(1):192–205.
20. Holland AE, Spruit MA, Troosters T, et al. An official European Respiratory Society/American Thoracic Society technical standard: field walking tests in chronic respiratory disease. *Eur Respir J.* 2014;44(6):1428–46.
21. Oga T, Nishimura K, Tsukino M, et al. Analysis of the factors related to mortality in chronic obstructive pulmonary disease: role of exercise capacity and health status. *Am J Respir Crit Care Med.* 2003;167(4):544–9.
22. Rathinam S, Oey I, Steiner M, et al. The role of the emphysema multidisciplinary team in a successful lung volume reduction surgery programme. *Eur J Cardiothorac Surg.* 2014;46:1021–26.

Current Optimized Medical Treatment and the Impact on Dynamic Hyperinflation

8

José R. Jardim

INTRODUCTION

Improving lung function in patients with chronic pulmonary obstructive disease (COPD) is the central objective of patient treatment. Better lung function must improve their quality of life, decrease dyspnea, and increase their ability for accomplishing their daily activities. Treatment should always be based on non-pharmacological and pharmacological approaches. Non-pharmacological treatment includes smoking cessation, education and self-management, exercise, nutritional support orientation, vaccination, and long-term oxygen therapy when needed. Pharmacological treatment includes two classes of bronchodilators, the anticholinergic agents blocking the muscarinic receptors and the beta-2 adrenergic agents directly promoting bronchodilation.

Dyspnea is the main symptom in COPD patients and should be evaluated at every visit. The ideal way is by comparing how much the patient is accomplishing his or her daily activities since the last visit. Dyspnea may be numerically evaluated by assigning it a score according to the MRC (or mMRC) Dyspnea Scale or by the COPD Assessment Test (CAT). Patients with a score equal to two or over in the mMRC are considered dyspneic. CAT scores cover eight domains (cough, dyspnea, self-confidence, sputum, limitation, energy, pressure on the chest, and sleep) with total score going from zero to 40 (the higher the score, the higher the impact of COPD on the patient); values over ten are considered abnormal.

There is no clear consensus if a patient with COPD should start his/her therapy on monotherapy or dual bronchodilation. However, in a real-world, study conducted in the United States with patients on

DOI: 10.1201/9781003251439-8

monotherapy bronchodilators, around 50% of patients with forced expiratory volume in the first second (FEV1) over 50% (mild and moderate bronchial obstruction) presented a mMRC of two or three, which is considered to be a symptomatic patient; in addition, around 60% of patients with a FEV1 under 50% (severe and very severe bronchial obstruction) had a mMRC of two, three, or four, showing that monotherapy may not be enough to treat dyspneic patients (1). A pan-European cross-sectional retrospective cohort study stratifying patients by levels of dyspnea demonstrated that dyspneic COPD patents (mMRC ≥2) had twice as much chance of having moderate or severe exacerbation than less dyspneic patients (mMRC 0–1), five more chances of hospital admissions, and four more chances of having emergency visits without hospitalizations (2).

RATIONALE FOR THE USE OF LAMA/ LABA COMBINATION

Classically, the airways are described to be distributed as central and distal airways – central airways largely innervated by cholinergic postganglionic parasympathetic nerves and distal or peripheral airways by the adrenergic sympathetic nerves.

One of the rationales for the use of a long-acting muscarinic antagonist (LAMA)/long-acting β_2-agonist (LABA) combination is based on airway innervation. The bronchial muscle tone of the central airways is regulated by the neurotransmitter acetylcholine (Ach). There are at least five acetylcholine or muscarinic receptors in the human body, three of them being expressed in human lungs: M1, which mediates the ganglionic neurotransmitter acetylcholine, and M3, which is located at the bronchial muscle and stimulates bronchial smooth muscle contraction. On the contrary, M2 muscarinic receptors are in the postganglionic nerve and function as an inhibitor of acetylcholine. Antimuscarinic receptor drugs inhibit the bronchial smooth muscle contraction by blocking the M1 and M3 muscarinic receptors; the M2 muscarinic receptors present a negative feedback mechanism for the acetylcholine release, but when blocked by an antimuscarinic molecule, will allow more acetylcholine to be released. Thus, the process of creating long-acting muscarinic antagonist molecules aims to develop molecules that have a long-blocking effect on M1 and M3 receptors and a short-blocking effect on M2 receptors.

Beta-2 adrenergic receptors are classically described as mainly expressed in the smooth muscle of the peripheral airways. The G protein coupled receptor when activated will activate Gs and stimulates adenyl cyclase activity, resulting in an increase of intracellular cyclic adenosine monophosphate (cAMP), leading to the activation of protein kinase A and relaxation of the bronchial smooth muscle. Contrary to the cholinergic pathway that is directly innervated by the vagus nerve, the sympathetic system is not directly innervated, and the receptor is stimulated by circulating sympathomimetic drugs like adrenaline. So, the airways may be dilated through direct beta-2 receptors stimulation or by inhibition of muscarinic antagonists, making sense to give a patient the two bronchodilators to equally bronchodilate the whole airway tree.

A second important point to consider about the use of dual bronchodilation comes from a Japanese study that compared the airways response to oxitropium and salbutamol on different days and observed that most of the individuals could answer to both drugs in a similar way. However, a subgroup of individuals presented either a better response to oxitropium or to salbutamol, denominated anticholinergic responders and adrenergic responders, respectively. From the patient perspective, as there is not a quick response test that decides which of the three classes the patient would fit in, the best approach is to give the patient the two drugs.

A third important point is that all studies have shown that dual bronchodilators have much better peak FEV1 or 24-hour-trough FEV1 responses compared with their monocomponents (3). Five meta-analyses have unequivocally demonstrated clinical benefits favoring the LAMA/LABA combination for the outcomes of moderate or severe exacerbations, dyspnea, lung function at three, six, and 12 months, and health-related quality of life (HRQL). In addition, for all evaluated adverse events (death, pneumonia, cardiac arrhythmias, cardiovascular adverse events), there are no statistical differences among the combination LAMA/LABA and LAMA, LABA, ICS/LABA, or placebo (4–8).

Recently, guidelines have stated that the most efficient initial bronchodilator treatment is LAMA/LABA combination. The American Thoracic Society Clinical Practice Guideline (2020) strongly recommends LAMA/LABA combination therapy over LABA or LAMA monotherapy for patients with COPD who complain of dyspnea or exercise intolerance (9). The National Institute for Health and Care Excellence (UK, 2019) also recommends the LAMA/LABA combination for spirometrically confirmed COPD patients with no asthmatic features, dyspneic, or having exacerbations despite using or been offered treatment for tobacco dependence, already under optimized non-pharmacological management, who have received adequate vaccination, and are making frequent use of a short-acting bronchodilator (10). GOLD (2024) has recommended that the initial treatment for the E subgroup (exacerbators independently of the level of symptoms of the patient) should be LAMA/LABA combination (11).

There are five LAMA/LABA combinations on the market: (1) olodaterol/tiotropium 2.5/2.5 µg via Respimat (two puffs once a day – mist); (2) umeclidinium/vilanterol 62.5/25 µg via Ellipta (once a day – dry powder); (3) glycopyrronium/indacaterol 50/110 µg via Breezehaler (once a day – dry powder); 4) aclidinium/formoterol 400/12 µg via Genuair/Pressair (twice a day – dry powder); (5) glycopyrrolate/formoterol 18/9.6 µg via Aerosphere (twice a day – metered-dose inhaler) (not all registered in all countries). There are just a few head-to-head studies evaluating LAMA/LABA combinations; however, all studies have proved their efficiency and safety versus their monocomponents.

LAMA/LABA INTERACTION

There is a complex interaction between LAMA/LABA receptors that is not yet completely understood. The stimulation of airway smooth muscle beta-2 receptors opens calcium-activated potassium channels (Kca), causing membrane hyperpolarization and consequently less release of acetylcholine. In animal studies, beta-2 receptor stimulation found that the inhibition of airway smooth muscle acetylcholine-induced contraction is associated with an increase in a protein kinase and inhibition of inositol phosphate accumulation. The inhibition of M3 receptors by muscarinic antagonists leads to a decrease in the activation of protein kinase C and phosphorylation of beta-2 receptors, inducing a larger bronchodilation. Thus, the evidence so far has shown that the LAMA/LABA combination may have some interactions resulting in bronchodilation that are more than just a combination of two independent mechanisms (12).

EXACERBATION IN PATIENTS ALREADY ON LAMA/LABA

Symptomatic COPD patients already on dual bronchodulators after a severe or moderate exacerbation should have inhaled corticosteroid added to their treatment. All large clinical trials that have compared the use of triple therapy (FF/UMEC/VIL [13], BUD/GLY/FOR [14], and DPB/GLY/FOR [15]) versus LAMA/LABA have shown significant reduction in the rate of moderate-to-severe exacerbations. However, the long-term use of an inhaled corticosteroid may present adverse events like oral candidiasis and hoarse voice. It should be avoided in patients that have had repeated pneumonias in the past, mycobacterial infections, or a blood eosinophil count under 100 cel/µL. There is some concern about the association of pneumonia and inhaled corticosteroid; however, inhaled corticosteroid-induced pneumonia usually has low morbidity and mortality. The ratio of exacerbation prevention over induced pneumonia favors the use of an inhaled corticosteroid based on the fact that up to 10% of patients with exacerbation may be hospitalized, some 10% of these patients may die in the first 30 days, and around 40% will be readmitted to hospital within three months.

It has been described in *in vitro* studies as an interesting molecular and possible synergic interaction mechanism between ICS and LABA: The corticosteroids increase beta-2 receptors, thus enhancing the bronchodilator effect, and, on the other hand, the beta-2 agonist increases the entry of corticosteroids into the cell, producing a larger anti-inflammatory effect.

There are two possibilities of providing triple therapy to patients: either through multiple inhalers (MITT), also known as open triple, or through one single inhaler (SITT), or closed triple. One study evaluated the action of single inhaler triple therapy versus multiple inhalers triple therapy using the Ellipta device (FF/UMEC/VIL) versus any non-Ellipta device according to the physician's choice. The primary objective was the proportion of CAT responders, considering a decreasing of ≤ 2 units in six months, and it was observed a significant greater response with FF/UMEC/VI (OR 1.31, 95% CI 1.13–1.51); in addition, the mean FEV_1 change from baseline was also significantly greater with FF/UMEC/VI (77 mL versus 28 mL). Adherence was not evaluated in this study, but others studies with multiple inhalers have shown that low adherence may be an issue for consideration (16).

INSPIRATORY FLOW AND THE ADEQUATE USE OF INHALER DEVICES

It is recognized that for the adequate use of inhalation devices, patients should be correctly educated. Inhaled medications are delivered in three different formulations, aerosol (metered-dose inhaler), powder, and mist, and it has been debated which is the most convenient one. Mist is the one with the lowest inspiratory resistance, but due to the technology in the device, it may be the most expensive in some countries. Aerosol demands good coordination of the patient to actuate the device and inspire at the same time. There are different powder devices with distinct inspiratory resistances, with some of them demanding a relatively high effort from the patient. Measurement of the real peak inspiratory flow rate is possible with the In Check Dial equipment, which makes it possible to check the necessary flow rate for the different device resistances provided by the equipment. An estimate of the peak inspiratory flow rate may be obtained from the inspiratory loop of the flow/volume curve, but it has to be taken into consideration that this inspiratory flow is obtained without inspiratory resistance. A third way to estimate the possibility of a patient adequately using a device is through clinical observation: Check if the patient is using his/her neck muscles and if the inspiration lasts for three to five seconds. It is considered that patients who are not able to generate a flow rate over 30 L/min should use medications delivered by mist or nebulization; those with a flow rate between 30 and 60 L/min may use any device but they should be well-oriented; and, finally, those able to generate flow rates over 60 L/min can use any device. From a practical point of view, most stable COPD patients may reach flow rates over 60 L/min no matter the severity of the disease.

DEFLATION AND IMPROVEMENT IN HEART FUNCTION

It is has been observed in several clinical trials that cardiac events are an important cause of mortality in COPD patients. In three years, for 6,000 patients in the TORCH Study, cardiac mortality accounted for 27% of the deaths, respiratory failure for 35%, and cancer 21% (17). The most frequent cardiac diseases asssociated with COPD are arterial blood hypertension, arrythmias, coronary isquemia, periphery arterial diseases, and heart failure. Overall, it is considered that around 25% to 30% of all COPD patients will develop a cardiac disease during the course of the respiratory disease. COPD exacerbation has been shown to incease the chance of a myocardial infarction by 2.7 times in the first five days, and the SUMMIT Study observed that the chances for heart disease after an exacerbation may be increased up to 12 months (18). The mechanism for the high occurence of heart disease in COPD patients is not fully understood, but it may be due to a common risk factor – cigarettes – or systemic COPD inflammation. Long-term hypoxia and lung vascular destruction in COPD patients may lead to pulmonary hypertension, which will impair right ventricular function.

Recently, diseases have been classified by phenotypes and patients have been categorized under treatable traits. Lung hyperinflation is associated with emphysematous phenotype patients and is physiologically characterized by increased residual volume, low inspiratory capacity/total lung capacity, and decreased vital capacity; clinically, emphysematous patients present dyspnea, usually low body mass index, and impaired heart function (19). In emphysematous patients, hyperinflation has been found to be associated with a reduction in the left ventricular filling, diastolic filling, stroke volume, and cardiac output (20). The mechanism for the interaction between heart impairment and lung hyperinflation is not completely understood, but preload reduction in patients with high intrathoracic pressure has been observed. High intrathoracic pressure compresses the pulmonary veins and decreases chamber sizes in the heart (19). In normal healthy young subjects, the development of incremental artificial dynamic hyperinflation induced by decreasing inspiratory capacity by 25%, 50%, and 75% progressively reduced left ventricular end-diastolic volume and left ventricular stroke volume, even at low levels. The occurrence of significant septal flattening highlights the fact that direct ventricular interaction may be responsible for the reduced left ventricular stroke volume during dynamic hyperinflation (21).

Deflation of the lungs should be a logical treatment for COPD hyperinflated patients. Bronchodilators have shown to decrease residual volume and improve dyspnea. One of first studies with the muscarinic antagonist tiotropium showed a remarkable decrease of over 500 mL in the functional residual capacity, what led some to refer to this decrease as a "pharmacological lung volume reduction surgery." In a small group of hyperinflated patients, the patients (mean residual volume of 153.7% of predicted normal) submitted to a single nebulization of the muscarinic antagonist glycopirronium. It was observed in a post-hoc analysis that there was a 0.446 L decrease in the residual volume, varying from 0.741 to 0.150 L, showing the bronchodilator drug effect on lung deflation (22).

A randomized 14-day study with the combination of one long-acting beta-2-agonist bronchodilator, vilanterol, with an inhaled corticosteroid, fluticasone furoate, versus placebo, compared with baseline, showed a significant deflation of 429 mL (p<0.001) in residual volume associated with an increase of 5.8 mL/m^2 (95% confidence interval, 2.74–8.91 [p< 0.001]) in the right ventricular end-diastolic volume index. In addition, left ventricular end-diastolic and left atrial end-systolic volumes increased by 3.63 mL/m^2 (p=0.002) and 2.33 mL/m^2 (p=0.002), respectively. In post-hoc analysis, right ventricular stroke volume increased by 4.87 mL/m^2 (p=0.003) and the right ventricular ejection fraction was unchanged (23).

It may be anticipated that bronchodilation with a muscarinic antagonist and beta-adrenergic combination would show a larger reduction in hyperinflation than bronchodilator monotherapy, resulting in a reduction of the compression of the pulmonary veins. Better blood flow through the microvasculature should improve left ventricular filling. A randomized study assigned 57 eligible COPD hyperinflated patients (residual volume >135% predicted) to test for the first time the cardiovascular response to a LAMA/LABA combination (glycopyrronium/indacaterol) versus placebo in a controlled crossover design. Patients under LAMA/LABA increased left ventricular end-diastolic volume from a mean 55.46 mL/m^2 (SD 15.89) at baseline to 61.76 mL/m^2 (95% CI 57.68–65.84), compared with a change from 56.42 mL/m^2 at baseline (13.54) to 56.53 mL/m^2 (52.43–60.62) after placebo (24).

REFERENCES

1. Dransfield MT, Bailey W, Crater G, Emmett A, O'Dell DM, Yawn B. Disease severity and symptoms among patients receiving monotherapy for COPD. *Prim Care Respir J.* 2011;20:46–53.

2. Punekar YS, Mullerova H, Small M, Holbrook T, Wood R, Naya I, Valle M. Prevalence and burden of dyspnea among patients with chronic obstructive pulmonary disease in five European countries. *Pulm Ther.* 2016;2:59–72.

3. Konno S, Makita H, Hasegawa M, Nasuhara Y, Nagai K, Betsuyaku T, Hizawa N, Nishimura M. Beta2-adrenergic receptor polymorphisms as a determinant of preferential bronchodilator responses to β2-agonist and anticholinergic agents in Japanese patients with chronic obstructive pulmonary disease. *Pharmacog Genomics.* 2011;21(11):687–93. doi: 10.1097/FPC.0b013e328349daa1.

4. Calzetta L, Rogliani P, Matera MG, Cazzola M. A systematic review with meta-analysis of dual bronchodilation with LAMA/LABA for the treatment of stable COPD. *Chest.* 2016;149(5):1181–1196. doi: 10.1016/j.chest.2016.02.646.

5. Huissman comparative efficacy of combination bronchodilator therapies in COPD: a network meta-analysis. *Int J COPD.* 2015;1863–1881.

6. Mills pharmacotherapies for chronic obstructive pulmonary disease: a multiple treatment comparison meta-analysis. 2011;107–129. doi: 10.2147/CLEP.S16235.

7. Tricco AC, Strifler L, Veroniki A-A, Yazdi F, Khan PA, Scott A, Straus SE. Comparative safety and effectiveness of long-acting inhaled agents for treating chronic obstructive pulmonary disease: a systematic review and network meta-analysis. 2015;1–14. doi: 10.1136/bmjopen-2015-009183.

8. Oba Y, Keeney E, Ghatehorde N, Dias S. Dual combination therapy versus long-acting bronchodilators alone for chronic obstructive pulmonary disease (COPD): a systematic review and network meta-analysis. *Cochrane Database Syst Rev.* 2018;12(12):CD012620. doi: 10.1002/14651858.CD012620.pub2.

9. Pharmacologic management of chronic obstructive pulmonary disease. An official American thoracic society clinical practice guideline. *Am J Respir Crit Care Med.* 2020;201(9):e56–e69. doi: 10.1164/rccm.202003-0625TH.

10. Hopkinson NS, Molyneux A, Pink J, Harrisingh MC. 09. Guideline Committee GC NICE. *BMJ.* 2019;366:l4486.

11. Global strategy or the diagnosis, management and prevention of chronic obstructive pulmonary disease (2023 Report). www.goldcopd.org, accessed November 15th, 2022.

12. Cazzola M, Molinard M. The scientific rationale for combining long-acting beta2-agonists and muscarinic antagonosts in COPD. *Pulm Pharmacol Therap.* 2010;23:257–267.

13. Lipson DA, Barnhart F, Brealey N, et al. Once-daily single-inhaler triple versus dual therapy in patients with COPD. *N Engl J Med.* 2018;378:1671–1680.

14. Martinez FJ, Rabe KF, Ferguson GT, Wedzicha JA, Singh D, Wang C, Rossman K, St Rose E, Trivedi R, Ballal S, Darken P, Aurivillius M, Reisner C, Dorinsky P. Reduced all-cause mortality in the ETHOS Trial of budesonide/glycopyrrolate/formoterol for chronic for chronic obstructive pulmonary disease. A randomized, double-blind, multicenter, parallel-group study. *Am J Respir Crit Care Med.* 2021 Mar 1;203(5):553–564. doi: 10.1164/rccm.202006-2618OC.

15. Papi A, Vestbo J, Fabbri L, Corradi M, Prunier H, Cohuet G, Guasconi A, Montagna I, Vezzoli S, Petruzzelli S, Scuri M, Roche N, Singh D. Extrafine inhaled triple therapy versus dual bronchodilator therapy in chronic obstructive pulmonary disease (TRIBUTE): a double-blind, parallel group, randomised controlled trial. *Lancet.* 2018 Mar 17;391(10125):1076–1084. doi: 10.1016/S0140-6736(18)30206-X. Epub 2018 Feb 9.

16. Halpin DMG, Worsley S, Ismaila AS, Beeh KM, Midwinter D, Kocks JWH, Irving E, Marin J, Martin N, Tabberer M, Snowise NG, Compton C. INTREPID: single- *versus* multiple-inhaler triple therapy for COPD in usual clinical practice. *ERJ Open Res.* 2021;7:00950–2020. doi: 10.1183/23120541.00950-202.

17. Calverley PM, Anderson JA, Celli B, Ferguson GT, Jenkins C, Jones PW, Yates JC, Vestbo J. Salmeterol and fluticasone propionate and survival in chronic obstructive pulmonary disease. *N Engl J Med.* 2007 Feb 22;356(8):775–789. doi: 10.1056/NEJMoa063070.

18. Vestbo J, Anderson JA, Brook RD, Calverley PM, Celli BR, Crim C, Martinez F, Yates J, Newby DE. Fluticasone furoate and vilanterol and survival in chronic obstructive pulmonary disease with heightened cardiovascular risk (SUMMIT): a double-blind randomised controlled trial. *Lancet.* 2016 Apr 30;387(10030):1817–26. doi: 10.1016/S0140-6736(16)30069-1.

19. Watz H, Waschki B, Meyer T, et al. Decreasing cardiac chamber sizes and associated heart dysfunction in COPD: role of hyperinflation. *Chest.* 2010;138(1):32–38. doi: 10.1378/chest.09-281017.

20. Barr RG, Bluemke DA, Ahmed FS, et al. Percent emphysema, airflow obstruction, and impaired left ventricular filling. *N Engl J Med.* 2010;362(3):217–227. doi: 10.1056/NEJMoa0808836.

21. Cheyne WS, Gelinas JC, Eves ND. Hemodynamic effects of incremental lung hyperinflation. *Am J Physiol Heart Circ Physiol.* 2018;315:H474–H481. doi: 10.1152/ajpheart.00229.2018.

22. Siler TM, Hohenwarter C, Xiong K, Sciarappa K, Sanjar S, Sharma S. Efficacy of nebulized glycopyrrolate on lung hyperinflation in patients with COPD. *Pulm Therapy.* 2021;7:503–516.

23. Stone IS, Barnes NC, James W-Y, Midwinter D, Boubertakh R, Follows R, John L, Petersen SE. Lung deflation and cardiovascular structure and function in chronic obstructive pulmonary disease. A randomized controlled trial. *Am J Respir Crit Care Med.* 2016;193:717–726.

24. Hohlfeld JM, Vogel-Claussen J, Biller H, Berliner D, Berschneider K, Tillmann HCn, Hiltl S, Bauersachs J, Welte T. Effect of lung deflation with indacaterol plus glycopyrronium on ventricular filling in patients with hyperinflation and COPD (CLAIM Study): a double-blind, randomised, crossover, placebo-controlled, single-centre trial. *Lancet Resp.* 2019. doi: 10.1016/s2213-26w00(18)30047-x.

Lung Volume Reduction Surgery

9

Technique, Tips, and Challenges

Andrew Akcelik and Charles T. Bakhos

INTRODUCTION

Chronic obstructive pulmonary disease (COPD) poses a great burden on a significant portion of the population. It is estimated that 328 million people worldwide suffer from COPD (1). In the United States, the economic burden of COPD was estimated to be US$49 billion in 2020 (2). Over the course of 20 years, surgical intervention for severe emphysema has found its place in the treatment algorithm.

Since the 1990s, lung volume reduction surgery (LVRS) has evolved to become an excellent modality for treating selected patients with severe emphysema. The pulmonary physiology following LVRS is not fully understood; however, the oldest concept involves an increase in elastic recoil and a reduction in lung volumes for optimal inspiratory muscle function (3). More recently, several studies have shown that following LVRS, improvements were observed in vital capacity and FEV1. Specifically, it is thought that the reduction in lung volume to an ideal size allows the thorax to accommodate itself. This in turn leads to an increased vital capacity, resulting in an increased FEV1 (4). The earliest report on a large series of patients who underwent lung volume reduction surgery was done at Washington University in the 1990s. Yusen et al. retrospectively analyzed 84 patients who had undergone bilateral lung volume reduction surgery (5). The operation yielded promising results, with significant increases in the average FEV1 of over 50% within the first year post-operatively, and an overall mortality of 6%. Later, Mckenna and colleagues found that patients with predominantly bilateral upper lobe emphysema benefitted the most from LVRS (6) with improvements in FEV1 of 73.2%, while patients with lower lobe/diffuse pattern had improvements of only 37.9%. These early results were promising, but they were mainly small retrospective series.

In 2003, the National Emphysema Treatment Trial (NETT) was published. This was a landmark multi-center randomized controlled trial analyzing 608 patients who underwent LVRS versus 610 who received medical therapy between 1998 and 2002 (7). Those with a predicted FEV1 of 20% or less and/or predicted carbon monoxide diffusing capacity of 20% or less were considered high risk and excluded from the operation. Additionally, those with a homogenous distribution of emphysema were excluded. Those

DOI: 10.1201/9781003251439-9

with predominantly upper lobe, lower lobe, and heterogeneous emphysema were included in the study. Of the 608 patients, 406 in the surgical group underwent median sternotomy while 174 patients underwent video-assisted thoracic surgery (VATS). The resections were bilateral stapled wedge resections with the objective of removing 20–35% of diseased lung. All patients who underwent LVRS were found to have a higher 90-day mortality (7.9%) compared with medical therapy (1.3%). Despite the overall mortality, this trial found a survival advantage in patients with a predominant upper lobe emphysema, with a risk ratio for death of 0.47 against medical therapy, based on a mean follow-up of 29.2 months. Additionally, a significant percentage of patients with predominant upper lobe emphysema had a more than 10-wattage improvement in maximal exercise for LVRS compared with medical therapy (30% versus 0% in the low exercise capacity group, and 15% versus 3% in those with high exercise capacity).

The NETT trial, however, did not specifically analyze lower lobe predominant emphysema and subsequent LVRS, as they combined the lower lobe group with diffuse emphysema and labeled this group as the non-upper lobe type (7). As such, the benefits of surgery for lower lobe LVRS were less well defined. One retrospective study analyzing 36 patients who underwent LVRS for lower lobe emphysema found short-term improvements in FEV1, and residual volume-to-total lung capacity ratios (8). These improvements, however, seemed to decrease with time from three to six months post-operatively, and data was not collected beyond 24 months.

Following the NETT trial, the pre-operative work-up and selection criteria continued to be refined. In 2010, Chandra and colleagues analyzed 284 patients with upper lobe predominant emphysema and lower exercise capacity who underwent perfusion scintigraphy (9). Of the 284 patients, 202 patients were found to have low upper zone perfusion (defined as less than 20% of total lung perfusion), while the remainder had high perfusion. Those with low upper zone perfusion had lower mortality with LVRS compared with medical therapy, with a risk ratio of 0.56.

Regarding the cost-effectiveness of LVRS versus medical treatment, the NETT trial found it to be $190,000 per quality-adjusted life year (QALY) at three years (10). An updated study by Ramsey and colleagues found that this ratio was lower for those with upper lobe emphysema and low exercise capacity, at $98,000 per QALY (11). Additionally, they extrapolated the data and found the cost-effectiveness to be $21,000 per QALY at ten years for this subgroup. Based on this, LVRS seems to become more cost effective compared with medical therapy over a longer period of time.

Furthermore, LVRS can be offered as a bridge therapy for those waiting to be transplanted. In fact, one large series in Europe analyzed 117 patients who underwent lung transplantation with 52 of those having previous LVRS (12). They found no statistically significant difference in mortality or median survival between lung transplant with or without prior LVRS.

PRE-OPERATIVE TESTING

The pre-operative work-up begins with a chest CT demonstrating heterogeneous emphysema (Figure 9.1) and spirometry. During spirometric analysis, appropriate surgical candidates ideally would have an FEV1 of 20-40% of predicted, residual volume greater than 200% of predicted, a total lung capacity greater than 120% predicted, and a residual volume-to-total lung capacity ratio of greater than 60% (13). Additionally, as described earlier, perfusion scintigraphy is obtained to assess the perfusion of the targeted areas of the lung. This is measured by the Q score, which is defined as the ratio of perfusion in the area of interest to the total lung perfusion. Patients must refrain from smoking and enroll in a pre-operative pulmonary rehabilitation program. They must also undergo cardiopulmonary exercise testing, an echocardiogram to exclude pulmonary hypertension, a nuclear stress test, and computed tomography with analysis of fissure integrity to exclude any suspicious nodules. Additionally, a multidisciplinary meeting is usually held that should include thoracic surgeons, pulmonologists, and radiologists.

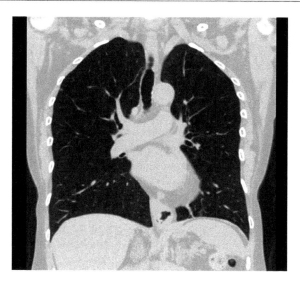

FIGURE 9.1   Coronal CT thorax demonstrating bilateral upper lobe predominant emphysema.

SURGICAL APPROACH

For LVRS, we typically perform VATS, and we favor a concomitant bilateral approach whenever indicated and feasible. We prefer a left-sided double lumen endotracheal intubation as it achieves a quicker and better lung isolation compared with a bronchial blocker, and we use epidural analgesia selectively. We begin by positioning the patient in the lateral decubitus position with the OR table flexed 30 degrees at the level of costal margin above the superior iliac crest. We typically start on the side with the better perfusion.

For upper lobe pneumectomies, the operation begins with placement of a port at the 7th intercostal space at the posterior axillary line. The pleural space is entered, and the lung is immediately deflated. Next, a 12 mm port is placed in the anterior axillary line at the 6th intercostal space, followed by another 15–20 mm port in the mid-axillary line in the 3rd intercostal space. A wound protector can be placed in that port to allow easier retrieval of the specimen. We typically do not insufflate CO_2 during LVRS.

When performing a right upper lobe pneumectomy, we begin by stapling off the emphysematous lung just above the minor fissure anteriorly (Figure 9.2), heading below the level of the azygous vein toward the superior segment of the right lower lobe. We prefer endoscopic medium thickness polyglycolic acid (PGA) reinforced staples (Figure 9.3), as they have been suggested to decrease the risk of post-operative air leak and subsequent parenchymal-pleural fistula (14). Deguchi and colleagues retrospectively analyzed 463 post-lobectomy patients for non-small cell lung cancer (NSCLC) and found a significant reduction in post-operative air leaks in the PGA reinforced stapler group compared with non-reinforced stapler group (9.6% and 22.4%, respectively). The specimen is then placed in an Endocatch bag and removed through the superior port site. In the back-table, we excise a portion of the specimen's staple line and send it for cultures (Figure 9.4). The specimen itself is weighed before sending it to pathology. A gentle mechanical pleurodesis is performed on the uppermost portion of the parietal pleura.

Before placing the patients on their opposite side to perform the contralateral LVRS, we make sure the thoracostomy tubes remain in position and do not get crushed by the bean bag. In our experience, most patients require at least one of the tubes to be placed on suction when proceeding with lung isolation on the opposite side.

The port placement for a left-sided LVRS is identical to the right. The left apical pneumectomy starts with stapling off above the lingula parenchyma anteriorly toward the posterior portion of the major

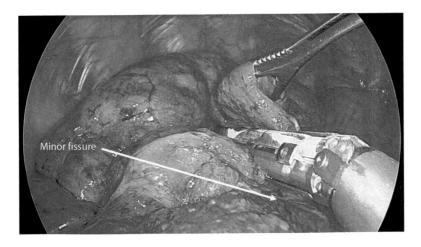

FIGURE 9.2   Right upper lobe thoracoscopic LVRS.

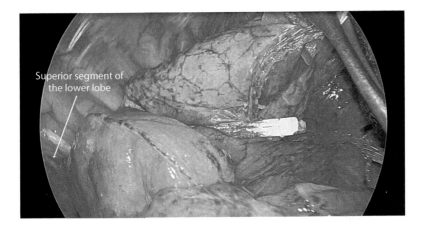

FIGURE 9.3   Reinforced staple line following right upper lobe LVRS.

fissure posteriorly. Again, when the specimen is removed, a portion of the staple line is excised and sent for cultures, and the lung tissue is weighed before being sent to pathology. A mechanical pleurodesis is performed again on the uppermost portion of the parietal pleura, and two apical chest tubes are placed.

Every effort is made to not delay extubation following the operation in order to decrease the severity of air leaks from positive pressure ventilation. Typically with small air leaks, we place our chest tubes in a water seal. If larger air leaks are present, we may elect to place them in −10 mmHg suction for the first 24 hours.

TECHNICAL TIPS

- Minimal handling of lung tissue that is not being resected.
- Use of reinforced staplers for parenchymal division.
- Judicious balancing of lysis of adhesions to allow full expansion of the remaining lung while minimizing the risk of prolonged air leakage.

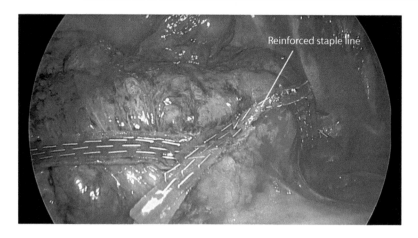

FIGURE 9.4   Final inspection of reinforced staple line.

- On the table – re-exploration if air leakage with lung re-expansion >20% of the set tidal volume is present.
- Careful examination of the parenchymal staple line(s) before placement of the chest tubes and lung re-ventilation.
- Avoidance of aggressive Valsalva maneuvers to expand the lungs.
- Judicious positioning of the two chest tubes with the tips at the apex of the pleural cavity.
- Gentle mechanical pleurodesis of the upper third of the parietal pleura.
- Judicious use of IV fluids during the procedure (<500 mL per one side of LVRS).

CONCLUSIONS

The management of severe emphysema/end-stage COPD has evolved significantly over the last several decades. As demonstrated by the NETT trial, LVRS has a clear benefit for those with low exercise capacity and upper lobe predominant emphysema. For this group of patients who are deemed at acceptable risk, LVRS is an excellent option that leads to improvements in quality of life and overall better survival without precluding future lung transplantation.

REFERENCES

1. Quaderi SA, et al. The unmet global burden of COPD. *Glob Health Epidemiol Genom*. (2018). doi: 10.1017/gheg.2018.1. PMID: 29868229; PMCID: PMC5921960.
2. Larsen DL, et al. The quality of care and economic burden of COPD in the United States: Considerations for managing patients and improving outcomes. American Health & Drug Benefits (2022).
3. Brantigan OC, et al. A surgical approach to pulmonary emphysema. *Am Rev Respir Dis*. (1959). doi: 10.1164/arrd.1959.80.1P2.194. PMID: 13670425.
4. Fessler HE, et al. Physiologic basis for improved pulmonary function after lung volume reduction. *Proc Am Thorac Soc*. (2008). doi: 10.1513/pats.200708-117ET. PMID: 18453348; PMCID: PMC2645312.
5. Yusen RD, et al. Results of lung volume reduction surgery in patients with emphysema. The Washington University Emphysema Surgery Group. *Semin Thorac Cardiovasc Surg*. (1996). PMID: 8679755.

6. McKenna RJ Jr, et al. Patient selection criteria for lung volume reduction surgery. *J Thorac Cardiovasc Surg.* (1997). doi: 10.1016/S0022-5223(97)70010-2. PMID: 9434691.

7. Fishman A, et al. National Emphysema Treatment Trial Research Group. A randomized trial comparing lung-volume-reduction surgery with medical therapy for severe emphysema. *N Engl J Med.* (2003). doi: 10.1056/NEJMoa030287. Epub 2003 May 20. PMID: 12759479.

8. Periklis P, et al. Long-term survival and symptomatic relief in lower lobe lung volume reduction surgery. *Eur J Cardiothorac Surg.* (2017). doi: 10.1093/ejcts/ezx242. PMID: 28950329.

9. Chandra D, et al. National Emphysema Treatment Trial Research Group. Perfusion scintigraphy and patient selection for lung volume reduction surgery. *Am J Respir Crit Care Med.* (2010). doi: 10.1164/rccm.201001-0043OC. Epub 2010 Jun 10. PMID: 20538961; PMCID: PMC2970864.

10. Marchetti N, et al. Surgical approaches to treating emphysema: Lung volume reduction surgery, bullectomy, and lung transplantation. *Semin Respir Crit Care Med.* (2015). doi: 10.1055/s-0035-1556064. Epub 2015 Aug 3. PMID: 26238644.

11. Ramsey et al. Updated evaluation of the cost-effectiveness of lung volume reduction surgery. *Chest.* 131(3) (2007). doi: 10.1378/chest.06-1790. PMID: 17356099.

12. Inci I, II, et al. Previous lung volume reduction surgery does not negatively affect survival after lung transplantation. *Eur J Cardiothorac Surg.* (2018). doi: 10.1093/ejcts/ezx318. PMID: 28957998.

13. Rathinam S, et al. The role of the emphysema multidisciplinary team in a successful lung volume reduction surgery programme. *Eur J Cardio-Thoracic Surg.* (2014). doi: 10.1093/ejcts/ezu129. PMID: 24771753.

14. Deguchi H, et al. Reduction of air leakage using linear staple device with bioabsorbable polyglycolic acid felt for pulmonary lobectomy. *Gen Thorac Cardiovasc Surg* (2020). doi: 10.1007/s11748-019-01207-2. PMID: 31541348.

Extending Candidacy for Lung Volume Reduction Surgery

10

Claudio Caviezel, Laurens Ceulemans and Walter Weder

INTRODUCTION

Chronic obstructive pulmonary disease (COPD) is a major health problem. The World Health Organization (WHO) reported a prevalence of 251 million cases globally in 2016, leading to about 3.17 million deaths in 2015, which was equal to 5% of all deaths globally that year [1].

Lung volume reduction (LVR) is the most effective palliative treatment option in patients with COPD and advanced emphysema [2]. Only lung transplantation can offer a more effective treatment for this widespread and severe condition. However, lung transplantation is restricted to a selected patient population, in general, to a much younger population than for LVRS. Furthermore, it is associated with a complex after treatment with some lifelong side effects.

In patients with emphysema, the lungs become hyperinflated and push down the diaphragm, which is the most important respiratory muscle. With LVR, the lungs are re-sized, which mainly results in a better functioning diaphragm [3]. Other positive consequences are the reopening of small collapsed airways and capillaries. This results in a better airflow and a lower pulmonary artery pressure. This effect can be achieved by either resecting the most emphysemateous and therefore most hyperinflated parts, which do not contribute much or anything to gas exchange (lung volume reduction surgery, LVRS) or by bronchoscopic procedures (bronchoscopic lung volume reduction, BLVR) [4]. The latter consists mainly of valves and coils. Valves are placed endobronchially and lead to an exclusion of the entire respective lobe (atelectasis) by allowing the air to exit the targeted lobe [5]. Valves are only effective in lung lobes that are fully separated by complete fissures. Otherwise, they will be filled with air through collateral ventilation despite perfect valve positions. Coils are placed far deeper in the smaller bronchi and produce shrinking of the targeted lung tissue [6]. However, their application is under critical review.

The initial identification of the subgroup with the highest mortality and, further on, the subgroup analysis of more successfully treated patients during the National Emphysema Treatment Trial (NETT)

DOI: 10.1201/9781003251439-10

[7, 8] led to an important step in emphysema treatment: the definition of indications and contraindications for LVRS.

Patients with emphysema are a vulnerable target population for surgery. Nevertheless, due to an overall shortage of donor lungs, other treatment options than transplantation are urgently needed.

The concept of LVRS consists of re-shaping the lungs to their original volume. In heterogeneous emphysema, the most hyperinflated and destroyed lung areas are targeted and resected. This has been proven to be successful within the classic, nowadays perhaps slightly conservative inclusion criteria [9, 10]. With experience since the mid-1990s [11–13], the so far gained knowledge has allowed a safe and innovative extension of the inclusion criteria by challenging old concepts based on a constant quality control. Therefore, during the last few years, these efforts have resulted in positive outcomes in borderline indication patients [14].

To date, only little evidence exists on LVRS in patients with alpha1-antitrypsin deficiency, with homogeneous emphysema, and for patients with previous LVR. The same is true for patients with mild pulmonary hypertension, diffusion capacity values lower than 20% predicted, and patients with advanced emphysema and concurrent early stage lung cancer.

ALPHA1-ANTITRYPSIN DEFICIENCY

Patients with alpha1-antitrypsin deficiency (A1-ATD) are usually younger when they are symptomatic than the classic smoker with often heterogeneous, upper-lobe predominant emphysema. In contrast, patients with A1-ATD present with heterogeneous, typically lower-lobe emphysema. A few single-center studies showed solid results but with particular drawbacks [15–18]. Beneficial in the short- and mid-term, lung functional improvements can be achieved after bilateral LVRS; however, the effects usually do not last as long in the classic heterogeneous emphysema population [16]. Regarding the selection of these patients, the surgeon should carefully inspect the CT scan for signs of chronic inflammation like scarring of the small bronchi and bronchiectasis, as these lesions usually hinder a beneficial course after LVRS. However, once A1AD patients are discussed at an emphysema board, there are few reasons to exclude them from LVRS if they are not showing any signs of above-mentioned chronic inflammation and presenting with severe hyperinflation, sometimes with a bridge-to-transplant concept.

HOMOGENEOUS EMPHYSEMA

While there is convincing and widespread evidence about LVRS in patients with severe hyperinflation and heterogeneous emphysema, the same is scarce in cases of homogeneous emphysema. Patients with purely homogeneous emphysema are often refused surgery, as there are only a handful of single-center studies dealing with this subgroup [19–22]. Being part of the subgroup with the highest mortality in early NETT results, patients with homogeneous emphysema should not be considered suitable LVRS candidates when FEV1 and/or DLCO values are <20% predicted [8]. However, in cases of severe hyperinflation and a preserved DLCO, these patients might profit from a bilateral LVRS, especially in cases of collateral interlobar ventilation precluding BLVR with valves [5]. The surgical approach consists of bilateral, apical, upper-lobe re-shaping as in upper-lobe predominant emphysema, preferably resecting not more than 20% of the upper part of the upper lobes [22]. Nevertheless, although the outcome can be promising regarding the improvement of lung function values, six-minute walking distance, and quality of life, its duration is again shorter compared with the results of LVRS homogeneous emphysema, usually lasting one to two years [20]. However, as shown in patients with homogeneous emphysema after BLVR coils or with valves,

the latter with the exclusion of even a whole lobe, the main benefit seems to derive from the reduction o
the residual volume (RV) [6].

PREVIOUS LVR

Today, more and more patients present with a history of LVR, either without favorable outcomes or loss o
its initial beneficial effect. The effects of LVRS in patients who initially had BLVR with valves have been
presented in retrospective papers from Heidelberg, Germany [21], with 20 patients and in a collaborative
work from Zurich, Switzerland, and Copenhagen, Denmark [22], with 34 patients. Both show safe and
favorable outcomes, although the lung functional benefit seems to be lower than after a primary LVRS -
this might be due to the natural progression of COPD. However, inclusion criteria are the same as in the
other patients eligible for LVRS. Non-functioning valves should be removed a few weeks before surgery
but left in situ in case of persisting atelectasis and a potential LVRS target zone on the contralateral side
to prevent a devastating increase of hyperinflation.

One study showed favorable outcomes regarding repeated LVRS on an already operated side [23]
These patients must present with the same inclusion criteria as for the first LVRS but have to be informed
about the possibly lesser effect and the higher duration of air leaks, as they might present with severe
adhesions [22].

PULMONARY HYPERTENSION

Patients with mean pulmonary artery pressures (mPAP) above 35 mmHg should be excluded from LVRS
[24]. However, there is a debate regarding patients with mild to moderate pulmonary hypertension (PH)
which is found in over half of all COPD patients [25–27]. While a few studies show no or minimally
impairing effects of LVRS on PAPs [28], there is some evidence that LVRS might even reduce PH [29, 30]
As LVRS reduces hyperinflation and air-trapping and improves arterial oxygen tension, it might ever
improve right ventricular function [31].

The authors recommend a transthoracic echocardiography for examining right and left ventricular
function and estimation of the RV/RA pressure. In case of RV/RA (or systolic PAP) >35 mmHg or other
signs of right ventricular dysfunction, a right heart catheter is indicated.

DLCO <20% PREDICTED

The preliminary published results from the NETT group [8] did not only identify the high-risk group for
LVRS, they also communicated one preoperative factor – again – to avoid: DLCO values below 20% predicted. Looking more precisely, this was only true and meaningful in patients with a combination with a
FEV1 <20% and/or homogeneous emphysema. In the latter, in combination with a very low DLCO, where
almost all lung parenchyma is equally destroyed, resection of lung tissue has indeed to be avoided. Ciccone
et al. (2003) already proved favorable results for a subgroup of 20 patients, provided that there are obvious heterogeneous target zones for LVRS [13]. The author and his colleagues reconfirmed these results
in a group of 33 patients [32]. There was no 90-day mortality and there was a significant improvement
in lung function. However, the duration of air leak was longer than usual. This significant postoperative

morbidity has to be taken into account, be it during preoperative informed consent or regarding postoperative management.

One might again realize that severe hyperinflation and an obvious target zone in heterogeneous emphysema are the true key factors to success, even in patients with very low DLCO.

CONCURRENT NSCLC

As COPD and emphysema with its usual smoking history go hand in hand with the occurrence of non-small lung cancer, many patients presenting at a multidisciplinary tumor and/or emphysema board show suspicious nodules [33, 34]. In cases of proven cancer or firm suspicion for malignancy, radiotherapy or resection is usually discussed. The latter offers the advantage of a complete histology including lymph node status, but in patients with severe COPD, it is often not feasible due to poor lung functional reserves. The European Society for Medical Oncology (ESMO) already lists in their guidelines evaluation for resection in potential LVRS candidates [35]. In an ideal case, the resection is complete, and the postoperative lung function even improves due to LVRS, which has been shown in several single-center studies [36–38]. It is of upmost importance to be alert during treatment decision discussions, keeping this surgical and lung function improving modality in mind.

WHEN TO EXTEND CANDIDACY FOR LVRS

Severe hyperinflation and well-planned target zones are the keys to success for most LVRS candidates. With this basic strategy, LVRS can even be offered to borderline candidates as mentioned earlier. Nevertheless, initial experience, especially when starting a new LVRS program, has to be gained with obvious, markedly heterogeneous emphysema patients with relatively preserved DLCO. Not only do the referring physicians have to be convinced about the potential success of LVRS, but their own team will also profit from more straightforward cases in the beginning. Finally, the more classic cases within strict criteria are treated, the more profit to the (borderline) patient, not forgetting that a multidisciplinary team approach, offering all modalities, including LVRS, BLVR, and even transplantation, is crucial.

REFERENCES

1. WHO. *Chronic obstructive pulmonary disease*. Fact Sheet 2017.
2. van Geffen WH, Slebos DJ, Herth FJ, Kemp SV, Weder W, Shah PL. Surgical and endoscopic interventions that reduce lung volume for emphysema: a systemic review and meta-analysis. *Lancet Respir Med* 2019;7:313–24.
3. Cassart M, Hamacher J, Verbandt Y, Wildermuth S, Ritscher D, Russi EW, et al. Effects of lung volume reduction surgery for emphysema on diaphragm dimensions and configuration. *Am J Respir Crit Care Med* 2001;163:1171–5.
4. Martini K, Caviezel C, Schneiter D, Milanese G, Opitz I, Weder W, et al. Dynamic magnetic resonance imaging as an outcome predictor for lung-volume reduction surgery in patients with severe emphysema. *Eur J Cardiothorac Surg* 2018.
5. Slebos DJ, Shah PL, Herth FJ, Valipour A. Endobronchial valves for endoscopic lung volume reduction: best practice recommendations from expert panel on endoscopic lung volume reduction. *Respiration* 2017;93:138–50.

6. Slebos DJ, Hartman JE, Klooster K, Blaas S, Deslee G, Gesierich W, et al. Bronchoscopic coil treatment fo patients with severe emphysema: a meta-analysis. *Respiration* 2015;90:136–45.
7. Fishman A, Martinez F, Naunheim K, Piantadosi S, Wise R, Ries A, et al. A randomized trial comparing lung volume-reduction surgery with medical therapy for severe emphysema. *N Engl J Med* 2003;348:2059–73.
8. National Emphysema Treatment Trial Research G, Fishman A, Fessler H, Martinez F, McKenna RJ Jr., Naunheim K, et al. Patients at high risk of death after lung-volume-reduction surgery. *N Engl J Med* 2001;345:1075–83.
9. Caviezel C, Franzen D, Inci I, Weder W. [Lung volume reduction surgery – State of the art 2016]. *Zentralb Chir* 2016;141(Suppl 1):S26–34.
10. Caviezel C, Franzen D, Weder W. [Lung volume reduction surgery]. *Pneumologie* 2018;72:64–78.
11. Bingisser R, Zollinger A, Hauser M, Bloch KE, Russi EW, Weder W. Bilateral volume reduction surgery fo diffuse pulmonary emphysema by video-assisted thoracoscopy. *J Thorac Cardiovasc Surg* 1996;112:875–82.
12. Brenner M, McKenna RJ, Jr., Chen JC, Serna DL, Powell LL, Gelb AF, et al. Relationship between amount o lung resected and outcome after lung volume reduction surgery. *Ann Thorac Surg* 2000;69:388–93.
13. Ciccone AM, Meyers BF, Guthrie TJ, Davis GE, Yusen RD, Lefrak SS, et al. Long-term outcome of bilateral lung volume reduction in 250 consecutive patients with emphysema. *J Thorac Cardiovasc Surg* 2003;125:513–25.
14. Caviezel C, Schneiter D, Opitz I, Weder W. Lung volume reduction surgery beyond the NETT selection crite ria. *J Thorac Dis* 2018;10:S2748–S53.
15. Gelb AF, McKenna RJ, Brenner M, Fischel R, Zamel N. Lung function after bilateral lower lobe lung volume reduction surgery for alpha1-antitrypsin emphysema. *Eur Respir J.* 1999 Oct;14(4):928–33.
16. Tutic M, Bloch KE, Lardinois D, Brack T, Russi EW, Weder W. Long-term results after lung volume reductio surgery in patients with alpha1-antitrypsin deficiency. *J Thorac Cardiovasc Surg* 2004;128:408–13.
17. Dauriat G, Mal H, Jebrak G, Brugière O, Castier Y, Camuset J, Marceau A, Taillé C, Lesèche G, Fournier M Functional results of unilateral lung volume reduction surgery in alpha1-antitrypsin deficient patients. *Int . Chron Obstruct Pulmon Dis.* 2006;1(2):201–6.
18. Stoller JK, Gildea TR, Ries AL, Meli YM, Karafa MT; National Emphysema Treatment Trial Research Group Lung volume reduction surgery in patients with emphysema and alpha-1 antitrypsin deficiency. *Ann Thorac Surg.* 2007 Jan;83(1):241–51.
19. Wisser W, Tschernko E, Wanke T, Senbaclavaci O, Kontrus M, Wolner E, Klepetko W. Functional improve ments in ventilatory mechanics after lung volume reduction surgery for homogeneous emphysema. *Eur . Cardiothorac Surg.* 1997 Oct;12(4):525–30.
20. Bloch KE, Georgescu CL, Russi EW, Weder W. Gain and subsequent loss of lung function after lung volume reduction surgery in cases of severe emphysema with different morphologic patterns. *J Thorac Cardiovasc Surg* 2002;123:845–54.
21. Weder W, Tutic M, Lardinois D, Jungraithmayr W, Hillinger S, Russi EW, Bloch KE. Persistent benefi from lung volume reduction surgery in patients with homogeneous emphysema. *Ann Thorac Surg.* 2009 Jan;87(1):229–36.
22. Weder W, Ceulemans LJ, Opitz I, Schneiter D, Caviezel C. Lung volume reduction surgery in patients with homogeneous emphysema. *Thorac Surg Clin.* 2021 May;31(2):203–209.
23. Eichhorn ME, Gompelmann D, Hoffmann H, Dreher S, Hornemann K, Haag J, Kontogianni K, Heussel CP Winter H, Herth FJF, Eberhardt R. Consolidating lung volume reduction surgery after endoscopic lung volume reduction failure. *Ann Thorac Surg.* 2021 Jun;111(6):1858–1865.
24. Mentzer SJ. Optimizing the selection of surgical candidates for lung volume reduction surgery. *Semin Thorac Cardiovasc Surg* 2007;19:151–6.
25. Nowak J, Hudzik B, Jastrzębski D, Niedziela JT, Rozentryt P, Wojarski J, Ochman M, Karolak W, Żegleń S Gierlotka M, Gąsior M. Pulmonary hypertension in advanced lung diseases: echocardiography as an importan part of patient evaluation for lung transplantation. *Clin Respir J.* 2018 Mar;12(3):930–938.
26. Eberhardt R, Gerovasili V, Kontogianni K, Gompelmann D, Ehlken N, Herth FJ, Grünig E, Nagel C Endoscopic lung volume reduction with endobronchial valves in patients with severe emphysema and estab lished pulmonary hypertension. *Respiration.* 2015;89(1):41–8.
27. Peinado VI, Pizarro S, Barberà JA. Pulmonary vascular involvement in COPD. *Chest.* 2008 Oct;134(4):808–814
28. Weg IL, Rossoff L, McKeon K, et al. Development of pulmonary hypertension after lung volume reductio surgery. *Am J Respir Crit Care Med* 1999;159:552–556.
29. Criner GJ, Scharf SM, Falk JA, et al. Effect of lung volume reduction surgery on resting pulmonary hemody namics in severe emphysema. *Am J Respir Crit Care Med* 2007;176:253–60.
30. Caviezel C, Aruldas C, Franzen D, Ulrich S, Inci I, Schneiter D, et al. Lung volume reduction surgery ir selected patients with emphysema and pulmonary hypertension. *Eur J Cardiothorac Surg* 2018.

31. Opitz I, Ulrich S. Pulmonary hypertension in chronic obstructive pulmonary disease and emphysema patients: prevalence, therapeutic options and pulmonary circulatory effects of lung volume reduction surgery. *J Thorac Dis.* 2018 Aug;10(Suppl 23):S2763–S2774.
32. Caviezel C, Schaffter N, Schneiter D, Franzen D, Inci I, Opitz I, et al. Outcome after lung volume reduction surgery in patients with severely impaired diffusion capacity. *Ann Thorac Surg* 2018;105:379–385.
33. de Torres JP, et al. Assessing the relationship between lung cancer risk and emphysema detected on low-dose CT of the chest. *Chest* 2007 Dec;132(6):1932–1938.
34. Celli BR, Wedzicha JA. Update on clinical aspects of chronic obstructive pulmonary disease. *N Engl J Med* 2019 Sep 26;381(13):1257–1266.
35. Postmus PE, Kerr KM, Oudkerk M, Senan S, Waller DA, Vansteenkiste J, et al. Early and locally advanced non-small-cell lung cancer (NSCLC): ESMO Clinical Practice Guidelines for diagnosis, treatment and follow-up. *Ann Oncol* 2017;28:iv1–iv21.
36. McKenna RJ Jr, Fischel RJ, Brenner M, et al. Combined operations for lung volume reduction surgery and lung cancer. *Chest* 1996;110:885–888.
37. Choong CK, Meyers BF, Battafarano RJ, et al. Lung cancer resection combined with lung volume reduction in patients with severe emphysema. *J Thorac Cardiovasc Surg* 2004;127:1323–1331.
38. Caviezel C, von Rotz J, Schneiter D, Inci I, Hillinger S, Opitz I, et al. Improved postoperative lung function after sublobar resection of non-small-cell lung cancer combined with lung volume reduction surgery in patients with advanced emphysema. *J Thorac Dis* 2018;10:S2704–S10.

The Interface between Lung Emphysema and Lung Cancer

11

Mario C. Ghefter, Ricardo Sales Santos and Luis C. Losso

INTRODUCTION

The importance of lung cancer among the main causes of global mortality is well known, in addition to being an important public health problem due to its high incidence. The estimated incidence and mortality rates standardized by age (world) for lung cancer in 2020, for both sexes, with ages between 50 and 79 years, was 96.8 and 77.1, respectively, which generates a case fatality rate per incidence of 79.6%.[1]

We can see the importance of these numbers when we compare them with the two most common neoplasms in the world, which are breast and prostate cancer, and which have much lower-case fatality rates per incidence of 30.6% and 17.2%, respectively, for the same age group mentioned.[1]

In almost all countries, lung cancer is among the leading causes of death, as is COPD. This is no coincidence, as several epidemiological studies have observed an important association between these two diseases and several mechanisms have been proposed to explain this relationship. Chronic inflammation due to tobacco exposure and lung repair mechanisms in COPD patients appear to be key features for the development of lung cancer. When these interrelated conditions are added together, they rank near the top of the leading causes of global mortality.

Based on the Burden of Obstructive Lung Diseases (BOLD) and other large-scale epidemiological studies, it is estimated that the global prevalence of COPD is 10.3% (confidence interval [CI] 8.2%–12.8%). With some caveats, there are approximately 3 million deaths from COPD per year, significantly surpassing the 1.8 million deaths per year from lung cancer. Hence, the importance of this lethal association. From now on, we will be referring to cigarette smoking COPD (COPD-C).[2]

When these linked conditions are added together, they come near the top of the leading causes of mortality.

In the last quarter of the 20th century, studies began proposing the increasing incidence and mortality of lung cancer associated with the presence of airway obstruction and changes in lung function,

DOI: 10.1201/9781003251439-11

demonstrating at the time that COPD was an independent factor associated with the incidence of small cell lung cancer. [3]

In a multifactorial proportional risk analysis, it was found that patients with mild ventilatory dysfunction were more likely to have lung cancer than those with moderate and severe dysfunction, and that these were more likely to develop lung cancer than those with normal lung function.[4]

Furthermore, acute exacerbation of COPD, GOLD I/II, advanced age, low BMI, and DLCO <80% were independent predictors of lung cancer.[5] Lung cancer, in turn, is a significant factor in morbidity and mortality of COPD.

Several epidemiological studies, including lung cancer screening studies, have found a two- to four-fold increase in the risk of patients with COPD when compared with individuals without airflow disturbance. Part of the risk attributed to airflow disturbance appears to derive from the presence of emphysema, which has proven to be an important risk factor for lung cancer in smokers without airflow disturbance and even in never-smokers. This evidence supports the idea of including patients with COPD and/or emphysema in lung cancer screening programs.[6]

Several mechanisms have been proposed to explain the association between COPD and lung cancer. These mechanisms include genetic susceptibility, deoxyribonucleic acid (DNA) damage and repair, epigenetics, specific microRNA downregulation, expression of hypoxia-induced pro-inflammatory genes, tumor growth factor B and integrins, telomere length and dysfunction, and immune responses. There is no definitive explanation for the association, and presumably interactions are present between many of them.

The evidence regarding the severity of emphysema and the risk of lung cancer is not consistent. In the PLuSS study, for example, Wilson and colleagues found that the risk of lung cancer was highest in individuals with mild emphysema, followed by those who had moderate-severe emphysema and trace emphysema, respectively.[7] On the other hand, Zulueta et al. found a linear trend between emphysema severity and lung cancer mortality, but the association was only significant for severe emphysema. A possible explanation for contradictory results may be the methodology used to determine the presence and amount of emphysema, as some studies use automated quantification of emphysema, and others use a visual assessment of emphysema.[8]

The presence of emphysema around the tumor region has also been the subject of study. The studies agree on the fact that lung cancer develops more frequently in areas of the lung with more emphysema. Bishawi and colleagues found a strong association for lung cancer to be located in the area with the highest degree of emphysema, generally in the right upper quadrant.[9]

Treatments such as immunotherapy and targeted therapy have become a reality, increasing disease-free survival and overall survival in various scenarios.[10] At the population level, three-year relative survival for all lung cancer stages combined increased from 22% for diagnoses during 2004 to 2006 to 33% for diagnoses during 2016 to 2018.[11] The gains not only reflect therapeutic improvement, but also the early detection of lung cancer and advances in staging and surgical procedures.[12, 13]

COPD AND LUNG CANCER: THE BIOLOGICAL INTERFACE

The connection between COPD and lung cancer is well known, and we can state that both diseases may share common causes, such as genetic polymorphisms and epigenetic changes. Recent studies have been carried out on people of different ethnicities suffering from COPD or lung cancer and have identified some genetic loci that may increase susceptibility to both diseases. Single nucleotide polymorphisms present in the nicotinic acetylcholine receptor genes CHRNA3, CHRNA4, and CHRNA5 have been associated with increased susceptibility and overlap between COPD and lung cancer. On the other hand, other single nucleotides appear to reduce the risk of these diseases. Of particular interest is the decreased expression of the VEGFR1 variant rs7326277C, which reduced lung inflammation and epithelial-mesenchymal transition, two known pathogenic features shared between COPD and lung cancer.[14]

We can also highlight that epigenetic changes, such as DNA methylation, histone modification, and miRNA expression, are important factors that increase the susceptibility of individuals with COPD to developing lung cancer. Studies have identified several miRNAs and genes, such as CCDC37 and MAP1B that are regulated differently in COPD patients who develop lung cancer. These miRNAs and genes are involved in regulating pathways associated with cancer development. Furthermore, bioinformatics analysis identified differentially expressed genes and miRNAs that can be used as biomarkers to stratify COPD patients more predisposed to developing non-small cell lung cancer (NSCLC).[14]

Other factors involved in the COPD–lung cancer interface are inflammation, oxidative stress, and DNA damage. Inflammation and oxidative stress in COPD can cause DNA damage and favor the development of lung tumors. The inflammatory process in COPD involves the activation of several immune cells that produce pro-inflammatory cytokines, chemokines, and reactive oxygen species. Tumor necrosis factor (TNF) is upregulated in individuals with COPD and appears to contribute to the formation of lung cancer. Leukotrienes, pro-inflammatory lipid mediators, have been found at increased levels in COPD patients and appear to be a critical component in the tumor microenvironment. Leukotriene B4 (LTB4) also has a critical role in the development of inflammation-induced tumors. Furthermore, among COPD patients, serum concentrations of higher molecular weight adiponectin were associated with the ratio of neutrophils to lymphocytes, a biomarker of systemic inflammation that has been implicated in lung cancer severity and response to treatment.[14]

Although the two diseases have points in common, they generally have very different paths. While lung cancer is mainly characterized by mutations in suppressor genes, cell proliferation, invasion increased angiogenesis, and metastasis, in COPD, airflow obstruction, infections, matrix degradation inflammation, decreased tissue repair, and mucociliary clearance represent the main characteristics.[14]

COPD AND LUNG CANCER SCREENING

Most lung cancer screening recommendation statements refer primarily to the NLST and NELSON studies to select high-risk groups based on age and smoking status. However, current recommendations regarding age group, amount of exposure to smoke, and time to quit smoking have not been fully established.[15,16] For example, the starting and ending ages of screening are 50 to 55 years and 70 to 80 years respectively. Smoking history varies from five pack-years to 30 pack-years, and the minimum time to quit smoking is five years. There is currently no evidence to support specific ages for starting and stopping screening. In 2020, the US Preventive Services Task Force revised lung cancer screening guidelines lowering the starting age for screening for high-risk groups from 55 to 50 years and reducing smoking exposure from 30 pack-years to 20 pack-years, allowing more people with lower exposure to smoke, but considered high risk, to benefit from screening.[17]

In England, those eligible for LDCT screening were considered individuals aged between 55 and 80 years, smokers (current or previous), and only those with a high risk of lung cancer, as calculated by the PLCOm2012 model (1.5%, 2.5%, or 5%), were invited for screening.[18]

In Germany, it has been established that individuals who should undergo screening are those aged between 50 and 75 years, smokers for more than 25 years, with exposure ≥15 pack-years, or ex-smokers <10 years.[19]

In China, recommendations consider local biological factors and characteristics. Therefore, the screening recommendation is for individuals aged between 50 and 80 years and must have one of the following conditions: (1) smoking ≥20 pack-years or passive smoking for ≥20 years; if stopping smoking now, the time to stop smoking should not exceed five years; (2) have a history of long-term occupational exposure to carcinogens (radon, arsenic, beryllium, chromium and their compounds, asbestos, chloromethyl ether, silicon oxide); and (3) first- and second-degree relatives with lung cancer and smokers ≥5 pack-years or passive smokers ≥5 years.[20]

In a recent publication, the Argentine consensus recommendation defined the risk population as the same as in the original NLST study.[21]

A consortium of experts from the Brazilian Society of Thoracic Surgery (SBCT), the Brazilian Society of Pulmonology (SBPT), and the Brazilian College of Radiology (CBR) recommends screening for lung cancer with a low dose computed tomography (LDCT) in adults aged 50 to 80 years who have a ≥20 pack-year smoking history or who currently smoke or have quit smoking within the last 15 years. Screening should be stopped when a person has not smoked for 15 years or develops a health problem that substantially limits life expectancy or the ability or willingness to undergo curative lung surgery.

In the most recent publication of the Global Initiative for Chronic Obstructive Lung Disease (GOLD), it is stated that a chest CT should be considered in COPD patients with persistent exacerbations, symptoms disproportionate to the severity of the disease on lung function tests, FEV1 less than 45% of predicted with significant hyperinflation and air trapping, or those who meet criteria for lung cancer screening.[2]

Another aspect is the incorporation of spirometry into screening programs. Bradley and colleagues investigated the prevalence of, and factors associated with, underdiagnosis and misdiagnosis of COPD in a high-risk lung cancer population who underwent spirometry along with LDCT for lung cancer screening. They concluded that spirometry offered alongside LDCT screening can potentially identify cases of undiagnosed and misdiagnosed COPD.[22]

Given the above evidence, there is debate in the literature about including the presence of COPD as an indication for lung cancer screening as the potential benefits of screening could be outweighed by the increased risk of death inherent in COPD and/or emphysema (especially if airflow obstruction or emphysema is severe) and its associated comorbidities.

De-Torres and colleagues explored the impact of screening in a sample of patients with mild and moderate COPD. Preliminary data from their group showed that it is in these subgroups that the risk of lung cancer is highest. When comparing lung cancer mortality in this group with that of a paired sample of COPD patients who were not screened, they observed that mortality was 30 times lower in the group that underwent screening (0.08 vs. 2.48 deaths per 100 person-years; p = 0.001). This analysis shows that the benefit of annual CT screening is greatest in those with normal lung function or only mild to moderate COPD.[23]

In a first pos- hoc analysis of NLST results (NLST-ACRIN), it was found that the presence of COPD had an important effect on screening results, showing a strong linear relationship between increasing severity of airflow limitation and the risk of lung cancer.[24] But in a more recent secondary analysis, it was found that although those with severe or very severe airway limitation (GOLD grade 3–4) have the highest risk of cancer, they also have the lowest rates of surgery (despite comparable staging), more aggressive histology, and higher rates of non-lung cancer deaths, suggesting that these factors may contribute to the lack of any apparent reduction in lung cancer mortality in this group after screening ("poor responders") and that their exclusion appears to improve screening efficiency. Another possible explanation for there being no benefit from screening in GOLD 3–4 individuals is that they die from other causes at a much higher rate in relation to their mortality rate from lung cancer. This may be attributed to higher rates of pre-existing respiratory illnesses and high rates of cardiorespiratory death during screening.[25]

We understand that the difficulty of including COPD patients in screening programs is accompanied by the inconvenience of including symptomatic individuals in the screened population, which violates a principle of a standard screening program, as described by Nielsen and Lang, when stating that: "The concept of screening usually refers to laboratory tests, physical examination, or radiologic tests performed on *asymptomatic* patients in the hope of discovering subclinical disease."[26] But perhaps here, specifically in the case of individuals with COPD, this inclusion should be made, creating specific criteria such as life expectancy due to COPD and the possibility of adequate cancer treatment in this population. We also understand that this population is already the target of individualized screening (i.e., recommending screening tests to patients in private clinical settings in a one-to-one manner). We must keep in mind that the main objective of a screening program is to save lives, and not just detect cases of cancer, or not miss cancers, but instead, find the cancer at an early and curable stage.

De-Torres and colleagues developed and validated a specific score for COPD with the aim of predicting the risk of lung cancer, the COPD-LUCSS (Table 11.1). Using the Pamplona International Early Lung

TABLE 11.1   Chronic obstructive pulmonary disease lung cancer screening score (COPD-LUCSS)

VARIABLE	SCORE (POINTS)	CATEGORIES
BMI <25	1	0–6 Low risk
>60 pack-years history	2	
Age >60 years	3	7–10 High risk
Radiologic emphysema	4	
Total	10	

BMI, body mass index.

Cancer Detection Program (P-IELCAP) and the Pittsburgh Lung Screening Study (PLuSS), they were able to propose two risk categories: low risk (scores 0–6) and high risk (scores 7–10). In comparison with low-risk patients, in both cohorts, lung cancer risk increased 3.5-fold in the high-risk category.[27]

This and other types of scores can be extremely useful in identifying COPD patients at increased risk of developing lung cancer.

Ethical principles must be considered when thinking about COPD as an inclusion criterion involved in lung cancer screening programs, or even in so-called individualized screening. Cancer screening is ethical when its effect has been validated in scientific studies and when the program takes ethical principles into account. Cancer screening where no effect has been found in previous scientific studies is unethical.[28]

In a screening program, the need for adequate and efficient treatment for early diagnosed forms of the disease is also implicit, which is true in lung cancer, with increasing evidence that newer surgical treatments, such as sublobar resections or lung volume reduction surgeries, or ablative treatments, such as stereotactic body radiotherapy (SBRT), that offer good long-term results in older patients, advanced patients, COPD, and/or emphysema. In any case, adequate patient selection is essential to reduce potential harm from screening to a minimum. Implementing a multidisciplinary approach and monitoring results as recommended will help overcome this potential problem.[29]

Patients with COPD and/or emphysema enrolled in screening programs could also benefit from smoking cessation treatments. In the DLCST, the authors found an overall increase in smoking cessation rate during the screening program, where greater motivation to quit at baseline predicted smoking abstinence in the final round of screening.[30] Positive CT results are especially associated with increased abstinence.[31] Achieving smoking abstinence in patients with COPD is especially useful as it is the most effective intervention to halt disease progression, as well as increasing survival and reducing morbidity, including the risk of lung cancer. If spirometry, a simple, inexpensive, and validated diagnostic test, were added to screening programs, smokers could also benefit from early diagnosis of COPD, an overwhelmingly underdiagnosed disease. Currently, screening for COPD is not recommended as there is no known benefit in treating asymptomatic patients. However, we can now have a major impact on mortality rates in COPD patients by detecting lung cancer, a leading cause of death in this population, in early and curable stages.

THE ROLE OF COPD IN THE TREATMENT OF LUNG CANCER

Surgery in limited stages

Prehabilitation

The concept of prehabilitation has been used for some years and reinforced with the implementation of ERAS-type protocols. This concept becomes extremely important in individuals with COPD, and should be started in the home environment, when smoking should be stopped at least four weeks before surgery. Prehabilitation should be considered for patients with borderline lung function or exercise capacity and other general measures.[32]

Preoperative pulmonary rehabilitation significantly improves the clinical status of COPD patients before lung resection. Improved lung function leads to increased exercise tolerance during rehabilitation, and the initial benefit tends to be more pronounced in patients with the worst pulmonary function and the weakest functional capacity.[33]

Sometimes, simple prehabilitation methods can improve clinical function in patients with mild to moderate COPD undergoing lobectomy, reducing postoperative pulmonary complications.[34]

In a recent prospective observational study, the authors found difficulties in completing a preoperative rehabilitation program due to the fact that the patient had multiple comorbidities, lived alone, and took a long time to start the program.[35]

There has been a strong trend in the literature to use preoperative rehabilitation (prehabilitation) in this patient population, as was amply demonstrated in the NETT study, and which has become a standard of action over the years.

When and how to resect a lung cancer?

We know that lung resection is the best therapeutic alternative for stage I and II lung cancer, which is being increasingly diagnosed due to screening programs and an active search for lung nodules. We have also had important changes in the understanding of what type of resection we can offer to patients with early disease with the publication of two randomized studies that concluded that sublobar resections, whether wedge resection or anatomical segmentectomy, are appropriate, which encourages us to think about these resections in patients with COPD. These studies had as a secondary outcome the evaluation of possible gains in lung function when performing sublobar resections in relation to lobectomy, which was not proven in either of the two studies.[36, 37, 38]

We must clinically evaluate risk factors for lung resection adequately and rigorously using stress tests, pulmonary function tests, and preoperative evaluation. Risk factors in their different degrees, from minor to major, must be taken into consideration.

Regarding surgical aspects, there is controversy over whether to perform an anatomical segmentectomy or just a wedge resection in cases of initial disease in high-risk patients, which can be defined, as in the ACOSOGZ4032 study, as those with FEV1 or DLCO≤50% (predicted) as major criteria. An ongoing study using these criteria is underway to define whether segmentectomy is superior to wedge resection in this population (JCOG1909), with regard to overall survival (primary endpoint), adverse events, postoperative respiratory function, relapse-free survival, proportion of local recurrence, operative time, and blood loss (secondary endpoints).[39, 40]

Another way of defining high-risk patients was proposed by Brunelli et al. In patients with lung cancer who were candidates for surgery, those considered at high risk were those according to a proposed functional algorithm, that is, PPO FEV1 or PPO D LCO <60% and VO2 max <10 mL/kg/min. The recommendation was that this group underwent pre- or postoperative pulmonary rehabilitation.[41]

It is well known that patients with heart disease and chronic lung diseases, both of which limit cardiopulmonary functional reserve, undergoing thoracic surgery are at increased risk, according to the patient's functional status and general health, with worsening of lung function, with increasing age, especially in those over 80 years old, and with the type of procedure, for example, a pneumonectomy.[42]

We can never fail to mention that the skill of the surgical and anesthetic team contributes to the good outcome of an operation, especially in this type of population.

The patient's clinical status is an important factor when deciding whether they are a candidate for lung resection. Therefore, the clinical factors that we must take into consideration start from the history of present illness to identify pulmonary risk factors. Some of the factors that should be evaluated are as follows: dyspnea at rest or on exertion, daily quantity and color of phlegm produced, frequent use of bronchodilators, a decline in exercise capacity, smoking history (active smoker or ex-smoker, duration of smoking), age (>80 years), poor nutritional status, obesity, continuous or periodic use of oxygen, ischemic heart disease, valve disease, cardiomyopathy, congestive heart failure, arrhythmias with dyspnea, and occupational history, such as exposure to asbestos, uranium, nickel, iron, coal, silica, and dust.

Since the rebirth of lung volume reduction surgery (LVRS) presented by Cooper in 1994,[43] interest in studying the risks involved in lung resections in patients with severe and very severe COPD has also increased. The NETT study was able to clearly stratify high-risk populations and even groups in which resection was prohibitive, such as in patients with emphysema who have a low FEV1 (20%) and either homogeneous emphysema or a very low carbon monoxide diffusing capacity (< 20%). These patients are at high risk for death after surgery and are unlikely to benefit from the surgery.[44]

The NETT trial was able to demonstrate that the survival benefit was limited to patients with predominantly upper lobe emphysema and a low baseline exercise capacity. However, functional benefits were noted in patients with predominantly upper lobe emphysema and a high baseline exercise capacity and in patients with non-upper lobe emphysema and a low baseline exercise capacity.[45] This leads us to understand that if lung cancer resection is possible in this population, in a target area for LVRS, this strategy may be beneficial from an oncological point of view.

Several intraoperative strategies can be used to perform a combined surgery (Table 11.2). The decision to perform a wedge resection or a lobectomy depends on the size and location of the tumor and the distribution and severity of the emphysema. A lobectomy is generally avoided in this population unless the tumor is within a lobe destroyed by emphysema. Otherwise, LVRS is chosen, encompassing the tumor with an adequate margin. If the tumor is in the middle lobe and the target areas for emphysema are in the upper lobes, it is possible to perform a middle lobectomy, associated with LVRS in the target areas. If the tumor is in a healthy area (other than the middle lobe), outside the target area, surgery will probably be contraindicated, or at most a wedge resection associated with LVRS will be performed. We must not forget that this approach must be accompanied by adequate exploration of the mediastinal lymph nodes.[46]

Postoperative period and complications

It has long been known that individuals with COPD who require any surgery have higher rates of postoperative complications. To this end, we seek not only to identify these patients, but also to offer minimally invasive approaches. There are a large series of studies comparing thoracotomy with video-assisted thoracoscopic surgery (VATS), but few specifically report on patients with COPD.

In a case-control study based on the STS General Thoracic Database, data from 12,970 patients who underwent anatomical lung resection (lobectomy or segmentectomy) by thoracotomy (n = 8,439) or VATS (n = 4,531) between 2000 and 2010 were analyzed. They found that thoracotomy was associated with a marked increase in pulmonary complications in patients with impaired lung function when compared with patients undergoing minimally invasive surgery.[47]

TABLE 11.2   The intraoperative strategies for a concomitant cancer resection and lung volume reduction surgery

LUNG CANCER LOCATION	TARGET AREA (EMPHYSEMA)	PROCEDURE OF CHOICE
Upper lobe	Severely destroyed upper lobe	Lobectomy
Upper lobe	Bilateral upper lobe with severely destroyed ipsolateral upper lobe	Lobectomy + contralateral LVRS
Upper lobe	Bilateral upper lobe	Bilateral LVRS
Upper lobe	Ipsolateral upper lobe	LVRS (large wedge resection)
Middle lobe	Ipso or contralateral upper lobe	Middle lobectomy + LVRS
Lower lobe	Ipso or contralateral upper lobe	Wedge resection + LVRS

Based on Choong et al.[46]

It is also a fact that better-preserved pulmonary function in the immediate postoperative period is strongly associated with lower pulmonary morbidity after lobectomy. Furthermore, VATS lobectomy allows for improved deep breathing, early expectoration, and postoperative ambulation, which contribute to reducing the risk of pulmonary morbidity.[48]

Meta-analyses demonstrated a significantly lower risk of pulmonary complications in patients undergoing VATS lobectomy compared with those undergoing open lobectomy (RR = 0.45; 95% CI, 0.30–0.67; p = 0.0001), as well as a tendency to reduce the risk of operative mortality in patients undergoing VATS lobectomy (RR = 0.51; 95% CI 0.24–1.06; p = 0.07).[49]

Optimizing patients for thoracic surgery can be challenging, especially for those with COPD. As surgical techniques evolve, as well as anesthetic and pre- and postoperative care, research will be needed to ensure that perioperative care continues to advance.

TREATMENT IN LOCALLY ADVANCED AND METASTATIC DISEASE

It is well known that COPD is a factor in worsening overall survival in patients with advanced lung cancer, just as COPD and smoking can negatively affect the efficacy and tolerability of systemic treatment in these patients.[50] COPD can also cause a decrease in lung capacity and carbon monoxide diffusion in patients with lung cancer treated with chemotherapy, surgery, or radiotherapy. It may even reduce the likelihood of patients receiving chemotherapy or radiation therapy in patients with severe and very severe COPD, as well as increase the risk of pneumonia and chemotherapy-induced febrile neutropenia.[51] COPD can influence the response to targeted therapy and immune checkpoint inhibitors in patients with lung cancer, being an important factor to be considered in decision-making.

COPD can modify the immune system and increase the number of CD8+ and CD4+ lymphocytes in the lung and tumor microenvironment, which may favor a response to immunotherapy with immune checkpoint inhibitors (ICIs). Furthermore, patients with COPD who received pembrolizumab had better overall and progression-free survival than patients without COPD. Smoking cessation is important to improve the quality of life and survival of patients with COPD and lung cancer, regardless of the stage of the disease.[52]

REFERENCES

1. https://gco.iarc.fr/today/online-analysis-multi-bars?v=2020&mode=cancer&mode_population=countries &population=900&populations=900&key=asr&sex=0&cancer=39&type=0&statistic=5&prevalence=0 &population_group=0&ages_group%5B%5D=0&ages_group%5B%5D=17&nb_items=5&group_cancer =1&include_nmsc=0&include_nmsc_other=1&type_multiple=%257B%2522inc%2522%253Atrue%252C %2522mort%2522%253Atrue%252C%2522prev%2522%253Afalse%257D&orientation=horizontal&type _sort=0&type_nb_items=%257B%2522top%2522%253Atrue%252C%2522bottom%2522%253Afalse%257D
2. COPD 2023 Gold Report. (2024). https://goldcopd.org/wp-content/uploads/2023/11/GOLD-2024_v1.0 -30Oct23_WMV.pdf.
3. Skillrud DM, et al. *Ann Intern Med.* (1986). doi: 10.7326/0003-4819-105-4-503
4. Carr LL, et al. *Chest.* (2018). doi: 10.1016/j.chest.2018.01.049
5. De Torres JP, et al. *Am J Respir Crit Care Med.* (2011). doi: 10.1164/rccm.201103-0430OC7
6. Gonzalez J, et al. *Ann Transl Med.* (2016). doi: 10.21037/atm.2016.03.57
7. Wilson DO, et al. *Am J Respir Crit Care Med.* (2008). doi: 10.1164/rccm.200803-435OC
8. Zulueta JJ, et al. *Chest.* (2012). doi: 10.1378/chest.11-0101

9. Bishawi M, et al. *J Surg Res.* (2013). doi: 10.1016/j.jss.2013.05.081
10. Gross ND, et al. *N Engl J Med.* (2022). doi: 10.1056/NEJMoa2209831
11. Forde PM, et al. *N Engl J Med.* (2022). doi: 10.1056/nejmoa2202170
12. Howlader N, et al. *N Engl J Med.* (2020). doi: 10.1056/nejmoa1916623
13. Potter AL, et al. *BMJ.* (2022). doi: 10.1136/bmj-2021-069008
14. Perrotta F, et al. *Minerva Medica.* (2022). doi: 10.23736/S0026-4806.22.07962-9
15. Aberle DR, et al. *N Engl J Med.* (2011). doi: 10.1056/NEJMoa1102873
16. de Koning HJ, et al. *N Engl J Med.* (2020). doi: 10.1056/NEJMoa1911793
17. Krist AH, et al. *JAMA.* (2021). doi: 10.1001/jama.2021.1117
18. https://view-health-screening-recommendations.service.gov.uk/document/625/download.
19. Vogel-Claussen J, et al. *Fortschr Röntgenstr.* (2023). doi: 10.1055/a-2178-2846
20. Chinese Expert Group on Early Diagnosis and Treatment of Lung Cancer and China Lung Oncology Group *Zhongguo Fei Ai Za Zhi.* (2023). doi: 10.3779/j.issn.1009-3419.2023.102.10
21. Boyeras I, et al. *BMJ Open.* (2022). doi: 10.1136/bmjopen-2022-068271
22. Bradley C, et al. *ERJ Open Res.* (2023). doi: 10.1183/23120541.00203-2023
23. De-Torres JP, et al. *Respir Med.* (2013). doi: 10.1016/j.rmed.2013.01.013
24. Hopkins RJ, et al. *Ann Am Thorac Soc.* (2017). doi: 10.1513/AnnalsATS.201609-741OC
25. Young RP, et al. *Thorax.* (2023). doi: 10.1136/thorax-2022-219334
26. Nielsen C, Lang RS. *Med Clin North Am.* (1999). doi: 10.1016/s0025-7125(05)70169-3
27. De-Torres JP, et al. *Am J Respir Crit Care Med.* (2015). doi: 10.1164/rccm.201407-1210OC
28. Törnberg SA. *Acta Oncol.* (1999). doi: 10.1080/028418699431834
29. Choong CK, et al. *J Thorac Cardiovasc Surg.* (2004). doi: 10.1016/j.jtcvs.2003.11.046
30. Ashraf H, et al. *Thorax.* (2014). doi: 10.1136/thoraxjnl-2013-203849
31. Slatore CG, et al. *Ann Am Thorac Soc.* (2014). doi: 10.1513/AnnalsATS.201312-460OC
32. Batchelor TJ, et al. *Eur J Cardiothorac Surg.* (2019). doi: 10.1093/ejcts/ezy301
33. Mujovic N, et al. *Arch Med Sci.* (2014). doi: 10.5114/aoms.2013.32806
34. Rispoli M, et al. *Tumori.* (2020). doi: 10.1177/0300891619900808
35. Catho E, et al. *BMJ Open.* (2021). doi: 10.1136/ bmjopen-2020-041907
36. Saji H, et al. *Lancet.* (2022). doi: 10.1016/S0140-6736(21)02333-3
37. Altorki N, et al. *N Eng J Med.* (2023). doi: 10.1056/NEJMoa2212083
38. Altorki N, et al. *J Thorac Cardiovasc Surg.* (2024). doi: 10.1016/j.jtcvs.2023.07.008
39. Fernando HC, et al. *J Clin Oncol.* (2014). doi: 10.1200/JCO.2013.53.4115
40. Shimoyama R, et al. *Jpn J Clin Oncol.* (2020). doi: 10.1093/jjco/hyaa107
41. Brunelli A, et al. *Chest.* (2013). doi: 10.1378/chest.12-2395
42. Shamji FM, et al. *Thorac Surg Clin.* (2021). doi: 10.1016/j.thorsurg.2021.07.004
43. Cooper JD, et al. *J Thorac Cardiovasc Surg.* (1995). doi: 10.1016/S0022-5223(95)70426-4
44. National Emphysema Treatment Trial Research Group. *N Engl J Med.* (2001). doi: 10.1056/NEJMoa011798
45. Fishman A, et al. *N Engl J Med.* (2003). doi: 10.1056/NEJMoa030287
46. Choong CK, et al. *Thorac Surg Clin.* (2009). doi: 10.1016/j.thorsurg.2009.04.004
47. Ceppa DP, et al. *Ann Surg.* (2012). doi: 10.1097/SLA.0b013e318265819c
48. Wang W, et al. *J Thorac Dis.* (2013). doi: 10.3978/j.issn.2072-1439.2013.08.23
49. Zhang R, Ferguson MK. *PLoS One.* (2015). doi: 10.1371/journal.pone.0124512
50. Lin H, et al. *Medicine* (Baltimore). (2019). doi: 10.1097/MD.0000000000014837
51. Dong W, Du Y, Ma S. *Int J Chron Obstruct Pulmon Dis.* (2018). doi: 10.2147/COPD.S182173
52. Lin H, et al. *Medicine* (Baltimore). (2019). doi: 10.1097/MD.0000000000014837

Bronchoscopic Lung Volume Reduction Innovations

12

Justin L. Garner and Pallav L. Shah

INTRODUCTION

The objective of lung volume reduction (LVR) is a reversal of the malign influence of pathological hyper-inflation (1) and restoring normal ventilatory mechanics and function (2, 3). Bronchoscopic lung volume reduction (BLVR) evolved from the established field of surgery (4) to offer a less invasive, less hazardous, and less costly approach. An estimated 1–2% of COPD sufferers (650,000 to 1,300,000 globally) are thought likely to benefit from LVR procedures (5). Five innovative endobronchial techniques have been developed: unidirectional valves, coils, airway bypass, thermal vapour ablation, and sealants. This chapter will review the evidence supporting these novel technologies, focusing on reports of randomised controlled trials (RCTs).

UNIDIRECTIONAL VALVES

One-way valves are implanted in the bronchi of selected lobes, those most severely diseased, collapsing them to achieve 'medical lobectomy', improving ventilatory mechanics and removing the impediment to potential functioning of healthier parts of the lungs. Their efficacy is critically dependent on the absence of inter-lobar collateral ventilation (CV). Intended as permanent implants, they can be revised or removed if necessary.

There are four marketed devices: the Zephyr® Endobronchial Valve (EBV) by Pulmonx, the Spiration® Valve System (SVS, formerly known as the Intrabronchial Valve, or IBV) by Olympus, the MedLung® Endobronchial Valve (EbV), and the Endobronchial Miyazawa Valve (EMV). The EBV and SVS have been the main subjects of research, and these will be discussed.

Zephyr® Endobronchial Valve

EBVs are inserted under sedation or general anaesthesia. After real-time endobronchial sizing of the air way, the selected valve is loaded into the proprietary catheter and deployed via a flexible bronchoscope. The self-customising nitinol frame adapts to secure it in its airway. The silicone skin duckbill mechanism occludes the airway during inspiration and opens in expiration to induce lobar atelectasis. Three to five are inserted per lobe (Figure 12.1).

Toma et al. performed the first in-human study in 2003 (6), and since then, the device has been evaluated in six RCTs and received regulatory approvals by the National Institute for Health and Care Excellence (NICE) 2017 and by the Food and Drug Administration (FDA) 2018 as a guideline therapy for selected individuals with severe emphysema and hyperinflation. The incremental cost-effectiveness ratio (ICER) is estimated at €39,000 (£33,425) per quality-adjusted life-year (QALY) at five years and €23,000 per QALY (£18,427) at ten years (7).

Clinical outcomes

Endobronchial Valve for Emphysema Palliation Trial (VENT), 2010, was a multi-centre RCT comparing unilateral lobar EBV treatment (220) to SoC (101) in patients with severe heterogeneous emphysema (defined using quantitative computed tomography [qCT] analysis converted to a Likert scale) and hyperinflation (8). At six months, EBV recipients experienced modest improvements in forced expiratory volume in one second (FEV1) +6.8% (95% CI, 2.1 to 11.5; p=0.005) and six-minute walk distance (6MWD) +5.8% (95% CI, 0.5 to 11.2; p=0.04) equivalent to a median +19.1 metres (95% CI, 1.3 to 36.8 p=0.02) – the co-primary efficacy endpoints – and St George's Respiratory Questionnaire (SGRQ) total score −3.4 points (95% CI, −6.7 to 0.2; p=0.04), likely explained by the small reductions in residual volume (RV) of −1.29±19.83% achieved. Over the course of 12 months, 31 subjects (14.1%) underwent valve removals for adverse events including migration (eight) or at their request (seven). Serious adverse events from early (within 90 days) and late periods (3–12 months) included pneumonia distal to the valve (0.9% and 3.3%), pneumothorax (4.2% and 1.0%), haemoptysis (5.6% and 6.1%), and exacerbations of COPD

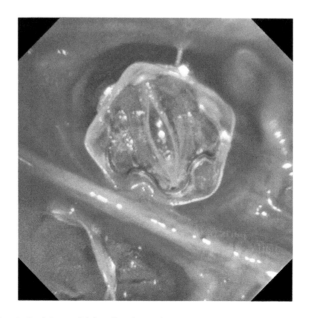

FIGURE 12.1   (A) Zephyr® Endobronchial Valve (EBV) by Pulmonx is available in four sizes: 4.0, 4.0 LP (low profile), 5.0, and 5.0 LP. The duckbill mechanism is closed during inspiration and open in expiration.

requiring hospitalisation (7.9%, EBV, vs. 1.1%, SoC; p=0.03 and 10.3%, EBV, vs. 9.2%, SoC; p=0.84). At 12 months, all cause death rate was 3.7%, EBV, and 3.5%, controls (log rank p=0.88) (Table 12.1).

The European arm of the trial lacked statistical power, but benefits were suggested in both heterogeneous and homogeneous disease (9). Post-hoc analyses identified individuals with CT evidence of fissure integrity (determined by visualisation as >90% complete), a surrogate for absent inter-lobar CV, and target lobar occlusion as predictors of therapeutic response (8, 9).

Bronchoscopic Lung Volume Reduction with Endobronchial Valves for Patients with Heterogeneous Emphysema and Intact Inter-Lobar Fissures (BeLieVeR-HIFi), 2015, was a single-centre, double-blind, sham-controlled study of 50 patients (1:1 assignment) with severe heterogeneous emphysema (assessed using the NETT study scoring system [4]), hyperinflation, and >90% visibly intact inter-lobar fissures (10). Subjects were also evaluated using the Chartis® System, a catheter-based tool detecting lobar expiratory airflow – however, no subject was denied treatment on the basis of a positive test for CV. The percentage change in FEV1 at three months increased by 24.77% (95% CI, 8.02 to 41.51) in EBV recipients compared with 3.87% (0.66–7.08) in controls. The EBV group also experienced statistically significant improvements in lung volumes, gas transfer, and 6MWD. Exclusion from the analysis of four patients who were CV positive on Chartis evaluation improved the responder rates to EBV treatment: FEV1 ≥15% – 47% (from 39%); RV ≥0.35 L reduction – 58% (48%), 6MWD ≥26 m – 63% (52%), SGRQ-C ≥4 points reduction – 58% (48%); CAT ≥2 points reduction – 68% (57%). At 90 days, COPD exacerbation was the most frequent adverse event but with no statistically significant difference between groups. Four recipients expectorated a valve (16%), two required valve removal (8%), two developed pneumonia (8%), two pneumothoraces (8%), and two died from respiratory complications (8%; respiratory failure and cor pulmonale).

Amalgamation of the data of individuals with intact inter-lobar fissures (Chartis negative), receiving EBVs in the first phase of an open-label cross-over RCT with those undergoing the procedure in the second phase (n=31), demonstrated consistently meaningful clinical outcomes at three months and confirmed the important role of intact fissures: FEV1 +27.3±36.4% (p<0.001), RV −0.49±0.76 litres (L; p=0.007), TLCO +3.62±5.16% (p<0.001), 6MWD +32.6±68.7 metres (m; p=0.01), CAT −4.1±8.5 points (p=0.03),

TABLE 12.1   Results of the randomised controlled trials

STUDY	DEVICE	PATIENTS TREATED, N	FOLLOW-UP, MONTHS	ΔFEV1, ML	ΔRV, ML	Δ6MWD, METRES	ΔSGRQ, POINTS
VENT	EBV	220	12	60*	–	19*	−3.4*
BELIEVER-HIFI	EBV	25	3	160	−370	33	−5.1†
STELVIO	EBV	34	6	191	−831	106	−14.7
TRANSFORM	EBV	65	6	230	−670	79	−6.5
LIBERATE	EBV	128	12	106	−522	39	−7.1
IMPACT	EBV	43	3	120	−480	40	−9.6
REACH	SVS	66	6	115	−370	36	−6.3
EMPROVE	SVS	113	12	0.099	−361*	6.9*	−9.5
RESET	LVRC	23	3	–	−310	64	−8.4
REVOLENS	LVRC	50	12	80	−360	21	−10.6
RENEW	LVRC	158	12	70	−310	14.6	−8.9
ELEVATE	LVRC	120	6	70	−460	–	−10.6
EASE	STENT	208	12	−10*	−61*	−7*	−2*
STEP-UP	BTVA	70	12	103	−237	3.6	−12.1
ASPIRE	AERISEAL	95	6	90	–	53	−9

Note: Δ, between-group difference (i.e., intervention minus control). †SGRQ-C questionnaire used. *Six-month data shown.

and SGRQ for COPD total score −8.5±20.2 points (p=0.05) (11). In this small cohort, the incidence of pneumothorax, considered a marker of an effective procedure, was 10.3% (including, however, one fatality), higher than in VENT (5%).

Endobronchial Valves for Emphysema without Inter-Lobar Collateral Ventilation (STELVIO), 2015, was a single-centre RCT of 68 patients (1:1 assignment) with severe emphysema (heterogeneous and homogeneous – assessed visually at baseline and after study completion using qCT at −950 Hounsfield units (HU) with a 15% threshold between target and ipsilateral lobes), hyperinflation, and no inter-lobar CV measured using the Chartis® System (12). At six months, improvements in FEV1, forced vital capacity (FVC), and 6MWD – the co-primary endpoints – were pronounced in the EBV group compared with controls: between-group differences in FEV1 +17.8% (95% CI, 7.6 to 28.0; p=0.001), FVC +14.4% (95% CI 4.4–24.3; p=0.005), and 6MWD +74 m (95% CI, 47 to 100; p<0.001). This was accompanied by clinically meaningful improvements in RV of −865 ml (95% CI, −1166 to −563), target lobe volume −1366 m (95% CI, −3604 to −28), and SGRQ −17.39 points (95% CI, −24.75 to −10.02) in treated patients. Those with heterogeneous emphysema benefitted the most. Repeat bronchoscopy was performed in 12 of 34 treated patients (35%): seven underwent permanent valve removal on account of unacceptable adverse events including torsion of the bronchus (two), recurrent pneumothorax (two), pneumonia distal to the valve (one), and worsening symptoms (two). Valve replacement for an implant-related event was permitted by the trial protocol and undertaken in four individuals (12%). Over six months, 22 respiratory-related serious adverse events (SAEs) were reported in the EBV group (three in SoC) including six pneumothoraces (18%), four COPD exacerbations (12%), three pneumonias (9%), and one death (3%).

A Multicentre Randomized Controlled Trial of Zephyr Endobronchial Valve Treatment in Heterogeneous Emphysema (TRANSFORM), 2017, was a study of 97 patients with severe heterogeneous emphysema (determined with qCT at −910 HU using a 10% difference between target and ipsilateral lobes), hyperinflation and inter-lobar CV excluded using the Chartis® System: EBV (65) and SoC (32) (13). At 45 days, EBV revision was undertaken if target lobe volume reduction (TLVR) <50% or incomplete lobar occlusion (*sic*) identified on CT; 55.4%, EBV, vs. 6.5%, SoC (p<0.001) achieved a ≥12% improvement in FEV1 at three months (intention-to-treat, ITT population) – the primary endpoint – durable to six months and accompanied by clinically meaningful benefits in RV of −0.67 L (95% CI, −1.09 to −0.25; p=0.002), 6MWD of +78.7 m (95% CI, 46.3 to 111.0; p<0.001), and SGRQ total score −6.5 points (95% CI, −12.4 to −0.6; p=0.031) favouring the EBV group. Repeat bronchoscopy was performed in 18 subjects: 17 underwent a revision and 12 achieved significant TLVR. Over six months, 44 respiratory-related SAEs occurred in 31 EBV recipients (47.7%) compared with four in three SoC subjects (9.4%) the majority within 30 days of the procedure including COPD exacerbation (48.8%, EBV, vs. 36.1%, SoC p=0.231), pneumothorax (30.3% EBV), dyspnoea (32.4% vs. 3.1%; p<0.001), and pneumonia (12.1% vs 3.1%; p=0.264). One patient was hospitalised for a pneumothorax and died from a cardiac arrest.

Pulmonx Endobronchial Valves Used in Treatment of Emphysema (LIBERATE), 2018, was a study of 190 patients with severe heterogeneous emphysema (defined on qCT at −910 HU as ≥15% difference in destruction scores between target and adjoining lobe), hyperinflation, and no inter-lobar CV on Chartis evaluation: EBV (128) and SoC (62) (14). To maximise treatment gains, post-procedure pulmonary rehabilitation was incorporated, and a revision procedure permitted at day 45 for TLVR <50% or incomplete lobar occlusion. At one year, 47.7%, EBV vs. 16.8%, SoC (ITT population) achieved the primary endpoint of a ≥15% improvement in FEV1 with a between-group difference of 31.0% (95% CI 18.0 to 43.9%; p<0.001). The proportion of responders for secondary outcomes favoured the EBV group RV ≥−310 ml (EBV, 61.6% vs. SoC, 22.4%), 6MWD ≥25 m (41.8% vs. 19.6%), and SGRQ total score ≥−4 points (56.2% vs. 30.2%). Improvements in multi-dimensional scores for breathlessness, activity, and psychosocial domains were also observed (15). These benefits could be correlated with the mean reduction in RV of 0.5 L, with 84.2% of EBV recipients achieving the minimal clinically important difference (MCID) in TLVR ≥350 ml at 12 months (14). Encouragingly, upper and lower lobe treatments afforded similar benefits. Two EBVs were expectorated and three migrated; 35 subjects underwent 54 additional procedures (including 11 adjustments, 28 removals and/or replacements following an adverse event, 12 clinical investigations, and three requested removals). During the treatment period (≤45 days), 35.2% of

EBV subjects compared with 4.8% of SoC experienced respiratory-related SAEs (p<0.001) – the majority pneumothoraces (26.6%, EBV) and COPD exacerbations (7.8% vs. 4.8%) – thereafter, the exacerbation rates were similar, 33.6% and 30.6%. Intriguingly, there was a small reduction in the rate of respiratory failure events and COPD exacerbations requiring hospitalisation in the longer term, although the study was not powered to confirm these changes. Five deaths occurred in the EBV group (three pneumothoraxes, one respiratory failure, one COPD exacerbation) and one death among the controls (cardiac arrhythmia).

The definitions of heterogeneous and homogeneous emphysema (and of lobar severity) have varied between studies, nevertheless VENT (European arm) and STELVIO suggested fewer pronounced benefits with the latter profile.

Endobronchial Valve Therapy in Patients with Homogeneous Emphysema (IMPACT), 2016, was a multi-centre RCT of 93 patients (EBV, 43 and SoC, 50) designed to address this problem (16). Homogeneous emphysema was defined as <15% difference at −910 HU between target and ipsilateral lobes and <20% difference in perfusion scintigraphy between right and left lungs. Inter-lobar CV was excluded with Chartis. The primary endpoint, change in FEV1 at three months, favoured treated patients (ITT population): +13.7±28.2%, EBV, and −3.2 ± 13.0%, SoC with a mean between-group difference of 17.0% (95% CI, 8.1 to 25.8%; p=0.0002). The EBV group also had a higher proportion of responders for secondary outcomes: RV ≥−430ml (EBV, 44.2% vs. 18.0%, SoC; p=0.006), 6MWD ≥26 m (50% vs. 14%; p=0.0002), and SGRQ ≥−4 points (56.8% vs. 25%; p=0.003), again reflecting the beneficial reduction in RV of 0.42±0.90 L. One valve was removed, and another was replaced, in a subject experiencing two migration events; 44.2%, EBV, vs. 12%, SoC, experienced respiratory-related SAEs, including pneumothorax (25.6%, EBV) and COPD exacerbation requiring hospitalisation (16.3% versus 12.0%); one death from nosocomial pneumonia occurred in the control group.

Combining the data from four RCTs (STELVIO, TRANSFORM, LIBERATE, IMPACT) for individuals who underwent Chartis evaluation (n=448), Hartman et al. estimated between-group differences in FEV1 of 17 to 29%, RV of −522 to −831ml, 6MWD of 39 to 79 m, and SGRQ of −6.5 to −14.7 points favouring the EBV over SoC at three to 12 months follow-up (17). However, revision bronchoscopy was required in 19–35% of patients and valve removal in 3–21%. Pneumothorax was the most common complication occurring in 18–34% of individuals and mainly within 72 hours of implantation, stressing the prudence of in-hospital monitoring during this peri-procedural period (18). Patients with a greater low attenuation volume percentage (LAV%) of the untreated ipsilateral lobe (i.e., more emphysematous) and a large residual volume are particularly vulnerable (19); however, the contribution of pleural adhesions is conflicting (19, 20). The mechanism is thought to be due to rapid conformational changes in lung architecture with redistribution of volume especially to the ipsilateral lobe inducing a tear or rupture of a bleb (21). Management with intercostal chest drainage is effective in the majority (21), and reassuringly, outcomes including survival out to five years are not adversely affected (22).

Longer-term data are accruing. In a case series of 256 patients, three-year responder rates for FEV1, RV, and 6MWD were highest in patients achieving complete lobar atelectasis: 10%, 79%, and 53%, respectively (23). Where bronchoscopic LVR is successful, significant survival benefits at five (22), six (24), and ten years (25) are observed.

Predictors of response

A crucial step in the assessment of an individual for EBV therapy is to quantify fissural integrity on high-resolution computed tomography (HRCT), a surrogate for absent CV (26). Koster et al. advised performing a Chartis test for individuals with a fissure completeness score (FCS) of 80–95%; those with >95% integrity could proceed directly to implantation while an FCS <80% should prompt consideration of alternative procedures including surgery or investigational treatments such as vapour or coils (27). Adoption of recommendations was predicted to reduce diagnostic bronchoscopies by 71% compared with a Chartis-only screening strategy and was embraced by best practice guidance published in 2019 (18). Subsequently in 2020, Klooster et al. proposed a modification to this algorithm – patients with incomplete oblique fissures (left FCS <80%, right <90%) could be excluded and a combined approach with Chartis suggested a right oblique FCS ≥90% (irrespective of horizontal fissure integrity) and a left oblique FCS 80% to 95% (28).

A recent update to the Chartis system software includes determination of a fraction of the expired gases, the volume during the last 20 seconds: VT20 ≤6 ml measured in an intubated and ventilated patient has been shown to reliably exclude CV and is particularly helpful in low flow states (29).

Finally, target lobar occlusion (9, 30) and complete atelectasis (23, 24) are predictors of therapeutic response, as is the occurrence of a pneumothorax (31).

Mechanism of action

The EBV works principally by inducing lung volume reduction (3). A beneficial impact on small airways function has also been described (32).

Emerging evidence

Chartis evaluation under general anaesthesia appears superior compared with sedation (33). Preliminary data suggest a potential role for EBVs in individuals with moderate hyperinflation (34), low gas transfer (35, 36), pulmonary hypertension (37), and alpha-1-antitrypsin deficiency (38, 39). Strategies are also emerging to mitigate post-procedural complications including, for example, COPD exacerbation by the prophylactic administration of antibiotics (40). In addition, the impact and optimal timing of pulmonary rehabilitation on EBV treatment are under evaluation (SOLVE – NCT03474471). Larger controlled trials are welcomed to support these findings and explore the impact and cost-effectiveness of EBVs on exacerbations, hospitalisations, and survival.

The problem with dependence of EBVs on fissure integrity is being addressed. Van der Molen et al have submitted convincing evidence for a genetic determination of CV (41). Studies are currently underway evaluating EBVs in patients whose CV channels are occluded with sealants – biological and synthetic (NCT04256408, NCT04559464). Meanwhile, a head-to-head trial of LVRS versus EBV implantation is in progress (CELEB - ISRCTN19684749).

The EBV has been shown to be a minimally invasive, safe, clinically efficacious, and cost-effective device that can be easily removed or replaced, and which may be combined with other interventional therapies.

Spiration® Valve System

The SVS adopts a flexible umbrella design to govern unidirectional airflow (Figure 12.2). Following pilot investigations, there have been four RCTs evaluating this device, which received US regulatory approval in 2018.

Clinical outcomes

To reduce the risk of pneumothorax, bilateral partial upper lobar occlusions were investigated in early RCTs. While well tolerated, outcomes were not clinically meaningful (42, 43). Subsequent studies have focused on achieving complete unilateral occlusion of a target lobe (44).

A Randomized Controlled Trial Assessing the Safety and Effectiveness of the Spiration® Valve System in the Treatment of Severe Emphysema (REACH), 2018, was a multi-centre study of 99 patients performed in China with severe heterogeneous emphysema (≥15% difference between target and ipsilateral lobes was visually assessed; discordance between reviewers was arbitrated using qCT at −920 HU), radiologically intact inter-lobar fissures (≥90%), and hyperinflation comparing the SVS (n=66) with SoC (n=33) (45). At three months, the treatment and control arms had mean FEV1 improvements, respectively, 0.104±0.178 and 0.003±0.147 L (p=0.001) – meeting the primary effectiveness endpoint – and durable to six months: FEV1 responder rate ≥15%, 41% versus 21%. At six months, the treatment group achieved

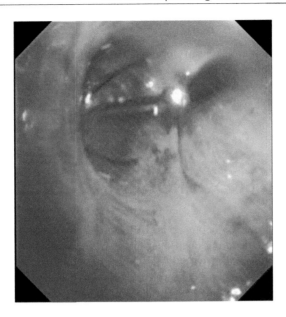

FIGURE 12.2   The Spiration® Valve System (SVS, formerly the Intrabronchial Valve, IBV) by Olympus is available in four sizes ranging from 5 mm to 9 mm.

mean TLVR of 757 ml (66.1% of recipients), reduction in RV of −0.42 L, and complete target lobar atelectasis in 28.8% (17 of 59 subjects) accompanied by relative improvements in 6MWT (15.5%) and SGRQ (−10.5 points); 14 additional bronchoscopy procedures in 12 treated patients (18.2%) were required for revision/replacement of valves. SAEs occurred in 33% of treated and 24.2% of control patients: the majority acute exacerbations of COPD (19.7%, SVS, versus 12.1%, SoC). Pneumothorax developed in only 7.6% of valve recipients. One death occurred in the control group.

Improving Lung Function in Severe Heterogenous Emphysema with the Spiration Valve System (EMPROVE), 2019, was a multi-centre RCT of 172 patients with severe heterogeneous emphysema (≥10% difference between target and ipsilateral lobes), radiologically intact inter-lobar fissures (≥90%), and hyperinflation comparing the SVS (n=113) with SoC (n=59) performed in the United States (46). At six months, between-group differences in mean FEV1 change of 0.101 L (95% Bayesian credible intervals, BCI: 0.060 to 0.141) – the primary efficacy endpoint – SGRQ −13.0 (95% BCI −17.4 to −8.5) and mMRC −0.6 (−0.9 to −0.3) favoured the treatment arm: responder rates for FEV1 ≥15% of 36.8% (10%, SoC), 6MWT ≥25 m of 32.4% (22.9%, SoC), and SGRQ ≥4 points of 54.3% (18%, SoC). SVS recipients attained a mean TLVR of 974 ml (MCID of −350 ml achieved in 75%) and a reduction in RV of 402 ml; complete target lobar atelectasis was achieved in 40%. Benefits in FEV1 and quality of life were durable to 12 months (physiological and radiological lung volume assessments were not undertaken at this time point). In contrast to the LIBERATE study, the impact on 6MWD (performed at the six-month visit only) was not statistically significant, and the authors attributed this to the lack of a post-treatment supervised pulmonary rehabilitation programme to capitalise on treatment gains. The primary safety endpoint, incidence of a pre-specified composite of thoracic SAEs over six months, was 31.0% in the treatment arm and 11.9%, SoC, the difference ascribable to a 12.4% rate of serious pneumothorax. In the longer term, there were no statistically significant differences between groups in the rates of thoracic and non-thoracic SAEs. Ten deaths (8.8%) of treated subjects and four (6.8%) controls were reported.

There are limited data on longer-term outcomes, predictors of response, and mechanism(s) of action.

Emerging evidence

A trial examining the efficacy of autologous blood instillation to seal an incomplete fissure in combination with SVS implantation is ongoing (NCT03010449).

Future directions and questions

Areas of enquiry include the optimal cut-off for target lobar emphysema destruction and determining the benefit of treating hyperinflation alone.

The hybridisation of treatments to target more than one phenotype of the disease is a realistic prospect, for example, combining valve implantation with modalities such as endobronchial coils (47–50) thermal vapour ablation (51, 52), targeted lung denervation (53–56), and radial metered cryospray (57).

ENDOBRONCHIAL COILS

Introduced in 2008, lung volume reduction coils (LVRCs) offer a therapeutic option for individuals with severe emphysema, hyperinflation, and inter-lobar CV (58, 59). Made from shape-memory nitinol, they are inserted into the subsegmental airways of the lung in a straight wire configuration. Upon release from the delivery catheter, they assume the form of a two-turn coil and gather the surrounding tissues. Approximately 12 coils are implanted in an upper lobe and 14 in a lower lobe to create a fan-shaped distribution within the middle third of the lung (60). Sequential bilateral (and typically symmetrical) treatments are undertaken four to eight weeks apart to reduce the risk of bilateral pneumothoraces (Figure 12.3). The proposed mechanisms of action include lung volume reduction (principally), increased elastic recoil, and re-tensioning of the airway network to improve gas emptying (61).

Clinical outcomes

Endobronchial Coils for the Treatment of Severe Emphysema with Hyperinflation: A Randomised Controlled Trial (RESET), 2013, was a multi-centre study of 47 patients with severe emphysema (heterogeneous and homogeneous characterised using qCT at −950 HU) and hyperinflation comparing LVRC (n=23) with SoC (n=24) (47). Sequential hemithorax treatments (including up to several lobes per lung) were separated by approximately one month to minimise the risk of bilateral pneumothoraces. At three months, the between-group difference in SGRQ change – the primary endpoint – was −8.36 (95% CI

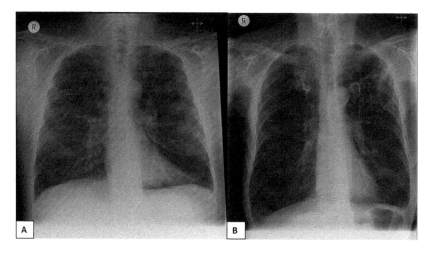

FIGURE 12.3   Lung volume reduction coil (LVRC) by PneumRx, BTG, is available in three sizes: 100 mm, 125 mm, and 150 mm (depicted). (A) Chest x-ray imaging depicts bilateral sequential coil implantation to the upper lobes. (B) Example of coil-associated opacity.

−16.24 to −0.47; p=0.04) favouring the coil arm. LVRC recipients also experienced clinically meaningful improvements in RV −0.51 (−0.20, SoC; p=0.03) and FEV1 +14.19% (+3.57%; p=0.03). During the first 30 days, six SAEs were reported in the LVRC group (two each of pneumothorax, COPD exacerbation, and lower respiratory tract infection) and one in SoC (COPD exacerbation) – the majority were self-limiting and resolved within seven days. From 30 to 90 days follow-up, three SAEs were experienced by each arm (exacerbations and chest infections). Similar benefits were observed in subjects who went on to receive open-label treatment and importantly, outcomes were durable to at least 12 months (48).

Lung Volume Reduction Coil Treatment versus Usual Care in Patients with Severe Emphysema (REVOLENS), 2016, was a multi-centre RCT of 100 patients with severe bilateral emphysema (heterogeneous and homogeneous graded using the NETT visual assessment score [62]) and hyperinflation: LVRC (n=50) and SoC (n=50) (63). LVRCs were implanted in only one lobe per lung in sequential hemithorax treatments separated by an interval of one to three months. The primary outcome was the responder rate for 6MWD of ≥54 m at six months achieved by 18 LVRC recipients (36%) and nine SoC subjects (18%; p=0.03). Improvements in FEV1 (+90 ml), RV (−370 ml), and SGRQ (−13.4 total points) favoured the coil arm and were durable to 12 months; 6MWD was modestly increased with a between-group difference of 21 m at both time points.

It is noteworthy the trial included individuals with greater disability (for example, 6MWD <140 m, DLCO <20%, α-1-antitrypsin deficiency) and set an almost two-fold higher MCID for the primary endpoint – furthermore, 6MWD was evaluated using one test with no supplemental oxygen contrary to ATS guidance, which may have impacted outcomes. Post-hoc analysis showed no difference in LVRC efficacy between emphysema profiles. Mild haemoptysis was the most common non-serious AE within 30 days (47%) and COPD exacerbation >30 days to 12 months (62%). Respiratory SAEs including COPD exacerbation (26%, LVRC, versus 22%, SoC; p=0.64), pneumonia (18%, LVRC, versus 4%, SoC; p=0.03), and pneumothorax (6%, LVRC, versus 2%, SoC; p=0.62) were reported during a 12-month follow-up. Four deaths occurred in the LVRC group (peritonitis, mesenteric ischaemia, COPD exacerbation; one cause was indeterminate) and three in SoC (p=0.99). Two-year follow-up showed LVRC therapy is associated with sustained volume reduction (albeit less pronounced), improved quality of life, and an acceptable safety profile (64) with a two-year incremental cost-effectiveness ratio (ICER) of €75,978/QALY (65).

Effect of Endobronchial Coils versus Usual Care on Exercise Tolerance in Patients with Severe Emphysema (RENEW), 2016, was a multi-centre assessor-blinded RCT of 315 patients with severe emphysema (heterogeneous, 23%, and homogeneous, 77%, using a semiquantitative visual assessment) and hyperinflation comparing bilateral sequential lobar coil implantation (n=158) with SoC (n=157) (50). The primary effectiveness endpoint, change in 6MWD at 12 months, was modest at 10.3 m for coil recipients, accompanied by improvements in RV (−410 ml), FEV1 (+3.8%), and SGRQ (−8.1 points) for coil recipients. Of note, the RV threshold was lowered from 225% to 175% following recruitment of 169 patients to include a broader population and, together with a predominant homogeneous emphysema profile of the cohort, may have impacted efficacy outcomes. The primary safety analysis was a comparison of the proportions of participants experiencing at least one of seven pre-specified major complications (death, pneumothorax requiring chest tube drainage >7 days, haemoptysis necessitating intervention beyond conventional bronchoscopy measures, hospitalisation for COPD exacerbation >7 days, lower respiratory tract infections [LRTIs] requiring intravenous antibiotics and/or corticosteroids, ventilatory support for respiratory failure, and secondary bronchoscopy to remove one or more coils for a device-related adverse event) – 34.8% of coil recipients compared with 19.1% SoC experienced SAEs (p=0.002). This was mainly attributable to an increased frequency of LRTIs (18.7%, LVRC, versus 4.5%, SoC; p<0.001), and in the coil arm, two cases of haemoptysis requiring intervention and two procedure-associated deaths (one pulmonary haemorrhage and one respiratory failure). A higher incidence of SAEs including pneumonia (LVRC, 20% and SoC, 4.5%; p<0.001), pneumothorax (9.7% versus 0.6%; p<0.001), and COPD exacerbation (27.7% versus 20.4%; p=0.15) was experienced by coil recipients.

Baseline predictors of response included a RV ≥200% predicted, heterogeneous emphysema, fewer comorbidities, and the development of a coil-associated opacity (CAO), thought to reflect a localised inflammatory response/structural parenchymal change. A recent post-hoc analysis identified additional predictors including an emphysema score of >20% low attenuation area (LAA) of treated lobes and absent airway disease (66).

Endobronchial Coil System vs. Standard-of-Care Medical Management in the Treatment of Subjects with Severe Emphysema (ELEVATE), 2021, was a prospective, multi-centre, open-label RCT (2:1) comparing LVRC (n=80) with SoC (40) – the projected enrolment of 210 individuals was stymied by premature study termination following the acquisition of PneumRx BTG by Boston Scientific for financial reasons. Cohort selection was refined using the aforementioned baseline predictors of response (50, 66); 120 patients were randomised (FEV1 29±7%, RV 251±41%, RV/TLC 67±6%, SGRQ 58±13 points) and 91 (57 LVRC and 34 SoC) had evaluable data at six months. The co-primary endpoints were the between-group differences in FEV1% and SGRQ total score at six months: +10.3% (+4.7 to +16.0 p=0.001) and −10.6 points (−15.9 to −5.4; p<0.001)), respectively, and accompanied by RV −460 ml (−716 to −203; p=0.001) favouring the LVRC. SAEs were reported in 30 coil recipients (most frequently: pneumonia 11%, COPD exacerbation 4.1%, pneumothorax 4.1%) and three SoC (all exacerbations). Five deaths occurred in the coil group (6.8%) – comparable to previously reported treatment arms (50, 63) – and none in the controls.

The potential for adverse influences of the different enrolment criteria, outcome thresholds, and coil sizes used in the above RCTs should be noted.

Identifying Responders and Exploring Mechanisms of Action of the Endobronchial Coil Treatment for Emphysema (REACTION), 2021, was a prospective non-randomised single-centre study of 24 patients with severe emphysema and hyperinflation undergoing bilateral sequential coil implantations (67). The principal mechanism of action of the LVRC was reduction of static hyperinflation accompanied by improved airways resistance. Efficacy was predicted by a higher RV, emphysema score of the treated lobes, and a lower physical activity level at baseline.

Longer-term data are limited. Patients enrolled in the first RCT, RESET, who achieved ≥10% reduction in RV at three months after completion of treatment (n=18) had a five-year transplant-free survival of 66.7% compared with 36.4% for non-responders (n=22; p=0.07) (49).

Similar lung tensioning strategies are currently under evaluation ([68] and NCT04520152).

AIRWAY BYPASS

Airway bypass creates transbronchial fenestrations at the segmental level, supported by self-expanding stents, to improve expiratory flow and reduce hyperinflation (69–74) and is intended as a minimally invasive treatment for patients with severe homogeneous emphysema. Up to six Exhale drug-eluting stents (DES; 1–2 per treated lobe) are placed using a proprietary catheter-based tunnelling system under general anaesthesia (Figure 12.4).

CLINICAL OUTCOMES

Bronchoscopic Lung-Volume Reduction with Exhale Airway Stents for Emphysema (EASE), 2011, was a prospective, multi-centre, randomised, double-blind, sham-controlled study of 315 patients with severe homogeneous emphysema (assessed using a semiquantitative approach): airway bypass, 208, versus sham control, 107 (75, 76). The co-primary efficacy endpoints were improvements of ≥12% in FVC and ≥1 point in mMRC at six months. Immediate (first day) benefits, improvements in FVC, FEV1, and RV, in the treated group, did not endure the first month. mMRC scores were lowered in both groups, out to 12 months, but at no time were clinically meaningful (SGRQ total score in bypass recipients at one month was however significantly improved). Bayesian analysis failed to show superiority of airway bypass with a posterior probability 0.749 (below the threshold of 0.965).

At six months, SAEs including major haemoptysis (≥200 ml, requiring transfusion or intervention); respiratory failure requiring ventilation >24 hours; pulmonary infection or exacerbation of COPD necessitating admission for >7 days; pneumothorax >7 days requiring drainage; or death

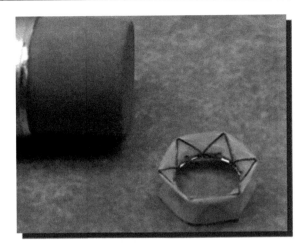

FIGURE 12.4 Exhale airway stent (Broncus Technologies, Mountain View, CA, USA).

– the composite primary safety endpoint – occurred in 14.4%, airway bypass, versus 11.2%, sham control, the procedure was judged non-inferior with a posterior probability of 1.00 (success threshold >0.95). Most events were COPD exacerbations or pulmonary infections; 12-month mortality was 6.7% in treated and 6.5% in control. The early loss of benefit has been attributed to a combination of factors: unsupported passages, expectorated stents, and importantly, loss of stent patency (despite paclitaxel elution). This RCT serves as proof of concept for the development of the device: Problems with anchorage and patency are to be addressed.

THERMAL VAPOUR ABLATION

Bronchoscopic thermal vapour ablation (BTVA; Uptake Medical Corporation, Tustin, CA, USA) delivers three to ten second bursts of steam to individual upper lobe segments (targeting the most diseased) in a two-staged procedure, inducing a local inflammatory reaction and healing with fibrosis to bring about volume reduction (77). The segmental approach addresses the recognised intra-lobar heterogeneity of disease and aims to preserve relatively functioning lung. Best practice guidance advises performing this procedure in the context of clinical studies and registries (78). Collateral ventilation is not an issue for this technique. (Figure 12.5).

Clinical outcomes

Segmental Volume Reduction Using Thermal Vapour Ablation in Patients with Severe Emphysema (STEP-UP), 2016, was the first multi-centre RCT of 70 patients with upper lobe-predominant disease (>15% difference between target and ipsilateral lobes) and hyperinflation comparing BTVA (n=46) with SoC (n=24) (51). One upper lobe segment was initially treated and up to two segments of the contralateral upper lobe 13 weeks later: The treatment time was calculated to deliver a target dose of 8.5 calories per gram of lung tissue. The co-primary efficacy endpoints were the between-group differences in FEV1 and SGRQ-C score at six months: +14.7% (7.8 to 21.5%; p<0.0001) and −9.7 points (−15.7 to −3.7; p=0.0021),

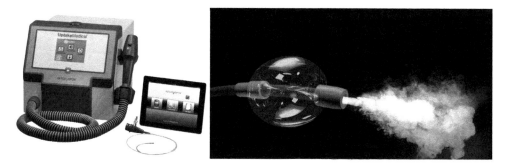

FIGURE 12.5 Bronchoscopic thermal vapour ablation (BTVA; Uptake Medical Corporation, Seattle, WA) system.

respectively, accompanied by improvement in RV (−302.5 ml; p=0.0145) favouring the BTVA group. qCT analysis revealed that targeted segments were reduced by 42% in volume with the re-expansion of adjacent healthier segments by 11%. SAEs included COPD exacerbation (24%, BTVA, vs. 4%, SoC), pneumonia/pneumonitis (18% vs. 8%), and one each (2%) of pneumothorax (no intervention), haemoptysis (requiring bronchoscopic tamponade), and death in the treated arm (the latter secondary to a COPD exacerbation judged possibly related to BTVA). Benefits were durable to 12 months (6MWD, however, was not significantly improved), and 17 of 24 (71%) respiratory-related SAEs occurred within the first 90 days (majority resolved using standard medical care), with equivalence between groups thereafter (52). A staged and limited therapeutic strategy might explain the comparatively low rate of pneumothorax and affords the opportunity for subsequent segmental treatment as the underlying disease progresses. NEXT STEP (NCT03670121) is currently evaluating BTVA in patients with homogeneous emphysema, and the results are eagerly awaited.

SEALANT

AeriSeal emphysematous lung sealant (ELS; Aeris Therapeutics, Inc. Woburn, MA, USA) is a synthetic foam (glutaraldehyde and polyvinylalcohol) administered to the subsegmental airways to cause inflammatory scar/absorption atelectasis (79–82) independent of CV (83) (Figure 12.6).

Clinical outcomes

A Randomised Trial of Lung Sealant vs. Medical Therapy for Advanced Emphysema (ASPIRE) 2015, was a multi-centre RCT of 95 patients with severe upper lobe-predominant emphysema (visually assessed) and hyperinflation comparing ELS (n=61) with SoC (n=34) (84). Prior to intervention, patients received a seven-day steroid taper and prophylactic antibiotic course to minimise the post-treatment acute inflammatory response (PAIR: fever, dyspnoea, cough, chest pain, and/or elevated inflammatory markers) observed in pilot studies (80). Two upper lobe subsegments in each lung were treated in a single session. Owing to a lack of funding, the study was terminated prematurely. Results were available for 34 patients at six months (despite a planned primary endpoint of change in FEV1% at 12 months): Improvements in FEV1 (18.9% and 100 ml, ELS, vs. 1.3% and 10 ml, SoC; p=0.043), 6MWD (31 m vs. −22 m; p=0.019), and SGRQ total score (−12 points vs. −3 points; p=0.0072) favoured the lung sealant group. Unfortunately, no record of volume reduction was published. The observed benefits were offset by a number of inflammatory-driven respiratory adverse events: 44%, ELS vs. 18%, SoC (p=0.0098). Three ELS-treated patients required

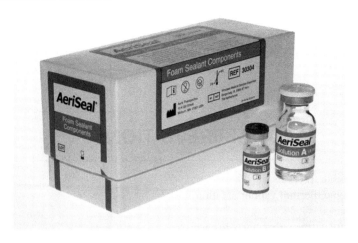

FIGURE 12.6 The AeriSeal® emphysema lung sealant (ELS) system.

invasive mechanical ventilation, with two subsequent tracheostomies. Two deaths occurred in the treatment group: one myocardial infarction 55 days after treatment and one from sepsis relating to pneumonia at the treatment site 65 days post-procedure. Pulmonx has since acquired the assets of ELS and is developing the product – ongoing trials include a modified staged treatment strategy (NCT02877459) to minimise inflammatory fallout, and combination with endobronchial valves (NCT04559464) to broaden eligibility in individuals with collateral ventilation.

CONCLUSION

Lung volume reduction has come of age with surgery and endobronchial valves now offered as standard-of-care therapies for patients with severe emphysema and hyperinflation, and the field continues to evolve with the development of novel technologies. Appropriate patient selection underpins therapeutic success – an algorithm is suggested in Figure 12.7. A combination of clinical (including exacerbation frequency, completion of pulmonary rehabilitation, and cardiovascular comorbidity), imaging (qCT and lung perfusion scintigraphy), and physiological (lung function and exercise capacity) metrics are considered by a multidisciplinary team (respiratory physician, thoracic surgeon, and radiologist), ensuring adoption of the procedure best suited to the individual patient. The design of large randomised controlled trials, where

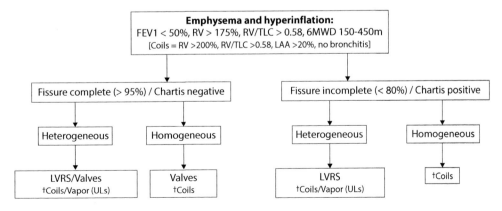

FIGURE 12.7 Suggested treatment algorithm.

possible incorporating double blinding and sham control, with extended follow-up periods and the utilisation of clinical registries, will help to clarify predictors of response, longer-term complications, durability of benefit, and survival impact of these treatments. The future of treating hyperinflation holds exciting prospects.

ABBREVIATIONS

BCI: Bayesian credible intervals
BTVA: Bronchoscopic thermal vapour ablation
CI: Confidence interval
COPD: Chronic obstructive pulmonary disease
CT: Computed tomography
CV: Collateral ventilation
DLCO: Gas transfer for carbon monoxide
EBV: Zephyr® Endobronchial Valve by Pulmonx
EbV: MedLung® Endobronchial Valve
ELS: Emphysematous lung sealant
EMV: Endobronchial Miyazawa Valve
FCS: Fissure completeness score
FDA: Food and Drug Administration
FEV1: Forced expiratory volume in one second
HRCT: High-resolution computed tomography
HU: Hounsfield units
ICER: Incremental cost-effectiveness ratio
IQR: Interquartile range
ITT: Intention-to-treat
L: Litre
LAA: Low attenuation area
LAV%: Low attenuation volume percentage
LRTI: Lower respiratory tract infection
LVR: Lung volume reduction
LVRC: Lung volume reduction coils
LVRS: Lung volume reduction surgery
m: Metres
MCID: Minimal clinically important difference
NICE: National Institute for Health and Care Excellence
PAIR: Post-treatment acute inflammatory response
qCT: Quantitative computed tomography
QoL: Quality of life
QALY: Quality-adjusted life-year
RCT: Randomised controlled trial
RV: Residual volume
SAE: Serious adverse event
SGRQ: St George's Respiratory Questionnaire
SGRQ-C: St George's Respiratory Questionnaire for COPD
SoC: Standard of care
SVS: Spiration® Valve System (formerly Intrabronchial Valve, IBV) by Olympus
TLC: Total lung capacity

TLCO: Gas transfer for carbon monoxide
TLVR: Target lobe volume reduction
T2RF: Type 2 respiratory failure
US: United States
VT20: Volume measured during the last 20 seconds using Chartis
6MWD: Six-minute walk distance

REFERENCES

1. O'Donnell DE, Webb KA, Neder JA. Lung hyperinflation in COPD: applying physiology to clinical practice. *COPD Research and Practice.* 2015;1(1):4.
2. Shah PL, Herth FJ, van Geffen WH, et al. Lung volume reduction for emphysema. *The Lancet Respiratory Medicine.* 2017;5(2):147–56.
3. van Geffen WH, Slebos DJ, Herth FJ, et al. Surgical and endoscopic interventions that reduce lung volume for emphysema: a systemic review and meta-analysis. *The Lancet Respiratory Medicine.* 2019;7(4):313–24.
4. Fishman A, Martinez F, Naunheim K, et al. A randomized trial comparing lung-volume-reduction surgery with medical therapy for severe emphysema. *The New England Journal of Medicine.* 2003;348(21):2059–73.
5. BLF. Lung volume reduction procedures for emphysema. 2021.
6. Toma TP, Hopkinson NS, Hillier J, et al. Bronchoscopic volume reduction with valve implants in patients with severe emphysema. *Lancet (London, England).* 2003;361(9361):931–3.
7. Hartman JE, Klooster K, Groen H, et al. Cost-effectiveness of endobronchial valve treatment in patients with severe emphysema compared to standard medical care. *Respirology (Carlton, Vic).* 2018;23(9):835–41.
8. Sciurba FC, Ernst A, Herth FJ, et al. A randomized study of endobronchial valves for advanced emphysema. *The New England Journal of Medicine.* 2010;363(13):1233–44.
9. Herth FJ, Noppen M, Valipour A, et al. Efficacy predictors of lung volume reduction with zephyr valves in a European cohort. *The European Respiratory Journal.* 2012;39(6):1334–42.
10. Davey C, Zoumot Z, Jordan S, et al. Bronchoscopic lung volume reduction with endobronchial valves for patients with heterogeneous emphysema and intact interlobar fissures (the BeLieVeR-HIFi study): a randomised controlled trial. *Lancet* (London, England). 2015;386(9998):1066–73.
11. Zoumot Z, Davey C, Jordan S, et al. Endobronchial valves for patients with heterogeneous emphysema and without interlobar collateral ventilation: open label treatment following the BeLieVeR-HIFi study. *Thorax.* 2017;72(3):277–9.
12. Klooster K, ten Hacken NH, Hartman JE, et al. Endobronchial valves for emphysema without interlobar collateral ventilation. *The New England Journal of Medicine.* 2015;373(24):2325–35.
13. Kemp SV, Slebos DJ, Kirk A, et al. A multicenter randomized controlled trial of zephyr endobronchial valve treatment in heterogeneous emphysema (TRANSFORM). *American Journal of Respiratory and Critical Care Medicine.* 2017;196(12):1535–43.
14. Criner GJ, Sue R, Wright S, et al. A multicenter randomized controlled trial of zephyr endobronchial valve treatment in heterogeneous emphysema (LIBERATE). *American Journal of Respiratory and Critical Care Medicine.* 2018;198(9):1151–64.
15. Dransfield MT, Garner JL, Bhatt SP, et al. Effect of zephyr endobronchial valves on dyspnea, activity levels, and quality of life at one year. Results from a randomized clinical trial. *Annals of the American Thoracic Society.* 2020;17(7):829–38.
16. Valipour A, Slebos DJ, Herth F, et al. Endobronchial valve therapy in patients with homogeneous emphysema. Results from the IMPACT Study. *American Journal of Respiratory and Critical Care Medicine.* 2016;194(9):1073–82.
17. Hartman JE, Vanfleteren LEGW, van Rikxoort EM, et al. Endobronchial valves for severe emphysema. *European Respiratory Review.* 2019;28(152):180121.
18. Herth FJF, Slebos DJ, Criner GJ, et al. Endoscopic lung volume reduction: an expert panel recommendation – Update 2019. *Respiration; International Review of Thoracic Diseases.* 2019;97(6):548–57.
19. Gompelmann D, Lim HJ, Eberhardt R, et al. Predictors of pneumothorax following endoscopic valve therapy in patients with severe emphysema. *International Journal of Chronic Obstructive Pulmonary Disease.* 2016;11:1767–73.

20. van Geffen WH, Klooster K, Hartman JE, et al. Pleural adhesion assessment as a predictor for pneumo thorax after endobronchial valve treatment. *Respiration; International Review of Thoracic Diseases* 2017;94(2):224–31.
21. Valipour A, Slebos DJ, de Oliveira HG, et al. Expert statement: pneumothorax associated with endoscopic valve therapy for emphysema--potential mechanisms, treatment algorithm, and case examples. *Respiration International Review of Thoracic Diseases*. 2014;87(6):513–21.
22. Gompelmann D, Benjamin N, Bischoff E, et al. Survival after endoscopic valve therapy in patients with severe emphysema. *Respiration; International Review of Thoracic Diseases*. 2019;97(2):145–52.
23. Gompelmann D, Heinhold T, Rotting M, et al. Long-term follow up after endoscopic valve therapy in patients with severe emphysema. *Therapeutic Advances in Respiratory Disease*. 2019;13:1753466619866101.
24. Hopkinson NS, Kemp SV, Toma TP, et al. Atelectasis and survival after bronchoscopic lung volume reduction for COPD. *The European Respiratory Journal*. 2011;37(6):1346–51.
25. Garner J, Kemp SV, Toma TP, et al. Survival after endobronchial valve placement for emphysema: a 10-year follow-up study. *American Journal of Respiratory and Critical Care Medicine*. 2016;194(4):519–21.
26. Garner JL, Desai SR. Lung fissural integrity: It's written in the genes. *American Journal of Respiratory and Critical Care Medicine*. 2021;204(7):750–2.
27. Koster TD, van Rikxoort EM, Huebner RH, et al. Predicting lung volume reduction after endobronchial valve therapy is maximized using a combination of diagnostic tools. *Respiration; International Review of Thoracic Diseases*. 2016;92(3):150–7.
28. Klooster K, Koster TD, Ruwwe-Glösenkamp C, et al. An integrative approach of the fissure completeness score and chartis assessment in endobronchial valve treatment for emphysema. *International Journal of Chronic Obstructive Pulmonary Disease*. 2020;15:1325–34.
29. Koster TD, Klooster K, McNamara H, et al. An adjusted and time-saving method to measure collateral ventilation with Chartis. *ERJ Open Research*. 2021;7(3).
30. Iftikhar IH, McGuire FR, Musani AI. Predictors of efficacy for endobronchial valves in bronchoscopic lung volume reduction: a meta-analysis. *Chronic Respiratory Disease*. 2014;11(4):237–45.
31. Gompelmann D, Herth FJ, Slebos DJ, et al. Pneumothorax following endobronchial valve therapy and its impact on clinical outcomes in severe emphysema. *Respiration; International Review of Thoracic Diseases* 2014;87(6):485–91.
32. Garner JL, Biddiscombe MF, Meah S, et al. Endobronchial valve lung volume reduction and small airway function. *American Journal of Respiratory and Critical Care Medicine*. 2021;203(12):1576–9.
33. Welling JBA, Klooster K, Hartman JE, et al. Collateral ventilation measurement using chartis: procedural sedation vs general anesthesia. *Chest*. 2019;156(5):984–90.
34. Klooster K, Hartman JE, van Dijk M, et al. Response to endobronchial valve treatment in emphysema patients with moderate hyperinflation. *Journal of Bronchology & Interventional Pulmonology*. 2021;28(1):e14–e7.
35. van Dijk M, Hartman JE, Klooster K, et al. Endobronchial valve treatment in emphysema patients with a very low DLCO. *Respiration; International Review of Thoracic Diseases*. 2020;99(2):163–70.
36. Lenga P, Ruwwe-Glösenkamp C, Grah C, et al. Endoscopic lung volume reduction with endobronchial valves in very low D (LCO) patients: results from the German Registry - Lungenemphysemregister e.V. *ERJ Open Res*. 2021;7(1).
37. Eberhardt R, Gerovasili V, Kontogianni K, et al. Effect of endoscopic lung volume reduction on established pulmonary hypertension in severe emphysema patients. *European Respiratory Journal*. 2014;44(Supp 58):P3711.
38. Tuohy MM, Remund KF, Hilfiker R, et al. Endobronchial valve deployment in severe α-1 antitrypsin deficiency emphysema: a case series. *The Clinical Respiratory Journal*. 2013;7(1):45–52.
39. Delage A, Hogarth DK, Zgoda M, Reed M. Endobronchial valve treatment in patients with severe emphysema due to alpha-1 antitrypsin deficiency. *European Respiratory Journal*. 2019;54(suppl 63):PA4800.
40. Abia-Trujillo D, Yu Lee-Mateus A, Garcia-Saucedo JC, et al. Prevention of acute exacerbation of chronic obstructive pulmonary disease after bronchoscopic lung volume reduction with endobronchial valves. *The clinical Respiratory Journal*. 2021.
41. Molen MCvd, Hartman JE, Vermeulen CJ, et al. Determinants of lung fissure completeness. *American Journa of Respiratory and Critical Care Medicine*. 2021;204(7):807–16.
42. Ninane V, Geltner C, Bezzi M, et al. Multicentre European study for the treatment of advanced emphysema with bronchial valves. *The European Respiratory Journal*. 2012;39(6):1319–25.
43. Wood DE, Nader DA, Springmeyer SC, et al. The IBV Valve trial: a multicenter, randomized, double-blind trial of endobronchial therapy for severe emphysema. *Journal of Bronchology & Interventional Pulmonology* 2014;21(4):288–97.

44. Eberhardt R, Gompelmann D, Schuhmann M, et al. Complete unilateral vs partial bilateral endoscopic lung volume reduction in patients with bilateral lung emphysema. *Chest.* 2012;142(4):900–8.

45. Li S, Wang G, Wang C, et al. The REACH trial: a randomized controlled trial assessing the safety and effectiveness of the Spiration(R) valve system in the treatment of severe emphysema. *Respiration; International Review of Thoracic Diseases.* 2019;97(5):416–27.

46. Criner GJ, Delage A, Voelker K, et al. Improving lung function in severe heterogenous emphysema with the spiration valve system (EMPROVE). A multicenter, open-label randomized controlled clinical trial. *American Journal of Respiratory and Critical Care Medicine.* 2019;200(11):1354–62.

47. Shah PL, Zoumot Z, Singh S, et al. Endobronchial coils for the treatment of severe emphysema with hyperinflation (RESET): a randomised controlled trial. *The Lancet Respiratory Medicine.* 2013;1(3):233–40.

48. Zoumot Z, Kemp SV, Singh S, et al. Endobronchial coils for severe emphysema are effective up to 12 months following treatment: medium term and cross-over results from a randomised controlled trial. *PloS One.* 2015;10(4):e0122656.

49. Garner JL, Kemp SV, Srikanthan K, et al. 5-year survival after endobronchial coil implantation: Secondary analysis of the first randomised controlled trial, RESET. *Respiration; International Review of Thoracic Diseases.* 2020;99(2):154–62.

50. Sciurba FC, Criner GJ, Strange C, et al. Effect of endobronchial coils vs usual care on exercise tolerance in patients with severe emphysema: the RENEW randomized clinical trial. *JAMA.* 2016;315(20):2178–89.

51. Herth FJ, Valipour A, Shah PL, et al. Segmental volume reduction using thermal vapour ablation in patients with severe emphysema: 6-month results of the multicentre, parallel-group, open-label, randomised controlled STEP-UP trial. *The Lancet Respiratory Medicine.* 2016;4(3):185–93.

52. Shah PL, Gompelmann D, Valipour A, et al. Thermal vapour ablation to reduce segmental volume in patients with severe emphysema: STEP-UP 12 month results. *The Lancet Respiratory Medicine.* 2016;4(9):e44–e5.

53. Slebos DJ, Shah PL, Herth FJF, et al. Safety and adverse events after targeted lung denervation for symptomatic moderate to severe chronic obstructive pulmonary disease (AIRFLOW). A multicenter randomized controlled clinical trial. *American Journal of Respiratory and Critical Care Medicine.* 2019;200(12):1477–86.

54. Pison C, Shah PL, Slebos DJ, et al. Safety of denervation following targeted lung denervation therapy for COPD: AIRFLOW-1 3-year outcomes. *Respiratory Research.* 2021;22(1):62.

55. Valipour A, Shah PL, Herth FJ, et al. Two-year outcomes for the double-blind, randomized, sham-controlled study of targeted lung denervation in patients with moderate to severe COPD: AIRFLOW-2. *International Journal of Chronic Obstructive Pulmonary Disease.* 2020;15:2807–16.

56. Slebos D-J, Degano B, Valipour A, et al. Design for a multicenter, randomized, sham-controlled study to evaluate safety and efficacy after treatment with the Nuvaira® lung denervation system in subjects with chronic obstructive pulmonary disease (AIRFLOW-3). *BMC Pulmonary Medicine.* 2020;20(1):41.

57. Garner JL, Shaipanich T, Hartman JE, et al. A prospective safety and feasibility study of metered cryospray for patients with chronic bronchitis in COPD. *The European Respiratory Journal.* 2020;56(6).

58. Herth FJ, Eberhard R, Gompelmann D, et al. Bronchoscopic lung volume reduction with a dedicated coil: a clinical pilot study. *Therapeutic Advances in Respiratory Disease.* 2010;4(4):225–31.

59. Slebos DJ, Klooster K, Ernst A, et al. Bronchoscopic lung volume reduction coil treatment of patients with severe heterogeneous emphysema. *Chest.* 2012;142(3):574–82.

60. Slebos DJ, ten ;Hacken NH, Hetzel M, et al. Endobronchial coils for endoscopic lung volume reduction: best practice recommendations from an expert panel. *Respiration; International Review of Thoracic Diseases.* 2018;96(1):1–11.

61. Palamidas AF, Kemp SV, Shen M, et al. Putative mechanisms of action of endobronchial coils. *American Journal of Respiratory and Critical Care Medicine.* 2017;196(1):109–15.

62. Fishman A, Fessler H, Martinez F, et al. Patients at high risk of death after lung-volume-reduction surgery. *The New England Journal of Medicine.* 2001;345(15):1075–83.

63. Deslee G, Mal H, Dutau H, et al. Lung volume reduction coil treatment vs usual care in patients with severe emphysema: the REVOLENS randomized clinical trial. *JAMA.* 2016;315(2):175–84.

64. Deslee G, Leroy S, Perotin JM, et al. Two-year follow-up after endobronchial coil treatment in emphysema: results from the REVOLENS study. *The European Respiratory Journal.* 2017;50(6).

65. Bulsei J, Leroy S, Perotin J-M, et al. Cost-effectiveness of lung volume reduction coil treatment in patients with severe emphysema: results from the 2-year follow-up crossover REVOLENS study (REVOLENS-2 study). *Respiratory Research.* 2018;19(1):84.

66. Slebos DJ, Cicenia J, Sciurba FC, et al. Predictors of response to endobronchial coil therapy in patients with advanced emphysema. *Chest.* 2019;155(5):928–37.

67. Hartman JE, Klooster K, Augustijn SWS, et al. Identifying responders and exploring mechanisms of action of the endobronchial coil treatment for emphysema. *Respiration; International Review of Thoracic Diseases.* 2021;100(5):443–51.
68. Hu Y, Cheng Y, Zhang H, et al. A new-designed lung-bending device for bronchoscopic lung volume reduction of severe emphysema: a feasibility study in pigs. *Respiration; International Review of Thoracic Diseases.* 2019;97(5):444–50.
69. Lausberg HF, Chino K, Patterson GA, et al. Bronchial fenestration improves expiratory flow in emphysematous human lungs. *The Annals of Thoracic Surgery.* 2003;75(2):393–7; discussion 8.
70. Choong CK, Macklem PT, Pierce JA, et al. Airway bypass improves the mechanical properties of explanted emphysematous lungs. *American Journal of Respiratory and Critical Care Medicine.* 2008;178(9):902–5.
71. Choong CK, Haddad FJ, Gee EY, Cooper JD. Feasibility and safety of airway bypass stent placement and influence of topical mitomycin C on stent patency. *The Journal of Thoracic and Cardiovascular Surgery.* 2005;129(3):632–8.
72. Choong CK, Phan L, Massetti P, et al. Prolongation of patency of airway bypass stents with use of drug-eluting stents. *The Journal of Thoracic and Cardiovascular Surgery.* 2006;131(1):60–4.
73. Rendina EA, De Giacomo T, Venuta F, et al. Feasibility and safety of the airway bypass procedure for patients with emphysema. *The Journal of Thoracic and Cardiovascular Surgery.* 2003;125(6):1294–7.
74. Cardoso PF, Snell GI, Hopkins P, et al. Clinical application of airway bypass with paclitaxel-eluting stents: early results. *The Journal of Thoracic and Cardiovascular Surgery.* 2007;134(4):974–81.
75. Shah PL, Slebos D-J, Cardoso PFG, et al. Design of the exhale airway stents for emphysema (EASE) trial: an endoscopic procedure for reducing hyperinflation. *BMC Pulmonary Medicine.* 2011;11(1):1.
76. Shah PL, Slebos DJ, Cardoso PF, et al. Bronchoscopic lung-volume reduction with Exhale airway stents for emphysema (EASE trial): randomised, sham-controlled, multicentre trial. *Lancet* (London, England). 2011;378(9795):997–1005.
77. Gompelmann D, Eberhardt R, Ernst A, et al. The localized inflammatory response to bronchoscopic thermal vapor ablation. *Respiration; International Review of Thoracic Diseases.* 2013;86(4):324–31.
78. Gompelmann D, Shah PL, Valipour A, Herth FJF. Bronchoscopic thermal vapor ablation: best practice recommendations from an expert panel on endoscopic lung volume reduction. *Respiration; International Review of Thoracic Diseases.* 2018;95(6):392–400.
79. Herth FJ, Gompelmann D, Stanzel F, et al. Treatment of advanced emphysema with emphysematous lung sealant (AeriSeal(R)). *Respiration; International Review of Thoracic Diseases.* 2011;82(1):36–45.
80. Herth FJ, Eberhardt R, Ingenito EP, Gompelmann D. Assessment of a novel lung sealant for performing endoscopic volume reduction therapy in patients with advanced emphysema. *Expert Review of Medical Devices.* 2011;8(3):307–12.
81. Kramer MR, Refaely Y, Maimon N, et al. Bilateral endoscopic sealant lung volume reduction therapy for advanced emphysema. *Chest.* 2012;142(5):1111–7.
82. Fruchter O, Fridel L, Kramer MR. The pathological features of bronchoscopic lung volume reduction using sealant treatment assessed in lung explants of patients who underwent lung transplantation. *Respiration; International Review of Thoracic Diseases.* 2013;86(2):143–4.
83. Magnussen H, Kramer MR, Kirsten AM, et al. Effect of fissure integrity on lung volume reduction using a polymer sealant in advanced emphysema. *Thorax.* 2012;67(4):302–8.
84. Come CE, Kramer MR, Dransfield MT, et al. A randomised trial of lung sealant versus medical therapy for advanced emphysema. *The European Respiratory Journal.* 2015;46(3):651–62.

Peri-Interventional Clinical Management of Endoscopic Emphysema Treatment

13

Johannes Wienker and Kaid Darwiche

INTRODUCTION

Advanced emphysema is the defining pathomorphological phenotype of severe chronic obstructive pulmonary disease (COPD) resulting in impaired lung function, exercise capacity, and quality of life due to excessive hyperinflation and insufficient gas exchange. COPD is an extremely challenging disease of modern medicine and one of the most common causes of death, especially in developed countries.

Initially smoking cessation, medical therapy, and rehabilitation programs can be sufficient to relieve the symptomatic burden. However, for patients with end-stage emphysema, these treatment modalities are limited, and surgical or interventional therapy options have been developed and evaluated in the last few years. These methods aim to reduce severely destructed emphysematous lung tissue, thereby reducing hyperinflation and improving elastic recoil together with diaphragm function.

Bronchoscopic lung volume reduction (BLVR), a minimal invasive approach, was developed in response to high mortality and morbidity rates in surgical lung volume reduction procedures (especially in patients with low forced expiratory volume in one second [FEV_1] and diffusing capacity of the lungs for carbon monoxide [DL_{CO}]) reported in the National Emphysema Treatment Trial (NETT) (Criner et al., 2011). Although varying in their mechanisms of action, the complication rates of most endoscopic procedures are considerably lower compared with the invasive surgical strategy (Franzen et al., 2018).

Treatment outcome does not solely depend on the interventional or surgical technique itself. Due to the increased risk of peri-interventional complications associated with the advanced stage of emphysema, together with frequent comorbidities, expertise in clinical patient management plays a significant role in achieving the best possible results. This concerns all actions before, during, and after the intervention.

DOI: 10.1201/9781003251439-13

TABLE 13.1   Current techniques used for BLVR

	EBV/IBV	COILS	BTVA	PLVR
Treatment side	Unilateral*	Bilateral	Unilateral*	Unilateral
Reversibility	Reversible	Irreversible	Irreversible	Irreversible
Fissure integrity	Complete	Incomplete	Incomplete	Incomplete
Mechanism of action	Occlusion	Distortion and compression	Inflammatory reaction	Inflammatory reaction, closure of fissure gaps
Major complication	Pneumothorax	COPD exacerbation, hemoptysis	Local/systemic inflammatory reaction, pneumonitis	Post-interventional pneumonia

*Bilateral in selected cases.
BLVR, bronchoscopic lung volume reduction; EBV, endobronchial valves; IBV, intrabronchial valves; COPD, chronic obstructive pulmonary disease; BTVA, bronchial thermal vapor ablation; PLVR, polymeric lung volume reduction.

Since the results of the first major randomized clinical trial (RCT) have been published (VENT, 2010) much has been learned and treatment protocols have been adapted (Sciurba et al., 2010). A differentiated patient selection with sophisticated diagnostical tools as well as profound knowledge of possible complications and their management is key to successful treatment.

BLVR TECHNOLOGIES

In the last decade, different approaches for bronchoscopic lung volume reduction were invented and implemented in clinical research (Table 13.1). Less promising techniques like airway by-pass stents led to high complication rates or non-significant clinical results (Shah et al., 2011). Endobronchial valves, coils, and vapor ablation are three methods that are used on a regular basis in emphysema care centers today. Lung volume reduction with a polymeric foam as a lung sealant (polymeric lung volume reduction [PLVR]) has initially not been considered to be clinically relevant enough, but after modification, the procedure is currently under evaluation in a clinical trial.

Endobronchial valves

Endobronchial valves (EBVs) are so-called blocking devices that only allow a unidirectional flow. Once a bronchus is successfully occluded, air is prevented from entering during inspiration while the residual-volume and secretions can gradually be exhaled. Eventually, this mechanism results in a reduction of hyperinflation and improvement in diaphragm function. Optimally, complete atelectasis is achieved so that the adjacent lobe(s), which are potentially less compromised from emphysematous remodeling, profit from more efficient ventilatory mechanics. The valves are placed in the segment or subsegment bronchi by using a delivery catheter via the working channel of a flexible bronchoscope.

Although, with intrabronchial valves (IBVs) and EBVs, there were initially two different kinds of valve-based blocking devices; EBVs showed better results with statistically significant and clinically meaningful improvements in major RCTs (BeLieVeR, Transform, STELVIO, IMPACT) (Davey et al., 2015; Kemp et al., 2017; Klooster et al., 2015; Valipour et al., 2016). However, head-to-head studies are not available.

EBVs (Zephyr, Pulmonx, Redwood City, California) are made of a silicone membrane and a nitinol frame with an elastic, soft lamellar closure mechanism ("fish mouth") that opens to air flow from expiration but remains closed during inspiration. Available in different sizes and lengths, they can be placed individually depending on the anatomical conditions and dimensions of the patient's bronchial system. If necessary, the valve can be removed in case of complications or lack of clinical improvements, which is a great advantage compared with other (irreversible) methods. In the first large RCT, only modest clinical improvements were observed. This was connected to the presence of interlobar fissures, small airway channels between the lobes, so that the unidirectional mechanism was disabled. Therefore, complete fissure integrity and careful patient selection are required for successful treatment. In aspects of safety, the most common adverse event after EBV placement is a pneumothorax, which can be seen in up to 26% of cases (Valipour et al., 2016).

Endobronchial coils

In contrast to the blocking approach with valves, endobronchial coils are a non-blocking and irreversible treatment option that does not depend on the absence of interlobar fissures. Consisting of nitinol, an alloy of nickel and titanium, they exhibit a shape-memory effect. Initially formed in a straight configuration, they are delivered to the site of lung parenchyma where the most severe emphysematous destruction is located. Once deployed, they take a double-looped form and within that loop retract parts of the surrounding tissue (Figure 13.1). Being available in different sizes, usually about ten to 14 coils on each lobe are implanted with an interval of four to six weeks between each treatment session. Endobronchial coils are an irreversible and permanent treatment, even though they might be removeable directly after implantation. So far, several randomized clinical trials have been published (e.g., REVOLENS, RESET, RENEW), showing significant clinical improvements for selected patients (Deslée et al., 2016; Sciurba et al., 2016; Shah et al., 2013), although they seem to have a significant rate of adverse events with major complications such as pneumothorax, COPD exacerbation, bleeding, and pneumonia requiring hospitalization after the procedure (Sciurba et al., 2016).

Bronchoscopic thermal vapor ablation

Bronchoscopic thermal vapor ablation (BTVA) is another technique that is based on the application of hot water steam via a disposable catheter to a defined lung segment. The principle behind this method is a local inflammatory stimulus causing acute tissue damage followed by scarring and fibrosis that finally causes shrinkage of tissue (Figure 13.2). Being able to target smaller segmental areas rather than complete lobes, vapor ablation is a very precise and selective method. In this regard, pre-interventional software-based

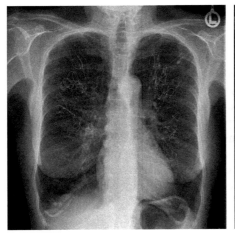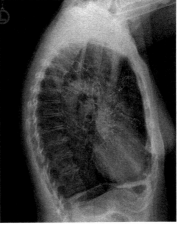

FIGURE 13.1 Chest X-ray of a 79-year-old female patient following the bilateral implantation of volume reduction coils.

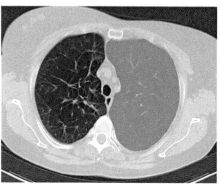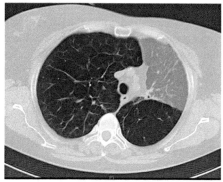

FIGURE 13.2 Chest CT scan of a 62-year-old male patient following BTVA of the left upper lobe (marked with following volume reduction and mediastinal shift.

target planning is performed to identify lung segments with the highest emphysema index and air trapping. A multicenter RCT (STEP-UP) showed significant changes in FEV_1 and SGRQ from baseline with an acceptable safety profile (Herth et al., 2016; Shah et al., 2016). More recent trials, for example, addressing lower lobe therapy, are lacking and are needed to estimate the exact value of the procedure.

Other techniques

Not being reliant on fissure integrity, PLVR (Aeriseal©) is a technique that irreversibly blocks small airways and channels for collateral ventilation to achieve lung volume reduction. Although not part of the clinical routine, this method is currently being investigated as part of the multicenter CONVERT trial. In this setting, lung sealant is intended as a pre-treatment to occlude collateral air channels, clearing the way for valve implantation as the definite therapy.

PATIENT SELECTION FOR INTERVENTIONAL PROCEDURES

As in most medical fields, careful preparation and profound treatment decision-making is extremely important to secure the best possible outcome. Especially in highly specialized clinical branches, such as interventional pulmonology, this needs particular attention. Optimal patient selection is a critical factor affecting the final result and is often course setting for further development of the patient's history It is important to mention that a bronchoscopic lung volume reduction should only be considered when patients continue to be highly symptomatic despite conservative treatment with optimal medical therapy pulmonary rehabilitation, and lifestyle adaptions according to the latest guidelines.

Potential candidates for lung volume reduction should be seen and preselected in an emphysema outpatient clinic before the start of the actual evaluation process. A mandatory criterion to continue is evidence of hyperinflation, which can be proven by prior lung function tests or sometimes needs to be confirmed by a simple chest X-ray and the trained eye of the clinician. Figure 13.3 gives a short idea of the patient selection and interventional process.

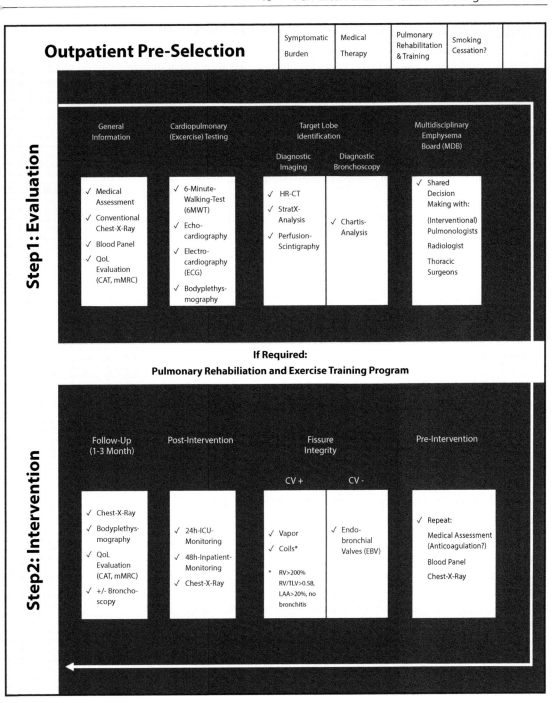

FIGURE 13.3 Process chart of patient evaluation and intervention; CAT, COPD Assessment Test; mMRC, Modified Medical Research Council Questionnaire; SPECT, Single Photon Emission Computed Tomography; PLVR, Polymeric Lung Volume Reduction.

Clinical characteristics: Inclusion criteria for BLVR

When symptoms due to worsened respiratory function and severe hyperinflation can no longer be con trolled via medication and supportive therapy, bronchoscopic lung volume reduction should be consid ered. Since the correlation of symptoms with impairments in lung function and physical condition i: highly individual in every patient, there is no one-path-to-follow option in the treatment decision-making process. Treatment options need to be discussed in a multidisciplinary board with (interventional) pulmo nologists, thoracic surgeons, and radiologists. Based on the results and insights of the clinical trials, there is, however, a widely accepted expert panel treatment algorithm that is continuously updated and provide: inclusion criteria for various BLVR techniques (Herth et al., 2019).

Generally, patients with the following clinical characteristics qualify for BLVR:

FEV_1	<45%
RV	>175% (>225% in coils)
RV/TLC	>0.58
6MWD	150–450 m

Further options are limited by the integrity of interlobar fissures, which can be directly analyzed with quantitative computed tomography and indirectly with the catheter-based Chartis© system:

Absence of interlobar fissure gaps (no collateral ventilation): Valves (vapor and coils)

Presence of interlobar fissures gaps (collateral ventilation): Vapor, coils, and PLVR For some patients, lung volume reduction surgery (LVRS) might still be a possible treatment modality, and lung transplantation should be considered in selected patients <65 years.

Clinical and technical evaluation

Clinical history, quality of life (CAT, SGRQ), and assessment of COPD exacerbations

It was already mentioned that interventional emphysema treatment should only be considered when medi cal therapy tailored to the individual clinical history of each patient did not relieve the symptomatic burden. It is important to ensure the patient's compliance to stick to the conservative treatment. In the daily clinical setting, it is often observed that, for example, inhalation devices are not used correctly (e.g. not inhaled deeply enough) or not according to the schedule. Patients should be informed about appro priate application. Therefore, obtaining a detailed clinical history, with special attention to exacerbation rates, is the basis for every further therapy planning. In this regard, specific standardized questionnaires like the COPD assessment test (CAT) or the Saint George Respiratory Questionnaire (SGRQ) can be used to evaluate the symptom severity. The assessment of comorbidities and the medication regime is another crucial factor that must be determined before every intervention. This affects, in particular, the implantation of coils and BTVA, as there are several exclusion criteria narrowing the application range for example, patients with anticoagulation therapy or hemorrhagic diathesis should not be considered for coils or BTVA.

---

* RV >200%, RV/TLV >0.58, LAA >20%, no bronchitis.

Pulmonary function (spirometry, plethysmography, DL$_{CO}$, 6MWT, echocardiography)

Testing the functional status of each patient should reveal obstruction in spirometry (FEV$_1$/FVC <0.7) with a FEV$_1$ predicted <50%. Also, very limited values of ≤20% may be considered at centers with expertise (Darwiche et al., 2016). Extensive hyperinflation and air trapping can be identified by plethysmography and the optimal RV should be >175% or even >225% when considering coil implantation. Furthermore, the DL$_{CO}$ has to be determined. Even though there is no absolute contraindication for DL$_{CO}$ values for BLVR, values <20% were associated with higher complication rates and a surgical approach as a possible alternative should no longer be considered. In order to examine physical fitness, the six-minute walk test (6MWT) is used as the standard protocol. Here, especially patients who will most likely not benefit from lung volume reduction can be identified. Patients with distances >450 m should be excluded since they are physically not limited to the extent where BLVR treatment could improve the symptomatic situation. On the other hand, patients with very low distances of <150 m also do not qualify as often cardiac comorbidities, musculoskeletal impairment, or obesity are the main problem. Pulmonary rehabilitation should be attempted first before the patient is re-evaluated. Regarding the cardiovascular function, every pre-interventional routine includes an echocardiography to assess cardiac function and screen for pulmonary hypertension, which can be a contraindication when the estimated pulmonary arterial systolic pressure (PAPsys) is >50 mm Hg.

Diagnostic imaging: CT scan, ventilation/perfusion scintigraphy

Further elements of the pre-interventional diagnostic protocol are imaging tests with a CT scan (optimally HR-CT) as the key technique. Not only can the severity and configuration of the emphysema be estimated but also comorbidities that display contraindications for BLVR like fibrosis, bronchiectasis, or even malignant processes can be ruled out. Furthermore, the anatomical topography can be studied, which aids the following endoscopic procedure. Ventilation/perfusion scintigraphy is a useful tool for the identification of the target lobe. Especially in patients where the emphysema is distributed more homogeneously over the lung, the lobe with the lowest perfusion rate is a good target when there is an ipsilateral lobe with good perfusion. Single photon emission computed tomography (SPECT) is a new imaging technology with the potential to improve target lobe selection.

Collateral ventilation assessment: QCT analysis, Chartis measurement

Complete lung fissures are required for the successful function of valves. Collateral ventilation can be assessed in two ways. Quantitative computed tomography analysis (established suppliers are StratX, Vida Diagnostics, or others) is a non-invasive method based on high-resolution CT scans. The analysis provides a more detailed evaluation of lobe volumes and emphysema heterogenicity next to the fissure. Preferably, the evaluation is completed with a second diagnostic tool: the catheter-based Chartis method. A balloon is inflated within a lobar bronchus identified earlier in the CT scan to occlude the lumen and expiratory flow together with inspiratory pressure as well as their ratio (= resistance), and the drained lobar volume is measured. Declining flow and a concomitant rise in resistance indicate CV negativity (Koster et al., 2016). Moreover, Chartis can be helpful for patient selection as the drained volume seems to be correlated with improvements in lung function, so patients with high volumes tend to show a better outcome (Wienker et al., 2020).

Rehabilitation and multidisciplinary board

COPD with emphysema is a multifactorial disease that is not limited to the lung but also causes physical impairment and inactivity. Together with respiratory muscle dysfunction and inefficient ventilatory mechanics, the symptomatic burden is even more aggravated. Therefore, improving exercise capacity is an important step in preparation for interventional lung volume reduction. Patients should be evaluated fo exercise capacity and limb muscle function and considered for special pulmonary rehabilitation program (Greulich et al., 2015).

At the end of the patient selection process, the final treatment decision should be discussed in a multidisciplinary board (MDB). Here, interventional pulmonologists together with thoracic surgeons and radiologists should discuss an individually adapted therapy based on the diagnostics run before.

Interventional treatment, patient, and complication management

Despite bronchoscopic lung volume reduction being a standard procedure in specialized emphysema care centers today, thorough treatment planning before every intervention is essential to minimize unwanted complications and unprepared conditions. The diagnostic recordings, especially CT scans, the patients routine medication, and comorbidities and contraindications should be reviewed in detail. For example antiplatelet and anticoagulant therapy that cannot be paused due to certain conditions is a contraindication for therapy with coils.

All mentioned procedures can be performed under general anesthesia or conscious sedation according to the standard routine of the clinic. If conscious sedation is favored by the examiner, rapid intubation and ventilation have to be secured. The airways can either be accessed via flexible bronchoscopy and positive pressure ventilation or with rigid bronchoscopy and jet ventilation. The procedure time is highly variable from patient to patient and depends on various factors such as anatomical accessibility, the physician's experience, the anesthesia technique, and, of course, unpredictable complications. The average time is about 15–25 minutes for valve, 30–45 minutes for coil placement, and <15 minutes for vapor application. The most common adverse events for each technique are listed in Table 13.2 (Gompelmann et al. 2018; Herth et al., 2017; Slebos et al., 2018).

Patients should be hospitalized for at least three nights for post-interventional observation, since a pneumothorax most likely occurs within the first two to three days after intervention (Gompelmann et al. 2014). Right after bronchoscopy, patients should be closely monitored, ideally within an intensive care setting for rapid pleural drainage in case of tension pneumothorax. To exclude the above-mentioned complications, a chest X-ray is routinely performed on the day of the intervention. When complications such as pneumothorax can be ruled out, cardiopulmonary stable patients can be discharged. Re-hospitalization is advised when there are signs of an exacerbation with increased frequency and severity of (productive coughing, worsened chest congestion, dyspnea, and wheezing.

TABLE 13.2   Most common adverse events

EBV/IBV	COILS	BTVA
1. Pneumothorax 20–30%	1. Pneumothorax 1–10%	1. COPD exacerbations 24%
2. COPD exacerbations	2. COPD exacerbations 10%	2. Pneumonia 18%
3. Pneumonia	3. Coil associated opacity 10%	3. Hemoptysis 3%
4. Valve migration	4. Minor hemoptysis 50%	4. Pneumothorax 3%
5. Airway kinking	5. Major hemoptysis 1%	

Note: EBV, endobronchial valve; IBV, intrabronchial valve; COPD, chronic obstructive pulmonary disease; BTVA, broncho scopic thermal vapor ablation.

Follow-up treatment

Varying from center to center, a follow-up examination is carried out at intervals of one to three months after BLVR. At this point, pulmonary function tests and a chest CT scan are repeated to control sufficient volume reduction of the target lobe and exclude valve dislocation or migration. The CAT or SGRQ should also be repeated to examine the extent of symptomatic relief. Care should also be taken to ensure that the patient continues to receive optimal supportive treatment and physical training, preferably as part of regularly coordinated and monitored training sessions.

REFERENCES

Come, C.E., Kramer, M.R., Dransfield, M.T., Abu-Hijleh, M., Berkowitz, D., Bezzi, M., Bhatt, S.P., Boyd, M.B., Cases, E., Chen, A.C., et al. (2015). A randomised trial of lung sealant versus medical therapy for advanced emphysema. *Eur Respir J 46*, 651–662.

Criner, G.J., Cordova, F., Sternberg, A.L., and Martinez, F.J. (2011). The National Emphysema Treatment Trial (NETT). *Am J Respir Crit Care Med 184*, 881–893.

Darwiche, K., Karpf-Wissel, R., Eisenmann, S., Aigner, C., Welter, S., Zarogoulidis, P., Hohenforst-Schmidt, W., Freitag, L., and Oezkan, F. (2016). Bronchoscopic lung volume reduction with endobronchial valves in low-FEV1 patients. *Respiration 92*, 414–419.

Davey, C., Zoumot, Z., Jordan, S., McNulty, W.H., Carr, D.H., Hind, M.D., Hansell, D.M., Rubens, M.B., Banya, W., Polkey, M.I., et al. (2015). Bronchoscopic lung volume reduction with endobronchial valves for patients with heterogeneous emphysema and intact interlobar fissures (the BeLieVeR-HIFi study): A randomised controlled trial. *Lancet 386*, 1066–1073.

Deslée, G., Mal, H., Dutau, H., Bourdin, A., Vergnon, J.M., Pison, C., Kessler, R., Jounieaux, V., Thiberville, L., Leroy, S., et al. (2016). Lung volume reduction coil treatment vs usual care in patients with severe emphysema: The REVOLENS randomized clinical trial. *JAMA 315*, 175–184.

Franzen, D., Straub, G., and Freitag, L. (2018). Complications after bronchoscopic lung volume reduction. *J Thorac Dis 10*, S2811–S2815.

Gompelmann, D., Herth, F.J.F., Slebos, D.J., Valipour, A., Ernst, A., Criner, G.J., and Eberhardt, R. (2014). Pneumothorax following endobronchial valve therapy and its impact on clinical outcomes in severe emphysema. *Respiration 87*, 485–491.

Gompelmann, D., Shah, P.L., Valipour, A., and Herth, F.J.F. (2018). Bronchoscopic thermal vapor ablation: Best practice recommendations from an expert panel on endoscopic lung volume reduction. *Respiration 95*, 392–400.

Greulich, T., Koczulla, A.R., Nell, C., Kehr, K., Vogelmeier, C.F., Stojanovic, D., Wittmann, M., and Schultz, K. (2015). Effect of a three-week inpatient rehabilitation program on 544 consecutive patients with very severe COPD: A retrospective analysis. *Respiration 90*, 287–292.

Herth, F.J.F., Slebos, D.-J., Criner, G.J., and Shah, P.L. (2017). Endoscopic lung volume reduction: An expert panel recommendation – Update 2017. *Respiration 94*, 380–388.

Herth, F.J.F., Slebos, D.-J., Criner, G.J., Valipour, A., Sciurba, F., and Shah, P.L. (2019). Endoscopic lung volume reduction: An expert panel recommendation – Update 2019. *Respiration 97*, 548–557.

Herth, F.J.F., Valipour, A., Shah, P.L., Eberhardt, R., Grah, C., Egan, J., Ficker, J.H., Wagner, M., Witt, C., Liebers, U., et al. (2016). Segmental volume reduction using thermal vapour ablation in patients with severe emphysema: 6-month results of the multicentre, parallel-group, open-label, randomised controlled STEP-UP trial. *Lancet Respir Med 4*, 185–193.

Kemp, S.V., Slebos, D.-J., Kirk, A., Kornaszewska, M., Carron, K., Ek, L., Broman, G., Hillerdal, G., Mal, H., Pison, C., et al. (2017). A multicenter randomized controlled trial of zephyr endobronchial valve treatment in heterogeneous emphysema (TRANSFORM). *Am J Respir Crit Care Med 196*, 1535–1543.

Klooster, K., ten Hacken, N.H.T., Hartman, J.E., Kerstjens, H.A.M., van Rikxoort, E.M., and Slebos, D.-J. (2015). Endobronchial valves for emphysema without interlobar collateral ventilation. *N Engl J Med 373*, 2325–2335.

Koster, T.D., van Rikxoort, E.M., Huebner, R.-H., Doellinger, F., Klooster, K., Charbonnier, J.-P., Radhakrishnan, S., Herth, F.J.F., and Slebos, D.-J. (2016). Predicting lung volume reduction after endobronchial valve therapy is maximized using a combination of diagnostic tools. *Respiration 92*, 150–157.

Sciurba, F.C., Criner, G.J., Strange, C., Shah, P.L., Michaud, G., Connolly, T.A., Deslée, G., Tillis, W.P., Delage, A., Marquette, C.-H., et al. (2016). Effect of endobronchial coils vs usual care on exercise tolerance in patients with severe emphysema: The RENEW randomized clinical trial. *JAMA 315*, 2178–2189.

Sciurba, F.C., Ernst, A., Herth, F.J.F., Strange, C., Criner, G.J., Marquette, C.H., Kovitz, K.L., Chiacchierini, R.P., Goldin, J., McLennan, G., et al. (2010). A randomized study of endobronchial valves for advanced emphysema. *N Engl J Med 363*, 1233–1244.

Shah, P.L., Gompelmann, D., Valipour, A., McNulty, W.H., Eberhardt, R., Grah, C., Egan, J., Ficker, J.H., Wagner, M., Witt, C., et al. (2016). Thermal vapour ablation to reduce segmental volume in patients with severe emphysema: STEP-UP 12 month results. *Lancet Respir Med 4*, e44–e45.

Shah, P.L., Slebos, D.-J., Cardoso, P.F.G., Cetti, E., Voelker, K., Levine, B., Russell, M.E., Goldin, J., Brown, M., Cooper, J.D., et al. (2011). Bronchoscopic lung-volume reduction with Exhale airway stents for emphysema (EASE trial): Randomised, sham-controlled, multicentre trial. *Lancet 378*, 997–1005.

Shah, P.L., Zoumot, Z., Singh, S., Bicknell, S.R., Ross, E.T., Quiring, J., Hopkinson, N.S., Kemp, S.V., and RESET trial Study Group. (2013). Endobronchial coils for the treatment of severe emphysema with hyperinflation (RESET): A randomised controlled trial. *Lancet Respir Med 1*, 233–240.

Slebos, D.-J., ten Hacken, N.H., Hetzel, M., Herth, F.J.F., and Shah, P.L. (2018). Endobronchial coils for endoscopic lung volume reduction: Best practice recommendations from an expert panel. *Respiration 96*, 1–11.

Valipour, A., Slebos, D.-J., Herth, F., Darwiche, K., Wagner, M., Ficker, J.H., Petermann, C., Hubner, R.-H., Stanzel, F., Eberhardt, R., et al. (2016). Endobronchial valve therapy in patients with homogeneous emphysema. Results from the IMPACT study. *Am J Respir Crit Care Med 194*, 1073–1082.

Wienker, J., Karpf-Wissel, R., Funke, F., Taube, C., Wälscher, J., Winantea, J., Maier, S., Mardanzai, K., and Darwiche, K. (2020). Predictive value of Chartis measurement for lung function improvements in bronchoscopic lung volume reduction. *Ther Adv Respir Dis 14*, 1753466620932507.

Bronchoscopic Lung Volume Reduction with One-Way Valves

14

Prevention and Management of Complications

T. David Koster, Hugo G. Oliveira and Dirk-Jan Slebos

INTRODUCTION

Bronchoscopic lung volume reduction (BLVR) with one-way endobronchial valves (Zephyr EBV [Pulmonx, Redwood City, CA, USA] or the Spiration® Valve System [SVS, Olympus, Redmond, WA, USA]) is a guideline treatment [1]. This treatment is an option for patients with severe emphysema and hyperinflation and aims to achieve a volume reduction of the treated target lobe, which leads to improvement of lung function, exercise tolerance, and quality of life [2–6].

The most important aspect of treating patients with valves is precise and adequate patient selection. This is important to achieve optimal effect and prevent possible complications. However, it is important to be aware of the potential risks and possible complications in this patient group. A patient should be able to tolerate the procedure itself and manage possible complications [7–9]. Therefore, it is important to review the expected benefits and possible risks before treatment and be aware of comorbidities and relevant medication. It is recommended that all patients be discussed with a multidisciplinary team to evaluate possible treatment options and their eligibility for treatment [7–9]. After implantation of valves, there are both short-term and long-term complications to be accounted for. The most important short-term complication is the occurrence of pneumothorax. A (post-obstruction) pneumonia or COPD exacerbation can occur shortly after the procedure, but this may also occur during follow-up. Long-term complications include the occurrence of granulation tissue and subsequent valve dislocation with loss of treatment effect.

DOI: 10.1201/9781003251439-14

This review summarizes the most important risk factors and possible short- and long-term complications after treatment. Furthermore, indications for revision bronchoscopy are described.

GENERAL CONSIDERATIONS BEFORE TREATMENT

Patients who are eligible for treatment are highly symptomatic COPD patients and should already receive optimal treatment for their COPD (smoking cessation, guideline pharmacological treatment, structured rehabilitation program, nutrition support, oxygen, and non-invasive ventilation if appropriate). If a patient is eligible for treatment, it is important to evaluate whether a patient is fit to receive treatment and be able to sustain possible side effects.

There are several comorbidities that are relative contraindications for treatment, mainly due to safety reasons. For example, patients with severe congestive heart failure (left ventricular ejection fraction <40%) and severe pulmonary hypertension (right ventricular systolic pressure >50 mmHg) are less eligible for treatment [8, 9]. Patients who are on anticoagulant therapy should be able to discontinue this for some time to be able to safely perform the procedure and handle complications (e.g., drainage for acute pneumothorax).

In general, patients with a low FEV_1 (≤20% of the predicted value) or a low diffusion capacity (DL_{co} ≤20% of the predicted value) have been excluded from most trials due to an expected higher risk of the procedure. Two recently published studies retrospectively showed that treatment could be performed safely and was effective in this patient group [10, 11]. Severe hypercapnia is also considered to be a higher risk for a complicated course. To date, there is little evidence regarding this subject. Two published abstracts show that patients with hypercapnia can be treated safely and effectively [12, 13]. In case of a good treatment target lobe and high expectation on improvement, lung volume reduction will improve the lung function ventilation, and therefore reduce the hypercapnia. An example of a successful treatment of a patient with a severe hypercapnia is shown in Figure 14.1. However, caution should be taken in case of a severe hypercapnia ($pCO2$ ≥8 kPa/≥60 mmHg) or hypoxemia ($pO2$ ≤6.0/≤45 mmHg), both because of peri-procedural and post-procedural risks, but foremost, outlier patients often do not have the right emphysema phenotype to treat. Potential risks and benefits are advised to be discussed with the patients [8, 9].

SHORT-TERM COMPLICATIONS, PREVENTION, AND TREATMENT

Pneumothorax

The most important acute and well known complication after treatment with valves is a pneumothorax and occurs in 4.2–34.4% of patients [2–5, 7, 14, 15]. The proposed mechanism is that due to the loss of volume in the treated lobe, there is redistribution of a part of the volume to the non-treated ipsilateral lobe. The subsequent expansion of this lobe may lead to a pneumothorax due to a rupture of blebs or bullae or a parenchymal rupture due to pre-existing pleural adhesions [7, 16]. A symptomatic pneumothorax may be life-threatening and requires immediate drainage.

A pleural rupture in the treatment target lobe due to the shift in position is usually self-limiting because the valves prevent an active air leak. Another manifestation of pneumothorax is the "pneumothorax ex vacuo." This is due to the increase in negative intrapleural pressure after the lobar collapse, gas

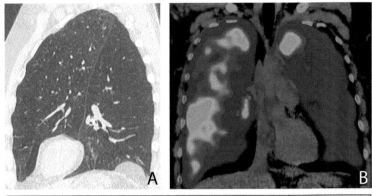

	Baseline	% pred	2 months FU	% pred	Difference
FEV$_1$ (L)	0.50	16	0.90	29	+80%/+ 0.40 L
FVC (L)	1.96	49	2.91	73	+48%/+ 0.95 L
RV (L)	5.82	283	4.46	216	-23%/- 1.36 L
pCO2 (kpa)	7.9		6.0		-24%/- 1.9 kPa

FIGURE 14.1 Example of a patient with severe hypercapnia who was treated successfully with endobronchial valves. Other than COPD, there were no other comorbidities. (A) CT scan revealed the left lower lobe as a potential treatment target lobe (quantitative CT scan analysis revealed a % voxel density <−950HU of 42%, with 100% complete left major fissure). (B) Single-photon emission computed tomography (SPECT) shows heterogeneous perfusion with lowest perfusion in the left lower lobe of 10%. (C) After treatment with a complete lobar atelectasis at two months follow-up, there is a large improvement of lung function and hypercapnia. FEV$_1$, forced expiratory volume in one second; FVC, forced vital capacity; RV, residual volume.

originating from ambient tissue, and blood drawn into the pleural space. In this case, there is no bronchopleural fistula, and drainage is usually not necessary.

Possible risk factors for the development of a pneumothorax after lung volume reduction include the presence of pleural adhesions, paraseptal emphysema, volume disbalance between target lobe and ipsilateral lobe, high emphysematous destruction of the ipsilateral non-target lobe, and homogeneous emphysema [16].

An expert statement regarding pneumothorax after lung volume reduction with valves has recently been published, but there is no consensus about strategies to reduce the risk of pneumothorax [16]. The majority of pneumothoraces develops within three days after valve treatment. Therefore, admission in the hospital during the first three nights after treatment is advised. Currently, there is only local practice on pneumothorax prevention management, ranging from adjustment of ventilator settings, cough suppression (lidocaine, opioids), bed rest after procedure, getting out of bed as soon as possible, provoked spirometry, sequential bronchoscopic procedures, more distal valve placement, and prophylactic chest-tube placement, all without any scientific evidence, but showing that dealing with the potential of a pneumothorax is serious enough [9, 16–19]. Furthermore, a staged placement of valves in two procedures has been reported to reduce the chance of a pneumothorax [17]. However, a staged treatment is currently not advised because this would significantly change the treatment regimen and this should be confirmed in an RCT first [16].

After occurrence of a pneumothorax, intercostal drainage is usually sufficient to manage the pneumothorax. In case of persistent high-flow air leak, removal of one or more valves can be considered to promote re-expansion of the treated lobe. Furthermore, thoracic surgery can be considered, depending on the patient's clinical status and local expertise. Extensive recommendations regarding treatment of a complicated pneumothorax after valve treatment have been described in the expert statement by van Dijk et al [16]

Pneumonia

Up to 8% of patients may develop a pneumonia in the first year after treatment with valve, which may be both in the treated lobe (post-obstruction pneumonia) and in the non-treated lobes [2–5, 7, 14, 15, 18]. To prevent a pneumonia shortly after treatment, a prophylactic course of antibiotics may be described and bronchial wash may guide antibiotic treatment if necessary. In case of a severe post-obstruction pneumonia, it is advised to remove the valves if there is no adequate response to treatment with antibiotics.

Risk factors to developing post-obstruction pneumonia after treatment with valves have not yet been described in the literature. In general, in studies, patients were excluded for treatment with valves in case of frequent COPD exacerbations or pneumonias, significant sputum production, or relevant bronchiectasis [4, 5]. Furthermore, maintenance immunosuppressive agents or prednisolone (>10 mg daily) is a relative contraindication for treatment [9]. In case of a good treatment target lobe, if there are local factors preventing valve placement (e.g., high dose immunosuppression), a video-assisted thoracoscopic surgery (VATS) lobectomy can be considered [7].

Hypoxemia

After treatment with valves, shunting with subsequent hypoxemia may develop due to decreased ventilation and intact perfusion. Usually, this is temporary because the pulmonary circulations show vasoconstriction in hypoxic areas of the lung (hypoxic pulmonary vasoconstriction). In some cases, vasoconstriction can be inhibited by medication such as calcium channel blockers [20]. Currently, there is no literature regarding the exact incidence and risk factors that may cause and prevent this. In general, if there is a low destruction score and relatively high perfusion of the treatment target lobe, this may be a contributing factor to hypoxemia, especially if baseline oxygenation is already marginal. Furthermore, hypoxic pulmonary vasoconstriction may cause or alter pulmonary hypertension [20, 21]. In case of persistent hypoxemia after valve treatment, medication that may inhibit vasoconstriction can be discontinued. Furthermore, it may be necessary to remove the valves if there is no clinical improvement after a few days of using oxygen and rest [7]

LONG-TERM COMPLICATIONS AND REVISION BRONCHOSCOPY

After treatment, follow-up is important to monitor the treatment effect and presence of atelectasis or lung volume reduction of the treated lobe, lack of initial effect after treatment, or loss of beneficial effect during follow-up.

If there is no initial effect after treatment with valves, or if there is loss of initial lung volume reduction, a CT scan and a subsequent revision bronchoscopy is advised to inspect and replace dysfunctioning valves. Other indications for revision bronchoscopy include the presence of recurring infections and exacerbations, hemoptysis, chronic and invalidating cough [7]

Currently, there are few studies regarding the frequency and success of follow-up bronchoscopies. Gompelmann et al. performed a retrospective analysis in patients who were treated with endobronchial valves [22]. In 76 of 449 patients (17%) who were treated between 2005 and 2013, the valves were removed. The most important indication for valve removal was treatment failure in 65 of 76 patients (86%); other indications included post-obstruction pneumonia (9%) and hemoptysis (4%). During this bronchoscopy, granulation tissue formation was observed in 40% of the patients. Another study by Gompelmann et al. described the removal of valves in 63 of 256 patients (25%) who were treated between 2006 and 2013. There is probably overlap in these patient groups [23]

Roodenburg et al. performed an analysis of patients who were treated with endobronchial valves between September 2016 and September 2019 [24]. Of the 179 patients who were included in the analysis, 74 (41%) underwent at least one revision bronchoscopy. The indications were mostly loss of initial treatment effect (N=32, 54%), no significant lung volume reduction after initial treatment (N=23, 31%), and hemoptysis, hypoxemia, persistent cough, and valve expectoration. The endoscopic diagnosis was granulation tissue in most patients (N=39, 53%), secretions, valve migration, or untreated subsegment and possible collateral ventilation (despite negative Chartis). In most patients, valves were replaced during the bronchoscopy, but in 24 patients (13%), valves were removed permanently. Replacement of dysfunctioning valves led to an improvement in lung function.

No initial effect after treatment with valves

If there is no initial effect at first follow-up (no target lobe volume reduction at CT scan, no improvement of lung function, and no clinical benefit), it is important to review the indication for valve treatment and the technical aspects of the first procedure. There are several causes that need to be reconsidered. The most important causes are presence of collateral ventilation and incomplete lobar occlusion due to valve misplacement [7]. Other causes include extensive pleural adhesions, temporary shunting, and airway folding [7]

In case of collateral ventilation between the target lobe and the ipsilateral lobe(s), there will be persistent flow in the treatment target lobe, which will prevent significant lung volume reduction [7, 25, 26]. Before treatment, the presence of collateral ventilation can be predicted based on the fissure completeness score between lobes [27–29]. However, even with nearly complete fissures (>95%), there is still a significant proportion of patients who will have collateral ventilation and thus no treatment effect [27, 28]. Therefore, it is advised to perform a Chartis measurement before treatment with valves in most patients [27]. In case there is no effect, the possibility of the presence of collateral ventilation can be considered based on a careful review for possible fissure defects of the baseline CT scan and review of the performed Chartis measurement. A Chartis measurement may come with several challenges (mucus plugging of the Chartis catheter, low flow pattern); if this was the case during the procedure, the measurement could have been a false negative [9, 30–32]

The correct placement of valves may be challenging due to local anatomy or patient factors (e.g., edema may lead to an undersizing of the valves). Therefore, it is possible that during the procedure, valves are slightly displaced, small subsegments have been missed, or the sizing of valves is not optimal. Furthermore, valves may migrate (spontaneously or in case of suboptimal sizing or placement) [7, 18]. This leads to persistent air leakage along the valves into the target lobe, preventing lung volume reduction.

If there is no effect after treatment, and a revision bronchoscopy did not resolve this, removal of valves should be considered.

Loss of initial treatment effect

If there is loss of initial effect after treatment with valves, a CT scan can show the re-inflation of the treated lobe and loss of previously achieved lung volume reduction. In general, this is caused by an incomplete occlusion of the target lobe by the valves due to different causes, which allows air to pass through or alongside the valves.

This may be due to valve dysfunction, for example, as a result of extensive mucus impaction. Furthermore, there may be an incomplete occlusion of the airways due to migration or dislocation of the valve. Although valves may migrate to the ipsilateral lobe or even the contralateral lung, in most cases, the extent of valve migration is limited to minor changes of the original position [7]

The formation of granulation tissue is the main cause of valve dysfunction after EBV treatment [7, 24]. However, the exact mechanism regarding the formation of granulation tissue is not known. A relationship between bacterial colonization has been proposed, but Roodenburg et al. found no difference between patients with and without granulation tissue formation, and evidence for a key role of microorganisms in the formation of granulation tissue formation is minimal [24, 33]. Furthermore, mucus impaction or smoking relapse may cause valve dysfunction (Figure 14.2). Other possible causes include the release of damage-associated molecular patterns (DAMPs), repetitive movement of the valve against the bronchial mucosa, and patient-related factors such as genetic susceptibility [7, 24, 33]

Revision bronchoscopy

In most cases, it is advised to perform a CT scan before revision bronchoscopy because this can show an indication of the possible cause of complaints (e.g., valve displacement or valve positioning, pneumonia, airway kinking) (Figure 14.3) [7, 34]. During revision bronchoscopy, there are several options. First, it is important to thoroughly inspect and clean the airways and valves. A bronchial wash for culture is advised in general and specifically in case of recurrent infections or exacerbations and hemoptysis to guide antimicrobiological treatment.

In case of hemoptysis, this might well be due to granulation tissue formation around the valves, or sometimes to the adjacent wall, as proof of repetitive trauma of the opposing wall to a valve (Figure 14.3 and Figure 14.4) [7]. However, a total endobronchial view is advised to exclude other causes of hemoptysis

Signs of valves displacement can be found in case of loss of initial effect or no treatment effect at all. During revision bronchoscopy, evaluation of the position of each separate valve is recommended. In some cases, valve displacement is clear and easy to see during bronchoscopy. However, in case of severe granulation tissue formation, it can be very challenging to determine which valve is dysfunctional. If a valve is dysfunctioning, air will leak alongside the valve. This can be tested during bronchoscopy by flushing saline at the valve location and checking for air bubbles outside the valve, or to show that saline or air is easily passed alongside the valve or pushes it aside.

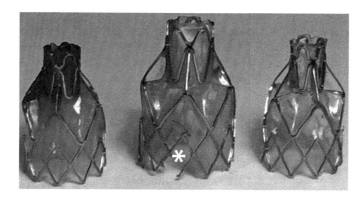

FIGURE 14.2 Example of a patient who was treated with endobronchial valves in the right lower lobe. After two years, there was an increase in dyspnea and loss of lung volume reduction. The subsequent bronchoscopy showed that due to a relapse in smoking, there is extensive soot on the valves and damage to the silicone part of the valve (*).

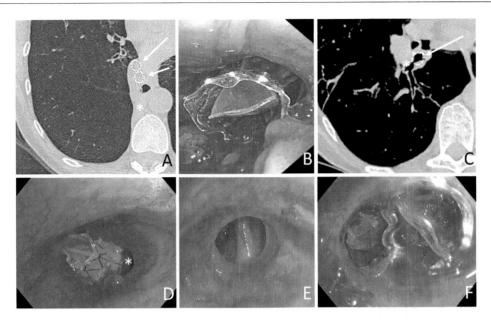

FIGURE 14.3 Revision after valve dislocation. This patient was treated eight years previously with endobronchial valves in the right lower lobe with a complete atelectasis at follow-up (A). (*Atelectasis of right lower lobe, arrows show two valves in situ.) Due to the increase of dyspnea, a CT scan was performed that showed loss of effect. A subsequent bronchoscopy revealed displacement of the valve in the superior segment of the right lower lobe (RB6), which was replaced with a new endobronchial valve (EBV 5.5LP) located in RB6 (B). However, after two months, the CT scan showed no atelectasis and there is dislocation of this valve (C). The valve (arrow) is located next to RB6 (*). It should have been located inside this segment. This was confirmed in a subsequent bronchoscopy that showed dislocation of this valve (D). The valve is now located above RB7-10 and RB6 is open (*). After removal of the valve (E), there is a clear view of RB6a and RB6b. Two new valves (EBV 4.0LP) were placed in RB6a and RB6b (F).

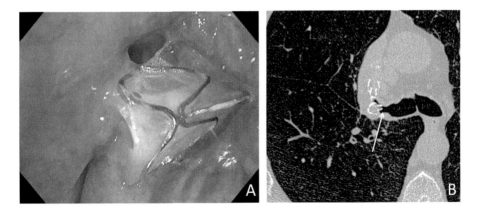

FIGURE 14.4 Evaluation of a patient with hemoptysis. (A) Endobronchial view of a patient with mild hemoptysis that shows a valve in the posterior segment of the right lower lobe (RB10), which shows that the proximal part of an endobronchial valve causes a granulation tissue reaction due to repetitive movement of the valve to the opposing airway wall. (B) A CT scan (axial view) shows the same endobronchial valve, showing the relationship of this valve to the adjacent wall (arrow).

Dysfunctional valves can be removed and replaced immediately during the same procedure. For replacement, the size of the valves can be adjusted if appropriate, and in general, it is advised to replace the valves more distally [7, 8]. Sometimes, the replacement of valves can be challenging due to severe granulation tissue formation. In this case, it is possible to remove the valves and wait 10–12 weeks before treatment to promote airway recovery. A course of corticosteroids and antibiotics before and after revision bronchoscopy can be prescribed to facilitate the ease of valve removal or airway healing after the removal of valves. Even though revision bronchoscopy can be successful, there is a chance of recurrence of granulation tissue formation. In case of severe granulation tissue formation or no successful revision, a VATS lobectomy can be considered, especially in cases where previous treatment with valves was successful.

CONCLUSION

In conclusion, treatment with valves is an important treatment option in patients with severe emphysema and hyperinflation. However, systematic and careful patient selection is important and a dedicated long term follow-up is crucial to monitor patients for possible side effects. The formation of granulation tissue is the cause of most long-term complications and loss of the initial treatment effects. A dedicated review of the CT scan and revision bronchoscopy are important to identify and manage most complications.

REFERENCES

1. Singh, D., et al., Global Strategy for the Diagnosis, Management, and Prevention of Chronic Obstructive Lung Disease: The GOLD Science Committee Report 2019. *Eur Respir J*, 2019. **53**(5).
2. Valipour, A., et al., Endobronchial Valve Therapy in Patients with Homogeneous Emphysema. Results from the IMPACT Study. *Am J Respir Crit Care Med*, 2016. **194**(9): p. 1073–1082.
3. Klooster, K., et al., Endobronchial Valves for Emphysema without Interlobar Collateral Ventilation. *N Engl J Med*, 2015. **373**(24): p. 2325–2335.
4. Kemp, S.V., et al., A Multicenter Randomized Controlled Trial of Zephyr Endobronchial Valve Treatment in Heterogeneous Emphysema (TRANSFORM). *Am J Respir Crit Care Med*, 2017. **196**(12): p. 1535–1543.
5. Criner, G.J., et al., A Multicenter Randomized Controlled Trial of Zephyr Endobronchial Valve Treatment in Heterogeneous Emphysema (LIBERATE). *Am J Respir Crit Care Med*, 2018. **198**(9): p. 1151–1164.
6. Criner, G.J., et al., Improving Lung Function in Severe Heterogenous Emphysema with the Spiration(R) Valve System (EMPROVE): A Multicenter, Open-Label, Randomized, Controlled Trial. *Am J Respir Crit Care Med* 2019.
7. Koster, T.D., et al., Endobronchial Valve Therapy for Severe Emphysema: An Overview of Valve-Related Complications and Its Management. *Expert Rev Respir Med*, 2020. **14**(12): p. 1235–1247.
8. Slebos, D.J., et al., Endobronchial Valves for Endoscopic Lung Volume Reduction: Best Practice Recommendations from Expert Panel on Endoscopic Lung Volume Reduction. *Respiration*, 2017. **93**(2): p. 138–150.
9. Klooster, K. and D.J. Slebos, Endobronchial Valves for the Treatment of Advanced Emphysema. *Chest*, 2020.
10. Darwiche, K., et al., Bronchoscopic Lung Volume Reduction with Endobronchial Valves in Low-FEV1 Patients. *Respiration*, 2016. **92**(6): p. 414–419.
11. Trudzinski, F.C., et al., Endoscopic Lung Volume Reduction Using Endobronchial Valves in Patients with Severe Emphysema and Very Low FEV1. *Respiration*, 2016. **92**(4): p. 258–265.
12. Trudzinski, F., et al., Endoscopic Lung Volume Reduction (eLVR) with Endobronchial Valves (EBV) in Patients with Hypercapnic Respiratory Failure. *Eur Respir J*, 2015. **46**.
13. Rötting, M., et al., Impact of Endoscopic Valve Therapy on Hypercapnia in Patients with Chronic Hypercapnic Failure Based on a Severe Lung Emphysema. *Eur Respir J*, 2020. **56**(Suppl. 64): p. 3777.

14. Li, S., et al., The REACH Trial: A Randomized Controlled Trial Assessing the Safety and Effectiveness of the Spiration(R) Valve System in the Treatment of Severe Emphysema. *Respiration*, 2019. **97**(5): p. 416–427.

15. Davey, C., et al., Bronchoscopic Lung Volume Reduction with Endobronchial Valves for Patients with Heterogeneous Emphysema and Intact Interlobar Fissures (the BeLieVeR-HIFi study): A Randomised Controlled Trial. *Lancet*, 2015. **386**(9998): p. 1066–1073.

16. van Dijk, M., et al., Expert Statement: Pneumothorax Associated with One-Way Valve Therapy for Emphysema: 2020 Update. *Respiration*, 2021: p. 1–10.

17. Egenod, T., et al., Two-Stage Bronchoscopic Endobronchial Valve Treatment Can Lead to Progressive Lung Volume Reduction and May Decrease Pneumothorax Risk. *Int J Chron Obstruct Pulmon Dis*, 2021. **16**: p. 1957–1965.

18. Fiorelli, A., et al., Complications Related to Endoscopic Lung Volume Reduction for Emphysema with Endobronchial Valves: Results of a Multicenter Study. *J Thorac Dis*, 2018. **10**(Suppl 27): p. S3315–S3325.

19. Klooster, K., et al., First in Human Experience of the Performance of the New 5.5-LP Size Zephyr Endobronchial Valve. *Respiration*, 2020. **99**(1): p. 50–55.

20. Ward, J.P.T. and I.F. McMurtry, Mechanisms of Hypoxic Pulmonary Vasoconstriction and Their Roles in Pulmonary Hypertension: New Findings for an Old Problem. *Curr Opin Pharmacol*, 2009. **9**(3): p. 287–296.

21. Sylvester, J.T., et al., Hypoxic Pulmonary Vasoconstriction. *Physiol Rev*, 2012. **92**(1): p. 367–520.

22. Gompelmann, D., et al., Endoscopic Valve Removal >180 Days since Implantation in Patients with Severe Emphysema. *Respiration*, 2018. **96**(4): p. 348–354.

23. Gompelmann, D., et al., Long-term Follow Up after Endoscopic Valve Therapy in Patients with Severe Emphysema. *Ther Adv Respir Dis*, 2019. **13**: p. 1753466619866101.

24. Roodenburg, S.A., et al., Revision Bronchoscopy After Endobronchial Valve Treatment for Emphysema: Indications, Findings and Outcomes. *Int J Chron Obstruct Pulmon Dis*, 2021. **16**: p. 1127–1136.

25. Herth, F.J., et al., Radiological and Clinical Outcomes of Using Chartis to Plan Endobronchial Valve Treatment. *Eur Respir J*, 2013. **41**(2): p. 302–308.

26. Koster, T.D. and D.J. Slebos, The Fissure: Interlobar Collateral Ventilation and Implications for Endoscopic Therapy in Emphysema. *Int J Chron Obstruct Pulmon Dis*, 2016. **11**: p. 765–773.

27. Klooster, K., et al., An Integrative Approach of the Fissure Completeness Score and Chartis Assessment in Endobronchial Valve Treatment for Emphysema. *Int J Chron Obstruct Pulmon Dis*, 2020. **15**: p. 1325–1334.

28. Koster, T.D., et al., Predicting Lung Volume Reduction after Endobronchial Valve Therapy Is Maximized Using a Combination of Diagnostic Tools. *Respiration*, 2016. **92**(3): p. 150–157.

29. de Oliveira, H.G., et al., Fissure Integrity and Volume Reduction in Emphysema: A Retrospective Study. *Respiration*, 2016. **91**(6): p. 471–479.

30. Gesierich, W., et al., Collapse Phenomenon during Chartis Collateral Ventilation Assessment. *Eur Respir J*, 2016. **47**(6): p. 1657–1667.

31. Welling, J.B.A., et al., Collateral Ventilation Measurement Using Chartis: Procedural Sedation vs General Anesthesia. *Chest*, 2019. **156**(5): p. 984–990.

32. Welling, J.B.A., et al., Temporary Right Middle Lobe Occlusion with a Blocking Device to Enable Collateral Ventilation Measurement of the Right Major Fissure. *Respiration*, 2020. **99**(6): p. 516–520.

33. Roodenburg, S.A., S.D. Pouwels, and D.J. Slebos, Airway Granulation Response to Lung-Implantable Medical Devices: A Concise Overview. *Eur Respir Rev*, 2021. **30**(161).

34. Koster, T.D., et al., Biodegradable Stent Placement for Airway Kinking after Bronchoscopic Lung Volume Reduction Treatment. *Ann Thorac Surg*, 2022. **113**(5): p. e375–e377.

Pulmonary Rehabilitation for COPD Patients

15

José R. Jardim

INTRODUCTION

Pulmonary rehabilitation is an individualized program offered to patients with chronic obstructive pulmonary disease (COPD) that aims to reduce dyspnea, increase day-to-day activities, and enhance quality of life. Initially, pulmonary rehabilitation (PR) was not a treatment strategy for patients with COPD because clinical improvement and structural muscle changes were not shown. In 1991, Casabury et al. demonstrated that patients with COPD should train using high loads; since then, this strategy has been considered a mandatory treatment for these patients. It has been shown that patients with COPD hospitalized due to a severe exacerbation and who started pulmonary rehabilitation within 90 days after discharge had lower mortality after one year than the patients who started rehabilitation after 90 days (7.3% versus 19.6%).[2] There is also an association between pulmonary rehabilitation and the reduction of rehospitalizations in patients with COPD.[3]

DEFINITIONS

Pulmonary rehabilitation

In 2013, the American Thoracic Society and the European Respiratory Society published a document on pulmonary rehabilitation and defined it as

> a comprehensive intervention based on a thorough patient assessment followed by patient tailored therapies that include, but are not limited to, exercise training, education, and behavior change, designed to improve

DOI: 10.1201/9781003251439-15

the physical and psychological condition of people with chronic respiratory disease and to promote the long-term adherence to health-enhancing behaviors.[4]

Physical activity

"Physical activity can be defined as any bodily movement produced by skeletal muscles that results in energy expenditure. Physical activity is a complex behavior that can be characterized by type, intensity, duration, patterns and symptom experience."[5]

Exercise

"Exercise is physical activity that is planned, structured, repetitive and purposeful. Physical activity also includes, but is not limited to, leisure-time, domestic and occupational activities."[5]

PULMONARY REHABILITATION INDICATION IN COPD

The physical limitations observed in a patient with COPD with a predominance of emphysema are closely linked to pulmonary hyperinflation. This condition is mainly related to reduced lung elastic recoil despite having a contribution of bronchial obstruction. During physical exertion, respiratory rate and tidal volume increase; however, the reduced lung elastic recoil hinders the full expiration before the next inspiration, resulting in remaining volume in the lungs. The repetition of this air retention leads to dynamic hyperinflation, which is added to the preexisting static hyperinflation. Dynamic hyperinflation imposes extra work on the inspiratory muscles, resulting in shortness of breath and respiratory discomfort. In addition, pulmonary hyperinflation may impair cardiac function. Moreover, exertional dyspnea limits the life of emphysematous patients with COPD, resulting in restricted efforts and a sedentary lifestyle. The exertional dyspnea, limitation of daily activities, and sedentary lifestyle result in a progressive descending spiral.[6-8] As a consequence of disease severity, emphysematous patients with COPD lose muscle mass due to their sedentary lifestyle and the ongoing systemic inflammatory process.[9]

Muscular alterations in patients with COPD can already manifest in the early stages of the disease.[10] Physical exercise enhances muscle capillarization, mitochondrial density, and oxidative capacity, and may accelerate the shift of type IIB fibers into type IIA fibers, which contain greater oxidative capacity.[11] A study demonstrated that physical exercise responds better to dyspnea, effort limitation, and quality of life than bronchodilators.[12]

PR should be recommended to patients with COPD at diagnosis, regardless of severity. Those with mild COPD must be instructed to maintain good physical condition to delay disease progression. In 2023, the American Thoracic Society (ATS) published *PR for Adults with Chronic Respiratory Disease*, a guideline based on six PICO questions (P = population, I = intervention, C = comparator, and O = outcome) and an extensive list of studies attesting that PR can improve dyspnea (Chronic Respiratory Disease Questionnaire, Transitional Dyspnea Index, and Medical Research Council), quality of life (Saint George Questionnaire), and exercise capacity (six-minute walk test, shuttle walk test, and peak work capacity).

The guideline also provides evidence that PR for patients with COPD recently hospitalized due to exacer bation reduces rehospitalizations and overall costs.[13]

Defining the Modern Pulmonary Rehabilitation

In 2021, the American Thoracic Society published the document *Defining the Modern Pulmonary Rehabilitation*, which addressed new pulmonary rehabilitation models, including telerehabilitation and home-based models (Tables 15.1 and 15.2).[14]

TABLE 15.1   Summary of the ATS document on PR (2021)

1. The definition of PR published in 2013 was maintained because it remains relevant.
2. The components of a PR program must come from clinical studies.
3. The components of the PR program can be adapted to local resources and health systems, and the needs, goals, and preferences of the patient can also be considered.
4. The future of PR will involve more options and greater customization.
5. Program customization should be based on a complete assessment.
6. The effectiveness and efficiency of the program must be regularly evaluated.
7. Alternative PR programs must be evaluated with the same standards as traditional rehabilitation centers.
8. The literature does not provide enough data to indicate which patients would best suit different rehabilitation models.
9. The success of a rehabilitation program should be assessed by the essential components or outcomes achieved.

TABLE 15.2   Components considered essential by ATS in modern PR

(a) Patient evaluation
1. Initial assessment conducted by a healthcare professional.
2. Exercise test during the initial assessment.
3. Field exercise test.
4. Measurement of quality of life.
5. Assessment of dyspnea.
6. Evaluation of nutritional status.
7. Assessment of occupational status.

(b) Program components
8. Endurance training.
9. Resistance training.

(c) Training method
10. Individually prescribed exercise program.
11. Exercise program with load individually adapted over time.
12. Presence of a healthcare professional with expertise in exercise prescription.

(d) Ensuring quality
13. Healthcare professionals are trained to provide the components of the described model.

GLOBAL EVALUATION OF THE COPD PATIENT

Ideally a PR center team should comprise a respirologist, physiotherapist, occupational therapist, nurse, social assistant, nutritionist, and psychologist, and each one should thoroughly evaluate the patient concerning their area.

Lung function

Spirometry assesses the severity of ventilatory impairment and the acute response to bronchodilators. Spirometry may also show the annual loss of lung function when repeated periodically. Patients with COPD and emphysema present a typical expiratory concave curve shape, demonstrating very low flows. Furthermore, by performing a cardiopulmonary test on a treadmill or cycle ergometer with continuous respiratory flow measurement, it is possible to evaluate the occurrence of dynamic hyperinflation.

The inspiratory peak flow may be obtained from the inspiratory loop. Patients with peak inspiratory flow over 60 liters/minute should not have difficulty inhaling medication from any device. However, this value must be interpreted cautiously as the inspiratory loop of the spirometry test is performed without resistance. In contrast, all inhaler devices present resistance to inspiratory flow. Airway resistance and conductance measurements indicate the degree of bronchoconstriction and may anticipate the response to bronchodilators. Patients with a predominance of emphysema may have normal airway resistance, contrary to bronchitis.

Patients with COPD and emphysema are typically hypoxemic but not hypercapnic, suggesting that they do not present alveolar hypoventilation. Therefore, arterial blood pH and gas values are essential for a comprehensive assessment. Blood oxygen pressure usually drops during exercise when COPD patients are exercising. Pulse oximetry is a simple test that reflects the ventilation-perfusion ratio while performing activities of daily living or during effort, such as walking, climbing stairs, carrying weight, or during a static walking test at a medical appointment. Nevertheless, lung diffusing capacity for carbon monoxide is a more accurate assessment for this variable.

Decreased respiratory muscle mass may increase dyspnea in patients with COPD and emphysema, requiring respiratory muscle training. Maximal inspiratory (MIP) and expiratory pressure (MEP) measurements can be obtained using handheld manovacuometers. However, low MIP and normal MEP values may indicate the shortening of inspiratory muscle fibers. Hand grip measurement also provides information about muscle strength mass and possible sarcopenia.

Physical capacity tests

The most used test worldwide for physical capacity is the six-minute walking test (6MWT). It should be performed in a 25 to 30 meter long space with the patient being stimulated to walk as fast as possible, and at the end of the test, the distance walked is measured. A walked distance of over 30 to 35 meters from baseline is considered as the minimal clinical important difference (MCDI) after any intervention.[15] The 6MWT performance reflects the overall exercise capacity as the test comprises ventilatory, cardiac, and muscle functions. Heart and respiratory rates and oximetry should be measured before and at the end of the test, which may give information about the effort of patients.[16]

The shuttle test is another test that may evaluate patients' physical capacity. It is performed with the patient walking up and down a ten meters long space with a progressively increased speed every minute. At the end of the test, the walked distance is measured. The most accurate test for physical capacity is the incremental cardiopulmonary test, but it requires technical expertise and specific and costly equipment. The test shows the systems that are contributing to patients' limitations: ventilatory, cardiac, or peripheral.

Functionality

The World Health Organization recommends that all patients should be evaluated on how they perform their activities of daily life to know the limits of each patient and how to prescribe a specific training program.

Psychology

It is not uncommon that patients with COPD may present symptoms and signals of anxiety and depression, usually because they feel themselves hopeless and/or feel they are a burden to their family. The Hospital Anxiety and Depression Scale is a simple, reliable, and quick tool to screen patients who should be referred for further investigation with a specialist.

Nutrition

Patients with COPD and predominantly emphysematous usually have lower weight and less muscle mass. Some of this muscle loss is due to systemic inflammation besides their sedentary life. Low muscle mass is associated with higher mortality in patients with COPD. Endurance and strength exercises are mandatory for these patients. Gain of muscle mass is enhanced by exercise, protein intake, and anabolics.[17] In case of male patients, prostate cancer must be ruled out before taking anabolics. Muscle mass may be quantified by anthropometry, bioelectrical impedance (BIA), or densitometry (dual-energy X-ray absorptiometry DEXA).[18]

Quality of life

Patients care more about their quality of life than lung function or cardiopulmonary test values. Quality of life is influenced by several factors, including income, freedom, climate, and own health status and of others; therefore, quality-of-life questionnaires have been redefined as health-related quality of life (HRQL) HRQL may be evaluated by questionnaires that have been developed to specifically look at a pulmonary disease (Saint George Respiratory, Chronic Respiratory Questionnaire) or generic questionnaires that may be applied to different diseases besides respiratory diseases (Short Form 36, Short Form 12). As these questionnaires are too long for routine use, they may be replaced by the COPD Assessment Test (CAT), an eight-question questionnaire that measures the impact of the disease on the patient.[19,20]

TRAINING PROGRAMS

A common finding in patients with COPD is a limitation in daily activities that require moderate/high capacity, like going up stairs or a low slope on a street, taking a shower, or even dressing up. In these situations, patients complain of breathlessness and/or muscle fatigue. These patients should be encouraged to follow a training program including strength and endurance exercises for upper and lower limbs.

Lower limb exercises

Lower limb training has been recognized as having 1A evidence by the American College of Chest Physicians (ACCP) and the American Thoracic Society/European Respiratory Society (ATS/ERS)[2] for its positive action on dyspnea, daily activities, and quality of life. No matter which muscle group is being trained, there are three specific requirements: intensity, duration, and frequency. *Intensity* is based on Casabury et al.'s study,[1] in 1991, which set the basis for the prescription of high load training after comparing two groups of patients with COPD trained with high and low load for eight weeks. Patients should be trained at 70–80% of maximal oxygen consumption tested in an incremental cardiopulmonary test, at 70–80% of the maximal heart rate obtained in a band or cycloergometer maximal test, or at a score of 5–6 on the Borg scale. *Duration* should last at least 30 minutes for each muscle group for oxidative metabolism to be activated. As for *frequency*, ideally, maximal results are reached with exercises being done every day, but patients should enjoy the exercises and not take them as boring and obligatory tasks. Patients may exercise four days a week, not necessarily on fixed days. Five minutes warm up and five minutes relaxing with a low load are recommended. Exercises may be performed on a cycloergometer or treadmill in a rehabilitation center being supervised by a multidisciplinary team. In case a rehabilitation center is not available, patients should conduct the walking exercise at home, in a park, or a community center

Upper limb exercises

It is considered that up to 80% of our daily activities are accomplished with some participation of the upper limbs. Muscles of the shoulder girdle carry a dual task: They have an antigravitational function, for instance, when the patient is holding a bag, lifting a cup, or storing an object on a high shelf; and they also have a ventilatory function, acting as accessory muscles when patients need to hyperventilate to carry out a heavy task. Upper limb training should follow the same rules concerning intensity, duration, and frequency. Arm cycle ergometry (ACE) is considered for many as the gold standard for upper limb exercises. However, ACE does not use all shoulder girdle muscles. Diagonal exercises, derived from Kabat's neuromuscular facilitation proprioceptive method, can use many of the shoulder girdle muscles. The exercise comprises two movements and they should be done with both arms (30 movements, twice) (Figure 15.1). Diagonal exercises seem to be more effective than ACE for maintaining better thoraco-abdominal synchrony and inducing fewer lung hyperinflations.[20] Hyperinflation is associated with respiratory discomfort and limited exercise endurance.[21–23] Exercises may be accomplished with halters, starting with 250 g and increasing by 250 g every two to three weeks up to the limit of the patient's capability.

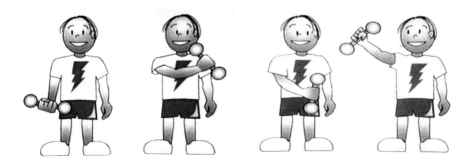

FIGURE 15.1   Diagonal exercises.

Strength exercises

After a long period when exercises were only aimed either for endurance or for strength, it is nowaday. recognized that both exercises should be included for patients with COPD. Strength exercises aim fo: gaining muscle mass and tone. Four simple and effective strength exercises are usually prescribed for the upper and lower limbs: (a) exercises for gran dorsal, brachioradialis, and rhomboid muscles; (b) vertica. supine for pectoralis major and anterior deltoid muscles; (c) abduction-adduction "pec deck" for the pec toralis major muscle; and (d) leg extensions for the quadriceps femoral muscle. Sessions should include two to three series of each exercise, with eight to ten repetitions of a load equivalent to 70% to 85% of . maximal load obtained through the one maximal repetition test.

Inspiratory muscle training

Inspiratory muscle training indication is restricted to COPD patients, and it is possible to show that inspi ratory muscle weakness is a contributing factor for their dyspnea. Flow or pressure generator equipmen should be used once a day for 15 minutes with 15–20 repetitions per minute.

When a rehabilitation center is not available

Globally, there are not enough rehabilitation centers in any country for all patients with COPD. In Lati. America, in 2021, there were 217 pulmonary rehabilitation centers, with four countries with no center eight with one or two centers; and just three countries with a large number of centers: Brazil (124). Argentina (45), and Colombia (24).[24] In this case, it is expected that the physician should be able to orien' the patient to a simple, low-cost, home-based pulmonary rehabilitation program adapted to real-life situ ations. Patients may walk for 40 minutes along a corridor at least 25 m long or be instructed to walk on the street or in a park (at a slow pace for the first five minutes, an increased pace for the next 30 minutes and a slow pace for the last five minutes), with a heart rate of 60–70% of the maximum heart rate for the subject's age (maximum heart rate = 220 − age). Subjects unable to walk for 40 minutes may start walking for 15 minutes during the first week and then gradually increase the time. After two weeks, the patients should do the walking exercise in the morning and go up and down a set of stairs in the afternoon. The stair exercise should gradually increase from five minutes a day to 15 minutes after two to three weeks After the second week, the patients should also add upper limb exercises, which may consist of diagona movements using up to 1 kg of load, for example, using an oil can.[25]

Education

It is essential for patients with COPD to understand their disease, how to manage their treatment, and the importance of complying with treatment. Education may be reached individually or in group discussion: (Table 15.3).

It is not expected that lung function or arterial blood oxygen will improve after an exercise program in patients with chronic lung disease. Exercise increases the muscle capillary network and mitochondria density as well as the change of glycolytic muscle fibers into oxidative metabolism. Chronic hypoxia ir patients with COPD induces adaptation processes resulting in the synthesis of hypoxia-inducible factor-▶ (HIF-1), responsible for oxygen homeostasis at cellular level, increasing the synthesis of proteins associ ated with angiogenesis through vascular endothelial growth factor (VEGF) and the erythropoietin.[26,27]

TABLE 15.3   Topics for discussion on education with the patients with COPD

1. Lung function
2. Importance of exercise
3. Where to exercise
4. Maintenance of exercise in post-rehabilitation
5. Oxygen therapy and benefits
6. Understanding medications
7. Correct use of inhaler medications
8. Pollution and smoking cessation
9. Energy conservation techniques for daily tasks
10. Breathing control strategies
11. Bronchial hygiene techniques
12. Recognizing exacerbations
13. Leisure, travel, and sexual activity
14. Panic and anxiety control, relaxation techniques, and stress management

REFERENCES

1. Casabury R, Patessio A, Ioli F, Zanaboni S, Donner CF, and Wasserman K. Reductions in exercise lactic acidosis and ventilation as a result of exercise training in patients with obstructive lung disease. *Amer Rev Respir Dis.* 1991;143. doi: 10.1164/ajrccm/143.1.9
2. Linden Auer K, Stefan MS, Pekow PS, Mazor KM, Priya P, Spitzer KA, Lagu TC, Quinn R, Pack RQ, Pinto-Plata VM, and ZuWallack R. Association between initiation of pulmonary rehabilitation after hospitalization for COPD and 1-year survival among medicare beneficiaries. *JAMA.* 2020;323(18):1813–1823. doi: 10.1001/jama.2020.4437
3. Stefan MS, Pekow PS, Priya A, ZuWallack R, Spitzer KA, Lagu TC et al. Association between initiation of pulmonary rehabilitation and rehospitalizations in patients hospitalized with chronic obstructive pulmonary disease. *Am J Respir Crit Care Med.* 2021;204:1015–1023.
4. Spruit MA, Singh SJ, Garvey C, ZuWallack R, Nici L, Rochester C et al. On behalf of the ATS/ERS Task Force on Pulmonary Rehabilitation. An official American Thoracic Society/European Respiratory Society statement: Key concepts and advances in pulmonary rehabilitation. *Amer J Respir Crit Care Med.* 2013.
5. Watz H, Pitta F, Rochester CL, Garcia-Aymerich J, ZuWallack R, Troosters T et al. An official European Respiratory Society statement on physical activity in COPD. *Eur Respir J.* 2014;44:1521–1537. doi: 10.1183/09031936.00046814
6. O'Donnell DE, and Webb KA. The major limitation to exercise performance in COPD is dynamic hyperinflation. *J Appl Physiol.* 2008;105:753–755; discussion 755 a 757.
7. Aliverti A, and Macklem PT. The major limitation to exercise performance in COPD is inadequate energy supply to the respiratory and locomotor muscles. *J Appl Physiol.* 2008;105:749–751; discussion 755 a 747.
8. Debigare R, and Maltais F. The major limitation to exercise performance in COPD is lower limb muscle dysfunction. *J Appl Physiol.* 2008;105:751–753; discussion 755 a 757.
9. Maltais F, Decramer M, Casaburi R, Barreiro E, Burelle Y, Debigaré R et al. An official American Thoracic Society/European Respiratory Society statement: Update on limb muscle dysfunction in chronic obstructive pulmonary disease. *Am J Respir Crit Care Med.* 2014;189(9):e15–e62. doi: 10.1164/rccm.201402-0373RD
10. Iamonti VC, Souza GF, Castro AAM, Porto EF, Cruz LGB, Colucci E, Colucci M, Sarmento A, Nascimento OA, and Jardim JR. Upper limb anaerobic metabolism capacity is reduced in mild and moderate COPD patients. *COPD.* 2022 May 20;19(1):265–273. doi: 10.1080/15412555.2022.2079485
11. Plotkin DL, Roberts MD, Haun CT, and Schoenfeld BJ. Muscle fiber type transitions with exercise training: Shifting perspectives. *Sports.* 2021;9:127. doi: 10.3390/sports9090127
12. Casabury R et al. JCOPD, pulmonary rehabilitation: Where we've succeeded and where we've failed. *COPD.* 2018;15(3):219–222. doi: 10.1080/15412555.2018.1503245

13. Rochester CL, Alison JA, Carli B, Jenkins AR, Cox NS et al. Pulmonary rahabilitation for adults with chronic respiratory disease. Thoracic society-An official American Practice Guideline. *Am J Respir Crit Car Med* 2023;208:e7–e27.

14. Holland AE, Cox NS, Houchen-Wolloff L, Rochester CL, Garvey C, ZuWallack R et al. Defining modern pulmonary rehabilitation an Official American Thoracic Society workshop report. *Ann Am Thorac Soc* 2021;18(5):e12–e29. doi: 10.1513/AnnalsATS.202102-146TH

15. Puhan MA, Mador MJ, Held U, Goldstein R, Guyatt GH, and Schunema HJ. Interpretation of treatment changes in 6-minute walk distance in patients with COPD. *Eur Respir J.* 2008;32:637–643. doi 10.1183/09031936.00140507

16. Casanova C, Celli BR, Barria P, Casas A, Cote C, de Torres JP, Lopez MV, Marin JM, Montes de Oca M Pinto-Plata V, Aguirre-Jaime A, and Jardim JR. The 6-min walk distance in healthy subjects: Reference standards from seven countries. *Eur Respir J.* 2010;37:150–156.

17. Ferreira IM, Verreschi IT, Nery LE, Goldstein RS, Zamel N, Brooks D, and Jardim JR. The influence of 6 months of oral anabolic steroids on body mass and respiratory muscles in undernourished COPD patients *Chest.* 1998 Jul;114(1):19–28. doi: 10.1378/chest.114.1.19

18. Lerário MC, Sachs A, Lazarettii MC, Saraiva IG, and Jardim JR. Body composition in patients with chronic obstrutive pulmonary disease: Which method to use in clinical practice. *Brit J Nutr.* 2006;96:86–92. doi 10.1079/BJN20061798

19. Jones PW, Harding G, Berry P, Wiklund I, Chen W-H, and Kline Leidy N. Development and first validation of the COPD Assessment Test. *Eur Respir J.* 2009;34:648–654.

20. Jardim JR, and Zillmer L. COPD Assessment Test: Rapid and easily applied test that promotes patient self management. *J Bras Pneumol.* 2014;39(4). doi: 10.1590/S1806-37132013000400001

21. Castro AAM, Porto EF, Feltrim MIZ, and Jardim JR. Asynchrony and hyperinflation in patients with chronic obstructive pulmonary disease during two types of upper limbs exercise. *Arch Bronconeumol* 2013;49(6):241–248.

22. Colucci M, Cortopassi F, Porto E, Castro A, Colucci E, Iamonti VC, Souza G, Nascimento O, and Jardim J. Upper Limb exercises using varied workloads and their association with dynamic hyperinflation in patient with COPD. *Chest.* 2010;138(1):39–46.

23. Porto EF, Castro AAM, Velloso M, Nascimento O, Dal Maso F, and Jardim JR. Exercises using the upper limbs hyperinflate COPD patients more than exercises using the lower limbs at the same metabolic demand *Monaldi Arch Chest Dis.* 2009;71(1):21–26.

24. Barreto GZ, Ivanaga IT, Chiavegato L, Gazzotti MR, Nascimento OA, and Jardim JR. Perspective of pulmonary rehabilitation centers in Latin America. *COPD.* 2021;18(4):401–405. doi: 10.1080/15412555.2021.193482

25. Pradella CO, Belmonte GM, Maia MN, Delgado CS, Luise AP, Nascimento OA, Gazzotti MR, and Jardim JR Home-based pulmonary rehabilitation for subjects with COPD: A randomized study. *Respir Care.* 2014. doi 10.4187/respcare.02994

26. Prabhakar NR, and Semenza GL. Adaptive and maladaptive cardiorespiratory responses to continuous and intermittent hypoxia mediated by hypoxia-inducible factors 1 and 2. *Physiol Rev.* 2012;92(3):967–1003. doi 10.1152/physrev.00030.2011

27. Semenza GL. Hypoxia-inducible factors in physiology and medicine. *Cell.* 2012;148(3):399–408. doi: 10.1016/j. cel

Results and Long-Term Follow-Up of Interventional Treatments for Lung Emphysema

Quality-of-Life Considerations

16

Alexey Abramov, Mark E. Ginsburg and Bryan P. Stanifer

INTRODUCTION AND BACKGROUND

Chronic pulmonary obstructive disease (COPD) is one of the most prevalent chronic respiratory diseases and the third leading cause of death worldwide ("WHO Global Health Estimates 2019" 2020; Vestbo et al. 2013). The most important risk factors for chronic respiratory diseases include tobacco use, exposure to indoor and outdoor pollutants, allergens, occupational exposures, poor nutrition, obesity, and physical inactivity ("WHO | Global Surveillance, Prevention and Control of Chronic Respiratory Diseases: A Comprehensive Approach" n.d.). Given our aging population and continuous exposure to risk factors, the incidence of chronic respiratory diseases is increasing worldwide. Indeed, a recent study on spatial and temporal global trends reports that chronic respiratory disease increased by 39% from 1990 to 2017 and was largely attributed to asthma and COPD (Xie et al. 2020).

While a comprehensive discussion of COPD pathophysiology is beyond the scope of this chapter, an overview of the relationship between risk factors and lung injury serves to illuminate the rationale behind historical and modern medical and surgical interventions. The etiology of COPD is an interaction of environmental influences, primary tobacco exposure, and genetic susceptibility (Li et al. 2018; Woodruff et al. 2016). Chronic inflammation leads to (1) narrowing of the small airways and (2) emphysematous

DOI: 10.1201/9781003251439-16

destruction of lung parenchyma and contributes to the progressive and irreversible limitation in airflow seen in COPD (Pauwels et al. 2001). Lung injury in COPD is associated with an imbalance of proteinases and anti-proteinases, coupled with oxidative stress induced by particle exposures and gases (Hogg 2004). As the resistance of small conducting airways increases, and/ or lung compliance increases due to lung injury, the volume of air that can be expired in one second $\left(FEV_1\right)$ and its ratio to forced vital capacity $\left(FEV_1 / FVC\right)$ decline. Post-bronchodilator FEV_1 and FEV_1 / FVC measurements inform clinicians to disease severity, as commonly assessed by the Global Initiative on Obstructive Lung Disease (GOLD) scoring system. Goals of managing COPD primarily include prevention of acute exacerbations, symptom relief, and slowing disease progression by improving lung function, overall health, exercise tolerance and quality of life (Adeloye et al. 2015). Staging disease severity plays an integral role in patient selection when considering appropriate interventions. COPD progression inevitably leads to severe dyspnea, and ultimately respiratory failure, which limits the patient's ability to perform activities of daily living and contributes to meaningful reductions in health-related quality-of-life measures (HRQOLs).

Figure 16.1 from the Genetic Epidemiology of COPD (COPDGene) study, an observational multi center longitudinal analysis of over 10,000 subjects, shows the complex interplay between patient char acteristics and exposures that drive disease progression. The impact of sex, race, and age have been well established and continue to be associated with a higher risk of poorer health outcomes. Female sex and African American (AA) race have been associated with an increased risk of acute episodes and may pres ent with more severe disease (Bowler et al. 2014; Han et al. 2011). Further, patients aged over 65 years old studied in the Evaluation of COPD Longitudinally to Identify Predictive Surrogate Endpoints (ECLIPSE) and GeneCOPD experienced worse lung function and exercise tolerance with more frequent use of long term oxygen therapy when compared with younger patients (Parulekar et al. 2017). Epidemiological

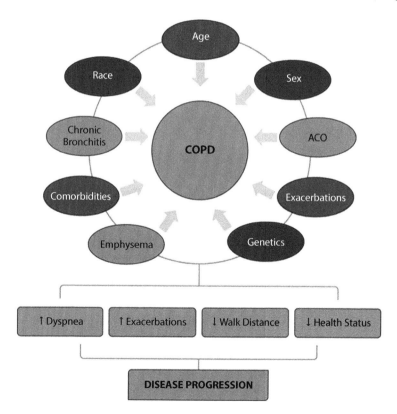

FIGURE 16.1 Complex and multifactorial influence of demographic characteristics, comorbidities, emphy-sema, chronic bronchitis, and genetics on the disease progression of COPD. ACO, asthma/COPD overlap (COPDGene https://www.ncbi.nlm.nih.gov/pmc/articles/PMC7198872/).

trends in COPD emerge as important considerations when evaluating patients for lung volume reduction interventions, with attention to relieving symptoms and improving heart-related quality-of-life measures.

Current effective medical therapies include pulmonary rehabilitation with exercise training, self-management education, smoking cessation, and pharmacologic therapies (Lindenauer et al. 2020). Smoking cessation is advised for all patients with underlying chronic respiratory diseases and typically consists of counseling in combination with varenicline, nicotine replacement therapy or bupropion (Tønnesen 2013; Stead et al. 2008; Panel 2008). Findings from the Lung Health Study of 5587 patients with mild COPD reported repeated smoking cessation for a period of five years was the most effective intervention in halting the progression of COPD, increasing survival, and reducing mortality (Simmons et al. 2005). Despite its efficacy in relieving dyspnea, significant patient and healthcare delivery barriers exist to widespread utilization of comprehensive pulmonary rehabilitation programs in the management of COPD, especially in rural communities (Spruit et al. 2013; McCarthy et al. 2015). When lifestyle modifications fail to stem disease progression, inhaled and oral pharmacologic therapies may be indicated (Calverley et al. 2007; Calzetta et al. 2020; Rehman et al. 2020). It should be noted that pulmonary rehabilitation and pharmacological interventions are not competitive but rather optimized to work together to result in more a successful outcome for the patient.

Despite receiving maximal medical therapy, most patients remain symptomatic and progress in their disease course. In properly selected patients, several surgical interventions have been found to be efficacious in relieving dyspnea and improving quality of life (Benditt 2006; Sciurba, Chandra, and Bon 2016; P. L. Shah et al. 2017; Herth et al. 2016). Indeed, a recent systematic review with meta-analysis on nearly 2800 patients supported the use of lung volume reduction intervention strategies in patients maximized on medical management (van Geffen et al. 2019). In this chapter, we describe the authors' approach to offering appropriate surgical interventions for patients with lung emphysema with attention to clinically meaningful outcomes and heart-related quality-of-life measures.

INDICATIONS FOR INTERVENTIONAL TREATMENT

Interventional treatments in lung emphysema are indicated when patients are refractory to maximal medical therapies as outlined by the GOLD guidelines and disease progression continues unabated. Lifestyle modifications with a multidisciplinary team-based approach include improved nutrition, definitive smoking cessation, and pulmonary rehabilitation with exercise training and/or a structured physical therapy program. Complementary pharmacological therapies include long-term oxygen therapy, inhaled long-acting bronchodilators, inhaled steroids, oral bronchodilators directed at decreasing airway resistance, antibiotics for acute and chronic infections, and preventive pneumococcal and influenza vaccinations (Calverley et al. 2007; Calzetta et al. 2020; Rawal and Yadav 2015). However, efficacy of multidisciplinary medical management in improving symptom management is stymied by the pathological hallmarks of COPD: irreversible air trapping from narrowing small airways and destroyed lung parenchyma. To date, there is no cure for this relentless disease. To address symptoms resulting from hyperinflation, several innovative surgical palliative procedures have been introduced with varying degrees of success (Naef 1997). More recently, breakthrough clinical trials evaluating the safety and efficacy of bronchoscopic or endoscopic lung volume reduction (ELVR) and operative lung volume reduction surgery (LVRS) have been conducted (Gompelmann, Sarmand, and Herth 2017; National Emphysema Treatment Trial Research Group 2003; Ginsburg et al. 2016).

Patients who remain highly symptomatic despite receiving optimal medical therapy typically stand to benefit the most from lung volume reduction interventions with endoscopic or minimally invasive operative approaches. Patients for consideration should have definitively quit smoking, completed a pulmonary rehabilitation and/or currently be participating in a structured physical therapy program, and maximized pharmacological therapy (Herth et al. 2017). Surgical evaluation includes a complete history and physical exam with lung function measurements with plethysmography, a multidetector computed tomography (MDCT) scan of the thorax, a six-minute walk test (6MWT), and cardiac risk stratification. Cardiovascular function should be assessed in consultation with a cardiologist with experience managing patients with COPD and routinely includes an echocardiogram to exclude the diagnosis of pulmonary hypertension. When an elevated right ventricular systolic pressure above 50 mm Hg is identified, a right heart catheterization should be performed. Properly selected patients with pulmonary hypertension may still be considered for endobronchial valve (EBV) placement after multidisciplinary discussion at experienced high-volume centers (Eberhardt et al. 2015).

Based on our center's experience and best available data, patients with severe and very severe airflow obstruction (i.e., GOLD Stage 3, 4, FEV_1 20–45%) who are highly symptomatic (grades C and D; modified Medical Research Council [mMRC] dyspnea score ≥ 2 , hyperinflation, i.e., residual volume [RV] $\geq 175\%$ or RV/total lung capacity ≥ 0.58); reduced six-minute walk distance (100–500 m) should be considered for lung volume reduction interventions. Acknowledging increased risks of post-operative mortality and morbidity, properly selected patients with an $FEV_1 \leq 20\%$ may still be considered for ELVR after multidisciplinary discussion. In these particularly difficult cases, patients are especially encouraged to clarify goals of care with their healthcare team.

HISTORY OF LUNG VOLUME REDUCTION SURGERY FOR EMPHYSEMA

With the advent of modern anesthetics and antiseptic surgical technique, mid-20th century surgeon scientists pioneered innovative and sometimes curious procedures for patients with diffuse lung emphysema. A glance to the past offers an opportunity here to better appreciate the evolution of lung volume reduction surgery and state-of-the-art surgical management. From an anatomic perspective, early approaches favored the chest wall, pleura, major airways, autonomous nervous system, or the lung parenchyma. As the lungs were clearly observed to be overinflated, initial operative techniques attempted to compress the lungs with a thoracoplasty or phrenicectomy. Conversely, others sought to encourage greater lung excursion with a costochondrectomy (Naef 1997). Predictably, both approaches failed to provide therapeutic benefit, and in fact worsened dyspnea.

In 1954, Nissen performed a tracheoplasty at the tracheobronchial bifurcation to manage expiratory airway collapse by suturing interpositional bone grafts, and later using a polytetrafluoroethylene prosthesis (Gore-Tex; W.L. Gore and Assoc, Flagstaff, AZ) (Nissen 1954). Further attempts to slow disease progression with surgery of the autonomous nervous system were with sympathectomy, vagotomy, stellate gangliectomy, and plexectomy in the 1940s and early 1950s (Reinhoff 1938; Blades, Beattie, and Elia 1950).

The term "lung volume reduction" is relatively modern when compared with its storied history dating to the early 1930s, when intracavity suction and bullectomy were performed on patients with extensive tuberculous cavities (Head and Avery 1949). The modern concept and technique of lung volume reduction is commonly credited to Otto Charles Brantigan (1904–1981), and later rediscovered and surgically refined by Joel Cooper in the mid-1990s. Brantigan presented data from his surgical practice at the 1958 symposium on emphysema in Aspen, Colorado. His technique of resecting the most distended and functionless areas of lung parenchyma was intended to reestablish what Brantigan understood to be the proper relationship between chest cavity and lung volume. By resecting diseased tissue, Brantigan hoped to encourage the re-expansion of unexploited but potentially functional lung (Brantigan, Mueller, and Kress 1959). The audience's reception of Brantigan's experience was, in a word, critical. Ultimately, his defense of resecting lung parenchyma in a disease understood to be characterized by relentless lung destruction was not fully understood or appreciated for decades. Indeed, nearly four decades later, Joel Cooper, a pioneering lung transplant surgeon, revisited Brantigan's technique and viewed lung volume reduction as a valuable and favorable alternative or bridge to lung transplantation for patients in his practice (Cooper et al. 1996).

ENDOSCOPIC LUNG VOLUME REDUCTION TREATMENTS

Over the course of the last decade, several innovative endoscopic interventions have been introduced to address symptom relief and are geared toward improving HRQOL measures in patients with severe lung emphysema. And, for appropriately selected patients, minimally invasive ELVR approaches have shown considerable promise (Gompelmann, Sarmand, and Herth 2017). While the surgical approach to LVRS is discussed later in this chapter, the fundamental physiologic principles underlying the LVRS procedure are equally relevant to ELVR. Table 16.1 provides a summary of techniques and goals of endoscopic therapeutic modalities, as well as notable physiologic considerations. Indeed, several ELVR techniques mimic the attempt in LVRS to correct perturbed respiratory mechanics. Targeted lung denervation (TLD) is a novel bronchoscopic intervention for selective ablation of parasympathomimetic innervation of the airways, with a desired effect similar to anticholinergic medications that remain under continued investigation (Slebos et al. 2015; Pison et al. 2021). The remainder of this section will examine two established endoscopic lung volume reduction techniques: (1) endobronchial valves and (2) endobronchial coils.

Endobronchial valves

Intervention with lung volume reduction endoscopic valve (LVRV) therapy involves the placement of a valve inside the bronchi to regulate airflow. The mechanics of the one-way valve permits flow of air out from a

TABLE 16.1   Interventional pulmonology in chronic obstructive pulmonary disease

ENDOSCOPIC TECHNIQUE	AIM	MECHANISM OF ACTION	DEGREE OF REVERSIBILITY	DEPENDENCE OF COLLATERAL VENTILATION
Endoscopic valve therapy	Lung volume reduction	Inducing lobar atelectasis	Reversible	Dependent
Endoscopic coil implantation	Lung volume reduction, improvement of lung elastic recoil	Leading to parenchymal compression	Partial irreversible	Independent
Polymeric lung volume reduction	Lung volume reduction	Inducing inflammatory reaction	Irreversible	Independent
Bronchoscopic thermal vapor ablation	Lung volume reduction	Inducing inflammatory reaction	Irreversible	Independent
Targeted lung denervation	Sustainable bronchodilation	Ablation of parasympathetic pulmonary nerves	Irreversible	Independent

Gompelmann et al. Current Opinion in Pulmonary Medicine 23(3):261–268, May 2017.

lobe's alveoli during expiration but prevents air inflow to the distal air spaces during inspiration. The lobe fo therapy (i.e., the most emphysematous lobe) is identified with a MDCT with specialized software. Attentio to interlobar collateral ventilation is essential as only those patients without collateral ventilation will benef from this intervention (Sciurba, Chandra, and Bon 2016; Herth et al. 2012). MDCT allows proper visualiza tion of the fissures and greater than 90% completeness on at least one axis is generally considered acceptabl to exclude collateral ventilation. An alternative methodology for assessing collateral ventilation has bee described using a catheter-based approach (Pulmonx, Inc., Neuchatel, Switzerland) by inflating a balloon i the lobe of interest and measuring the reduction in airflow (Schuhmann et al. 2015). Commercially availabl endobronchial (Zephyr, Pulmonx, Inc., Neuchatel, Switzerland) and intrabronchial (Spiration, Olympus Tokyo, Japan) valves differ in sizes but perform similarly.

The result of proper LVRV placement inside the bronchi is target lobar volume reduction (TLVR) principally by iatrogenic atelectasis. Outcomes from more than seven randomized controlled trials (RCTs and retrospective observational studies are now available for examination. The Euro-VENT trial dem onstrated promising results with an FEV_1 improvement of 26%±24% and 6MWT by 22%±38% in th intervention group (Herth et al. 2012). More recently, the Endobronchial Valve Therapy in Patients wit Homogenous Emphysema (IMPACT) study revealed patients assigned to the intervention had an FEV improvement of 13.7%±28.2% at the three-month timepoint. Post-procedure, the most common complica tion of EBV therapy is pneumothorax, reported at a rate of 18–26% (Valipour et al. 2016; Herzog et al 2015; van Geffen et al. 2019). Small studies with long-term survival data in patients treated with EBV als show a potential survival benefit (Hopkinson et al. 2011; Garner et al. 2016). In summary, LVRV present a viable therapeutic option for appropriately selected patients with severe emphysema with absent col lateral ventilation (Figure 16.2).

Endobronchial coils

The implantation of lung volume reduction endobronchial coils (LVRC) with a bronchoscope and fluoroscopi guidance may be performed unilaterally, or more commonly bilaterally, over the course of two separate proce dures. The technique employs commercially available LVR coils (Lung Volume Reduction Coils, PneumRx Inc., Mountain View, CA, USA) to reduce the size of damaged lobar parenchymal tissue. Coil lobar com pression achieves TLVR by reducing hyperinflation, increases elastic recoil, and redirects preferential airflow filling from injured tissue to healthier tissue. Briefly, the procedure is performed as follows: First, the airway is measured with a guidewire and fluoroscopic markers, the operator pulls the catheter back, and deploys th nitinol coils by releasing the forceps. Target lobes for intervention are identified by MDCT imaging. LVR therapy is not dependent on absent collateral ventilation (as discussed in the LVRV procedure) (Kontogianni e al. 2014). Health-related quality-of-life outcomes, including an improved FEV_1 and 6MWT, come from thre RCTs and more retrospective observational cohort studies performed in patients with heterogenous emphysem with incomplete fissures. The Effect of Endobronchial Coils vs. Usual Care on Exercise Tolerance in Patient with Severe Emphysema (RENEW) trial randomized 315 patients and reported 7% improvement in media FEV_1 and a 6MWT of 10.3 meters between study groups (Sciurba et al. 2016). Additional studies corroborate these findings and supported LVRC in properly selected patients with more severe disease: lower 6MWT, lowe FEV_1, and larger residual volumes and total lung capacities. In summary, EVRC may be offered in experi enced centers as a feasible intervention for patients with severe emphysema, with special attention to those wit collateral ventilation. As we await longer term survival data, clinical outcomes from this novel interventio suggest improved exercise tolerance and lung function (Figure 16.3).

Operative interventions

In the mid-1990s, LVRS was reestablished by Cooper as an effective procedure for patients with end-stag emphysema (Cooper et al. 1996). The operative technique confronts the destructive pathophysiology o

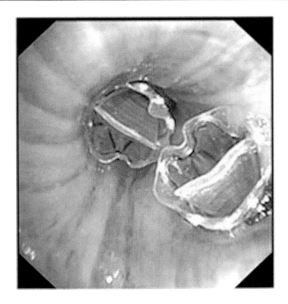

FIGURE 16.2 Interventional pulmonology in chronic obstructive pulmonary disease (Gompelmann et al. *Current Opinion in Pulmonary Medicine* 23(3):261–268, May 2017).

COPD head-on to correct the profound aberrations in respiratory mechanics. Overexpansion of distal air spaces leads to hyperinflation, which is observed directly in the operative field or radiographic studies and quantified by pulmonary function tests. Clinically, progressive increases in thoracic volume contribute to diaphragmatic dysfunction, leading to increased work of breathing, dyspnea, and exercise intolerance. Here we discuss operative approaches toward palliating this incurable disease. First, we make mention of a relatively rare but fascinating disease pathology of giant bullous emphysema and later focus our attention on the LVRS procedure and its durable impact on improving patient-centered health-related quality of outcomes.

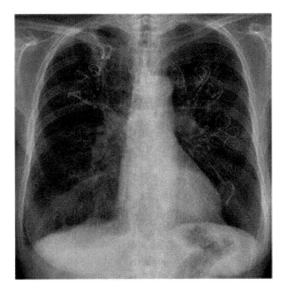

FIGURE 16.3 Interventional pulmonology in chronic obstructive pulmonary disease (Gompelmann et al. *Current Opinion in Pulmonary Medicine* 23(3):261–268, May 2017).

Giant bullous emphysema

A bulla is defined as an air-filled space measuring 1 cm or greater in diameter within the lung parenchyma. In rare circumstances, one or several bullae may enlarge to a point where they occupy more than a third of the hemithorax, and this disease is termed giant bullous emphysema (GBE). As the patient inspires, airflow is preferentially directed to fill this highly compliant reservoir. As air fills into the bulla and progressively expands its size, giant bulla overdistention causes normal healthy surrounding lung parenchyma to collapse (Morgan et al. 1989; Ting, Klopstock, and Lyons 1963). Resultant hyperinflation limits gas exchange and contributes to the already familiar respiratory symptoms of dyspnea and exercise intolerance. Limited case series report GBE complications of pneumothorax, prolonged air leaks, and infection or hemorrhage that warrants urgent surgical intervention.

Demographics of patients with GBE suggest a strong association between tobacco exposure and underlying COPD (Krishnamohan et al. 2014). Indeed, in a 12-year retrospective observational cohort study conducted at the Mayo Institute from 1988 to 2010, only 63 patients underwent treatment for this disease (Krishnamohan et al. 2014). Since the late 1940s, many pioneering surgeons have proposed surgical interventions for GBE, namely Monaldi's two-stage endocavitary aspiration (Monaldi 1947), Brompton's one-stage endocavitary aspiration with sclerosis and pleurodesis (S. S. Shah and Goldstraw 1994), plication (BENFIELD et al. 1966), and bullectomy and lobectomy (Laros et al. 1986; Pearson and Ogilvie 1983; FitzGerald et al. 1974). Today, GBE is commonly approached with video-assisted thoracic surgery (VATS) or open thoracotomy to perform a bullectomy or lobectomy, and less frequently, a bulla plication (Krishnamohan et al. 2014). The most common post-operative complications of bullectomy or lobectomy for GBE include persistent air leaks, atrial fibrillation, and pneumonia, and reassuringly operative mortality (3–7.3%) is low (Krishnamohan et al. 2014; Palla et al. 2005).

Most patients with GBE present with dyspnea and exercise intolerance; these symptoms emerge as the principal considerations for patient-centered quality-of-life measures. Pre-operatively, patients are encouraged to undertake a pulmonary rehabilitation program, when possible. Work-up for surgical intervention in GBE includes confirmatory radiographic imaging with MDCT of nonfunctioning bullae with compression of the normal lung that is amenable to a surgical intervention, and routine pulmonary function testing. Ideal surgical candidates who stand to benefit the most are patients with localized disease and vascular crowding, compression of otherwise healthy normal lung parenchyma, and an FEV_1 less than half of their predicted value. In the Mayo Clinic series, over 70% of patients experienced resolution of their symptoms or substantial improvement in their perceived quality of life post-surgery (Krishnamohan et al. 2014). Retrospective observational studies report that patients with severe reductions in FEV_1 and those with underlying severe COPD less than 40% did not benefit considerably from bullectomy (Palla et al. 2005; Gunstensen and McCormack 1973; Nakahara et al. 1983). In summary, symptomatic patients with giant bullous emphysema and favorable pre-operative criteria should be offered a bullectomy or lobectomy with VATS or open thoracotomy, as determined by surgeon preference.

Lung volume reduction surgery

Our up-to-date and enriched understanding of COPD led to a warmer reception when Cooper reintroduced his modernized LVRS technique in 1996. Advances from translational bench-side to bedside research demonstrated that COPD pathophysiology is not solely characterized by relentless and irreversible lung parenchymal destruction, but also exacerbated by unfavorable airflow mechanics that exacerbate existing ventilation to perfusion mismatches. As air is preferentially directed toward highly compliant distal air spaces with limited capacity for diffusion, healthier lung tissue still capable of efficient gas exchange participates in respiration less. The LVRS procedure expanded the lung surgeon's armamentarium and focused our attention on optimizing gas exchange in these untapped respiratory units.

Pre-operative work-up for LVRS includes a full functional and radiographic assessment with PFTs, MDCT and quantitative perfusion scan, 6MWT, and cardiac risk stratification. Similar to other interventions, patients are maximized medically according to GOLD guidelines (Vestbo et al. 2013)

Multidisciplinary COPD care programs at experienced centers have been shown to effectively optimize pre-operative therapies, reduce operative risk with risk stratification, and improve post-operative follow-up care (McCarthy et al. 2015).

The procedure is classically described as a median sternotomy or bilateral thoracotomy approach followed by serial resection of grossly abnormal hyperinflated peripheral wedges with a linear stapler with the goal of excising damaged and nonfunctional lung parenchyma (Cooper et al. 1996). More recently, safe and effective minimally invasive VATS techniques have also been described (Ginsburg et al. 2016). Using a left-sided double-lumen endotracheal tube provides isolated ventilation to either lung, and a thoracic epidural catheter reduces the amount of narcotics administered to permit extubation at the end of most cases. Post-operatively, thoracostomy tubes are kept water sealed, when possible, to mitigate against excessive suction that introduces further risk for developing prolonged air leaks. The most common complications following LVRS are prolonged air leak, pneumothorax, and hemorrhage. Cooper's published experience on 150 patients reported a 4% all-cause operative mortality at 90 days and actuarial survive to 93% at one year and 92% at two years (Cooper et al. 1996).

In response to the rapid uptake of LVRS in centers as part of end-stage COPD management, the National Emphysema Treatment Trial (NETT) was conducted to rigorously evaluate the safety and efficacy of LVRS. The multicenter trial enrolled 1218 patients with heterogenous and homogenous forms of emphysema. The patients were randomized to LVRS or continued medical management. The primary outcomes of mortality and maximal exercise capacity were shown two years after randomization (National Emphysema Treatment Trial Research Group 2003). Results from NETT show that patients who underwent surgery were more likely to have improved exercise tolerance. Further, the trial clarified that appropriately selected patients with upper-lobe emphysema considerably benefited from operative intervention. The trial determined that patients with other variants of emphysema did not considerably benefit from the LVRS procedure. Long-term analysis to five years after randomization also supported mid-term study results and showed durable health-related quality-of-life benefits to patients with upper-lobe predominant emphysema (Naunheim et al. 2006).

After the discouraging results of NETT, adoption of LVRS decreased in centers in the United States. While the trial was well intentioned to examine the treatment effect of LVRS, critics contend that randomizing patients with homogenous emphysema, a variant of disease least likely to benefit from surgical intervention introduced selection bias. Further, the trial was carried out prior to technical refinements, such as minimally invasive approaches with improved clinical outcomes. The decline of LVRS procedures was further compounded by patients seeking less invasive endoscopic alternatives. And while less endoscopic interventions such as LVRV appeared less risky, larger studies with a longer follow-up demonstrated that LVRV was associated with higher mortality than LVRS. Indeed, a recent single-institution ten-year experience retrospective study on 91 patients undergoing LVRS reported 0% surgical mortality at six months, survival of 78% at five years, and considerable improvements in FEV_1 and exercise tolerance (Ginsburg et al. 2016). Following this was the largest LVRS series to date, with 111 patients. The authors report six-month and one-year mortality of 0% and 1%, respectively (Stanifer and Ginsburg 2018). Virtually all functional outcomes improved and the 6MWT remained improved at five years as well. These data, among other reports from high-volume centers, support that LVRS is an effective procedure in properly selected patients that can be safely performed with a minimally invasive VATS approach at experienced centers (van Geffen et al. 2019).

QUALITY-OF-LIFE CONSIDERATIONS

Lung emphysema is a progressive, relentless, and debilitating disease without a cure. Clinically, most patients present with dyspnea and exercise intolerance, which profoundly affects their ability to perform activities of daily living. Multidisciplinary approaches toward medical management with smoking cessation, pulmonary rehabilitation with structured physical therapy programs, and pharmacological therapies with timely vaccinations have been proven to be effective in slowing disease progression. However, disease progression with irreversible destruction of delicate gas exchange units in the lung parenchyma continues unabated. Lung volume reduction interventions, such as LVRS, geared to preferentially redirecting airflow toward available healthier tissues and optimizing gas exchange have shown durable clinical benefits and improved quality-of-life scores (van Geffen et al. 2019). While endoscopic techniques such as LVRV offer patients relatively less operative risk than LVRS, long-term quality-of-life and survival benefits appear to be inferior when compared with surgical intervention at this time (Garner et al. 2016; Stanifer and Ginsburg 2018; van Geffen et al. 2019). Large series with long-term follow-ups at experienced surgical centers demonstrate that operative interventions in properly selected patients offer considerable returns in terms of quality-of-life and survival benefits (Stanifer and Ginsburg 2018).

Meaningful interventions, be they endoscopic or operative, derive value from the direct improvement of measurable health-related quality-of-life outcomes. Patient-reported tools such as the disease-specific St. George Respiratory Questionnaire (SGRQ) and the genetic EuroQol Five-Dimension Health Utility Questionnaire (EQ-5D) are designed to assess a patient's health status and inform on the efficacy of various interventions in large clinical trials, which lay the foundation for further innovation and improvements in global population health (Meguro et al. 2007; Ringbaek et al. 2008).

REFERENCES

Adeloye, Davies, Stephen Chua, Chinwei Lee, Catriona Basquill, Angeliki Papana, Evropi Theodoratou, Harish Nair, et al. 2015. "Global and Regional Estimates of COPD Prevalence: Systematic Review and Meta-Analysis." *Journal of Global Health* 5 (2): 020415. https://doi.org/10.7189/jogh.05-020415.

Benditt, Joshua O. 2006. "Surgical Options for Patients with COPD: Sorting Out the Choices." *Respiratory Care* 51 (2): 173–82.

Benfield, John R., Edna M. Cree, John R. Pellett, Robert Barbee, John T. Mendenhall, and Robert C. Hickey. 1966. "Current Approach to the Surgical Management of Emphysema." *Archives of Surgery* 93 (1): 59–70. https://doi.org/10.1001/archsurg.1966.01330010061009.

Blades, Brian, Edward J. Beattie, and William S. Elias. 1950. "The Surgical Treatment of Intractable Asthma." *Journal of Thoracic Surgery* 20 (4): 584–97. https://doi.org/10.1016/S0096-5588(20)31686-X.

Bowler, Russell P., Victor Kim, Elizabeth Regan, André A. A. Williams, Stephanie A. Santorico, Barry J. Make, David A. Lynch, et al. 2014. "Prediction of Acute Respiratory Disease in Current and Former Smokers with and without COPD." *Chest* 146 (4): 941–50. https://doi.org/10.1378/chest.13-2946.

Brantigan, Otto C., Eugene Mueller, and Milton B. Kress. 1959. "A Surgical Approach to Pulmonary Emphysema." *American Review of Respiratory Disease* 80 (1P2): 194–206. https://doi.org/10.1164/arrd.1959.80.1P2.194.

Calverley, Peter M. A., Julie A. Anderson, Bartolome Celli, Gary T. Ferguson, Christine Jenkins, Paul W. Jones, Julie C. Yates, Jørgen Vestbo, and TORCH investigators. 2007. "Salmeterol and Fluticasone Propionate and Survival in Chronic Obstructive Pulmonary Disease." *The New England Journal of Medicine* 356 (8): 775–89. https://doi.org/10.1056/NEJMoa063070.

Calzetta, Luigino, Beatrice Ludovica Ritondo, Maria Gabriella Matera, Mario Cazzola, and Paola Rogliani. 2020. "Evaluation of Fluticasone Propionate/Salmeterol for the Treatment of COPD: A Systematic Review." *Expert Review of Respiratory Medicine* 14 (6): 621–35. https://doi.org/10.1080/17476348.2020.1743180.

Cooper, Joel D., G. Alexander Patterson, R. Sudhir Sundaresan, Elbert P. Trulock, Roger D. Yusen, Mary S. Pohl, and Stephen S. Lefrak. 1996. "Results of 150 Consecutive Bilateral Lung Volume Reduction Procedures in Patients with Severe Emphysema." *The Journal of Thoracic and Cardiovascular Surgery* 112 (5): 1319–30. https://doi.org/10.1016/S0022-5223(96)70147-2.

Eberhardt, Ralf, Vasiliki Gerovasili, Konstantina Kontogianni, Daniela Gompelmann, Nicola Ehlken, Felix J. F. Herth, Ekkehard Grünig, and Christian Nagel. 2015. "Endoscopic Lung Volume Reduction with Endobronchial Valves in Patients with Severe Emphysema and Established Pulmonary Hypertension." *Respiration* 89 (1): 41–48. https://doi.org/10.1159/000368369.

FitzGerald, Muiris X., Patrick J. Keelan, David W. Cugell, and Edward A. Gaensler. 1974. "Long-Term Results of Surgery for Bullous Emphysema." *The Journal of Thoracic and Cardiovascular Surgery* 68 (4): 566–87. https://doi.org/10.1016/S0022-5223(19)39855-1.

Garner, Justin, Samuel V. Kemp, Tudor P. Toma, David M. Hansell, Michael I. Polkey, Pallav L. Shah, and Nicolas S. Hopkinson. 2016. "Survival after Endobronchial Valve Placement for Emphysema: A 10-Year Follow-Up Study." *American Journal of Respiratory and Critical Care Medicine* 194 (4): 519–21. https://doi.org/10.1164/rccm.201604-0852LE.

Geffen, Wouter H. van, Dirk-Jan Slebos, Felix J. Herth, Samuel V. Kemp, Walter Weder, and Pallav L. Shah. 2019. "Surgical and Endoscopic Interventions That Reduce Lung Volume for Emphysema: A Systemic Review and Meta-Analysis." *The Lancet Respiratory Medicine* 7 (4): 313–24. https://doi.org/10.1016/S2213-2600(18)30431-4.

Ginsburg, Mark E., Byron M. Thomashow, William A. Bulman, Patricia A. Jellen, Beth A. Whippo, Cody Chiuzan, Shing Lee, Dan Bai, and Joshua Sonett. 2016. "The Safety, Efficacy, and Durability of Lung-Volume Reduction Surgery: A 10-Year Experience." *The Journal of Thoracic and Cardiovascular Surgery* 151 (3): 717–24.e1. https://doi.org/10.1016/j.jtcvs.2015.10.095.

Gompelmann, Daniela, Nilab Sarmand, and Felix J. F. Herth. 2017. "Interventional Pulmonology in Chronic Obstructive Pulmonary Disease." *Current Opinion in Pulmonary Medicine* 23 (3): 261–68. https://doi.org/10.1097/MCP.0000000000000373.

Gunstensen, J., and R. J. McCormack. 1973. "The Surgical Management of Bullous Emphysema." *The Journal of Thoracic and Cardiovascular Surgery* 65 (6): 920–25.

Han, MeiLan K., Douglas Curran-Everett, Mark T. Dransfield, Gerard J. Criner, Lening Zhang, James R. Murphy, Nadia N. Hansel, et al. 2011. "Racial Differences in Quality of Life in Patients with COPD." *Chest* 140 (5): 1169–76. https://doi.org/10.1378/chest.10-2869.

Head, Jerome R., and Edward E. Avery. 1949. "Intracavitary Suction (Monaldi) in the Treatment of Emphysematous Bullae and Blebs." *Journal of Thoracic Surgery* 18 (6): 761–76. https://doi.org/10.1016/S0096-5588(20)31301-5.

Herth, Felix J. F., Marc Noppen, Arschang Valipour, Sylvie Leroy, Jean-Michel Vergnon, Joachim H. Ficker, Jim J. Egan, et al. 2012. "Efficacy Predictors of Lung Volume Reduction with Zephyr Valves in a European Cohort." *European Respiratory Journal* 39 (6): 1334–42. https://doi.org/10.1183/09031936.00161611.

Herth, Felix J. F., Dirk-Jan Slebos, Gerard J. Criner, and Pallav L. Shah. 2017. "Endoscopic Lung Volume Reduction: An Expert Panel Recommendation - Update 2017." *Respiration* 94 (4): 380–88. https://doi.org/10.1159/000479379.

Herth, Felix J. F., Arschang Valipour, Pallav L. Shah, Ralf Eberhardt, Christian Grah, Jim Egan, Joachim H. Ficker, et al. 2016. "Segmental Volume Reduction Using Thermal Vapour Ablation in Patients with Severe Emphysema: 6-Month Results of the Multicentre, Parallel-Group, Open-Label, Randomised Controlled STEP-UP Trial." *The Lancet. Respiratory Medicine* 4 (3): 185–93. https://doi.org/10.1016/S2213-2600(16)00045-X.

Herzog, Dominik, Alexander Poellinger, Felix Doellinger, Dirk Schuermann, Bettina Temmesfeld-Wollbrueck, Vera Froeling, Nils F. Schreiter, et al. 2015. "Modifying Post-Operative Medical Care after EBV Implant May Reduce Pneumothorax Incidence." *PLOS ONE* 10 (5): e0128097. https://doi.org/10.1371/journal.pone.0128097.

Hogg, James C. 2004. "Pathophysiology of Airflow Limitation in Chronic Obstructive Pulmonary Disease." *The Lancet* 364 (9435): 709–21. https://doi.org/10.1016/S0140-6736(04)16900-6.

Hopkinson, N. S., S. V. Kemp, T. P. Toma, D. M. Hansell, D. M. Geddes, P. L. Shah, and M. I. Polkey. 2011. "Atelectasis and Survival after Bronchoscopic Lung Volume Reduction for COPD." *The European Respiratory Journal* 37 (6): 1346–51. https://doi.org/10.1183/09031936.00100110.

Kontogianni, Konstantina, Vasiliki Gerovasili, Daniela Gompelmann, Maren Schuhmann, Claus Peter Heussel, Felix J. F. Herth, and Ralf Eberhardt. 2014. "Effectiveness of Endobronchial Coil Treatment for Lung Volume Reduction in Patients with Severe Heterogeneous Emphysema and Bilateral Incomplete Fissures: A Six-Month Follow-Up." *Respiration* 88 (1): 52–60. https://doi.org/10.1159/000358441.

Krishnamohan, Pradheep, K. Robert Shen, Dennis A. Wigle, Mark S. Allen, Francis C. Nichols, Stephen D. Cassivi, William S. Harmsen, and Claude Deschamps. 2014. "Bullectomy for Symptomatic or Complicated Giant Lung Bullae." *The Annals of Thoracic Surgery* 97 (2): 425–31. https://doi.org/10.1016/j.athoracsur.2013.10.049.

Laros, C. D., H. J. Gelissen, P. G. M. Bergstein, J. M. M. Van Den Bosch, R. G. J. R. A. Vanderschueren, C. J. J. Westermann, and P. J. Knaepen. 1986. "Bullectomy for Giant Bullae in Emphysema." *The Journal of Thoracic and Cardiovascular Surgery* 91 (1): 63–70. https://doi.org/10.1016/S0022-5223(19)38482-X.

Li Xingnan, Victor E. Ortega, Elizabeth J. Ampleford, R. Graham Barr, Stephanie A. Christenson, Christopher B. Cooper, David Couper, et al. 2018. "Genome-Wide Association Study of Lung Function and Clinical Implication in Heavy Smokers." *BMC Medical Genetics* 19 (1): 134. https://doi.org/10.1186/s12881-018-0656-z.

Lindenauer, Peter K., Mihaela S. Stefan, Penelope S. Pekow, Kathleen M. Mazor, Aruna Priya, Kerry A. Spitzer, Tara C. Lagu, Quinn R. Pack, Victor M. Pinto-Plata, and Richard ZuWallack. 2020. "Association between Initiation of Pulmonary Rehabilitation after Hospitalization for COPD and 1-Year Survival among Medicare Beneficiaries." *JAMA* 323 (18): 1813–23. https://doi.org/10.1001/jama.2020.4437.

McCarthy, Bernard, Dympna Casey, Declan Devane, Kathy Murphy, Edel Murphy, and Yves Lacasse. 2015. "Pulmonary Rehabilitation for Chronic Obstructive Pulmonary Disease." *The Cochrane Database of Systematic Reviews*, no. 2 (February): CD003793. https://doi.org/10.1002/14651858.CD003793.pub3.

Meguro, Makiko, Elizabeth A. Barley, Sally Spencer, and Paul W. Jones. 2007. "Development and Validation of an Improved, COPD-Specific Version of the St. George Respiratory Questionnaire." *Chest* 132 (2): 456–63. https://doi.org/10.1378/chest.06-0702.

Monaldi, V. 1947. "Endocavitary Aspiration: Its Practical Applications." *Tubercle* 28 (11): 223–28. https://doi.org/10.1016/S0041-3879(47)80060-1.

Morgan, M. D., C. W. Edwards, J. Morris, and H. R. Matthews. 1989. "Origin and Behaviour of Emphysematous Bullae." *Thorax* 44 (7): 533–38. https://doi.org/10.1136/thx.44.7.533.

Naef, A. P. 1997. "History of Emphysema Surgery." *The Annals of Thoracic Surgery* 64 (5): 1506–8. https://doi.org/10.1016/S0003-4975(97)00864-3.

Nakahara, K., K. Nakaoka, K. Ohno, Y. Monden, M. Maeda, A. Masaoka, K. Sawamura, and Y. Kawashima. 1983. "Functional Indications for Bullectomy of Giant Bulla." *The Annals of Thoracic Surgery* 35 (5): 480–87. https://doi.org/10.1016/s0003-4975(10)60419-5.

National Emphysema Treatment Trial Research Group. 2003. "A Randomized Trial Comparing Lung-Volume-Reduction Surgery with Medical Therapy for Severe Emphysema." *New England Journal of Medicine* 348 (21): 2059–73. https://doi.org/10.1056/NEJMoa030287.

Naunheim, Keith S., Douglas E. Wood, Zab Mohsenifar, Alice L. Sternberg, Gerard J. Criner, Malcolm M. DeCamp, Claude C. Deschamps, et al. 2006. "Long-Term Follow-Up of Patients Receiving Lung-Volume-Reduction Surgery Versus Medical Therapy for Severe Emphysema by the National Emphysema Treatment Trial Research Group." *The Annals of Thoracic Surgery* 82 (2): 431–43.e19. https://doi.org/10.1016/j.athoracsur.2006.05.069.

Nissen, R. 1954. "Tracheoplastik Zur Beseitigung Der Erschlaffung Des Membranosen Teils Der Intrathorakalen Luftroehre." *Schweiz.Med.Wochenschr* 84: 219–21.

Palla, Antonio, Massimiliano Desideri, Giuseppe Rossi, Giulio Bardi, David Mazzantini, Alfredo Mussi, and Carlo Giuntini. 2005. "Elective Surgery for Giant Bullous Emphysema: A 5-Year Clinical and Functional Follow-Up." *Chest* 128 (4): 2043–50. https://doi.org/10.1378/chest.128.4.2043.

Panel, Tobacco Use and Dependence Guideline. 2008. *Treating Tobacco Use and Dependence: 2008 Update.* US Department of Health and Human Services.

Parulekar, Amit D., Carlos Martinez, Chu-Lin Tsai, Nicholas Locantore, Mustafa Atik, Abebaw M. Yohannes, Christina C. Kao, et al. 2017. "Examining the Effects of Age on Health Outcomes of Chronic Obstructive Pulmonary Disease: Results from the Genetic Epidemiology of Chronic Obstructive Pulmonary Disease Study and Evaluation of Chronic Obstructive Pulmonary Disease Longitudinally to Identify Predictive Surrogate Endpoints Cohorts." *Journal of the American Medical Directors Association* 18 (12): 1063–68. https://doi.org/10.1016/j.jamda.2017.09.028.

Pauwels, R. A., A. S. Buist, P. M. Calverley, C. R. Jenkins, S. S. Hurd, and GOLD Scientific Committee. 2001. "Global Strategy for the Diagnosis, Management, and Prevention of Chronic Obstructive Pulmonary Disease. NHLBI/WHO Global Initiative for Chronic Obstructive Lung Disease (GOLD) Workshop Summary." *American Journal of Respiratory and Critical Care Medicine* 163 (5): 1256–76. https://doi.org/10.1164/ajrccm.163.5.2101039.

Pearson, M. G., and C. Ogilvie. 1983. "Surgical Treatment of Emphysematous Bullae: Late Outcome." *Thorax* 38 (2): 134–37. https://doi.org/10.1136/thx.38.2.134.

Pison, Christophe, Pallav L. Shah, Dirk-Jan Slebos, Vincent Ninane, Wim Janssens, Thierry Perez, Romain Kessler, et al. 2021. "Safety of Denervation Following Targeted Lung Denervation Therapy for COPD: AIRFLOW-1 3-Year Outcomes." *Respiratory Research* 22 (1): 62. https://doi.org/10.1186/s12931-021-01664-5.

Rawal, Gautam, and Sankalp Yadav. 2015. "Nutrition in Chronic Obstructive Pulmonary Disease: A Review." *Journal of Translational Internal Medicine* 3 (4): 151–54. https://doi.org/10.1515/jtim-2015-0021.

Rehman, Anees ur, Mohamed Azmi Ahmad Hassali, Sameen Abbas, Irfhan Ali Bin Hyder Ali, Sabariah Noor Harun, Jaya Muneswarao, and Rabia Hussain. 2020. "Pharmacological and Non-Pharmacological Management of COPD; Limitations and Future Prospects: A Review of Current Literature." *Journal of Public Health* 28 (4): 357–66. https://doi.org/10.1007/s10389-019-01021-3.

Reinhoff, William Francis. 1938. "Treatment of Intractable Bronchial Asthma by Bilateral Resection of the Posterior Pulmonary Plexus." https://jamanetwork.com/journals/jamasurgery/article-abstract/543697.

Ringbaek, Thomas, Eva Brøndum, Gerd Martinez, and Peter Lange. 2008. "EuroQoL in Assessment of the Effect of Pulmonary Rehabilitation COPD Patients." *Respiratory Medicine* 102 (11): 1563–67. https://doi.org/10.1016/j.rmed.2008.06.016.

Schuhmann, Maren, Philippe Raffy, Youbing Yin, Daniela Gompelmann, Ipek Oguz, Ralf Eberhardt, Derek Hornberg, Claus Peter Heussel, Susan Wood, and Felix J. F. Herth. 2015. "Computed Tomography Predictors of Response to Endobronchial Valve Lung Reduction Treatment. Comparison with Chartis." *American Journal of Respiratory and Critical Care Medicine* 191 (7): 767–74. https://doi.org/10.1164/rccm.201407-1205OC.

Sciurba, Frank C., Divay Chandra, and Jessica Bon. 2016. "Bronchoscopic Lung Volume Reduction in COPD: Lessons in Implementing Clinically Based Precision Medicine." *JAMA* 315 (2): 139–41. https://doi.org/10.1001/jama.2015.17714.

Sciurba, Frank C., Gerard J. Criner, Charlie Strange, Pallav L. Shah, Gaetane Michaud, Timothy A. Connolly, Gaëtan Deslée, et al. 2016. "Effect of Endobronchial Coils vs Usual Care on Exercise Tolerance in Patients With Severe Emphysema: The RENEW Randomized Clinical Trial." *JAMA* 315 (20): 2178–89. https://doi.org/10.1001/jama.2016.6261.

Shah, Pallav L., Felix J. Herth, Wouter H. van Geffen, Gaetan Deslee, and Dirk-Jan Slebos. 2017. "Lung Volume Reduction for Emphysema." *The Lancet. Respiratory Medicine* 5 (2): 147–56. https://doi.org/10.1016/S2213-2600(16)30221-1.

Shah, Samir S., and Peter Goldstraw. 1994. "Surgical Treatment of Bullous Emphysema: Experience with the Brompton Technique." *The Annals of Thoracic Surgery*, Thirty-first Annual Meeting of the Society of Thoracic Surgeons 58 (5): 1452–56. https://doi.org/10.1016/0003-4975(94)91934-8.

Simmons, M. S., J. E. Connett, M. A. Nides, P. G. Lindgren, E. C. Kleerup, R. P. Murray, W. M. Bjornson, and D. P. Tashkin. 2005. "Smoking Reduction and the Rate of Decline in FEV1: Results from the Lung Health Study." *European Respiratory Journal* 25 (6): 1011–17. https://doi.org/10.1183/09031936.05.00086804.

Slebos, Dirk-Jan, Karin Klooster, Coenraad F. N. Koegelenberg, Johan Theron, Dorothy Styen, Arschang Valipour, Martin Mayse, and Chris T. Bolliger. 2015. "Targeted Lung Denervation for Moderate to Severe COPD: A Pilot Study." *Thorax* 70 (5): 411–19. https://doi.org/10.1136/thoraxjnl-2014-206146.

Spruit, Martijn A., Sally J. Singh, Chris Garvey, Richard ZuWallack, Linda Nici, Carolyn Rochester, Kylie Hill, et al. 2013. "An Official American Thoracic Society/European Respiratory Society Statement: Key Concepts and Advances in Pulmonary Rehabilitation." *American Journal of Respiratory and Critical Care Medicine* 188 (8): e13–64. https://doi.org/10.1164/rccm.201309-1634ST.

Stanifer, B. Payne, and Mark E. Ginsburg. 2018. "Lung Volume Reduction Surgery in the Post-National Emphysema Treatment Trial Era." *Journal of Thoracic Disease* 10 (Suppl 23): S2744–47. https://doi.org/10.21037/jtd.2018.05.135.

Stead, L. F., R. Perera, C. Bullen, D. Mant, and T. Lancaster. 2008. "Nicotine Replacement Therapy for Smoking Cessation." *The Cochrane Database of Systematic Reviews*, no. 1 (January): CD000146. https://doi.org/10.1002/14651858.CD000146.pub3.

Ting, Er Yi, Robert Klopstock, and Harold A. Lyons. 1963. "Mechanical Properties of Pulmonary Cysts and Bullae." *American Review of Respiratory Disease* 87 (4): 538–44. https://doi.org/10.1164/arrd.1963.87.4.538.

Tønnesen, Philip. 2013. "Smoking Cessation and COPD." *European Respiratory Review* 22 (127): 37–43. https://doi.org/10.1183/09059180.00007212.

Valipour, Arschang, Dirk-Jan Slebos, Felix Herth, Kaid Darwiche, Manfred Wagner, Joachim H. Ficker, Christoph Petermann, Ralf-Harto Hubner, Franz Stanzel, and Ralf Eberhardt. 2016. "Endobronchial Valve Therapy in Patients with Homogeneous Emphysema. Results from the IMPACT Study." *American Journal of Respiratory and Critical Care Medicine* 194 (9): 1073–82. https://doi.org/10.1164/rccm.201607-1383OC.

Vestbo, Jørgen, Suzanne S. Hurd, Alvar G. Agustí, Paul W. Jones, Claus Vogelmeier, Antonio Anzueto, Peter J. Barnes, et al. 2013. "Global Strategy for the Diagnosis, Management, and Prevention of Chronic Obstructive Pulmonary Disease: GOLD Executive Summary." *American Journal of Respiratory and Critical Care Medicine* 187 (4): 347–65. https://doi.org/10.1164/rccm.201204-0596PP.

"WHO Global Health Estimates 2019." 2020. Factsheet. World Health Organization. https://www.who.int/news-room/fact-sheets/detail/the-top-10-causes-of-death.

"WHO | Global Surveillance, Prevention and Control of Chronic Respiratory Diseases: A Comprehensive Approach." n.d. WHO. World Health Organization. Accessed December 14, 2021. https://www.who.int/gard/publications/GARD_Manual/en/.

Woodruff, Prescott G., R. Graham Barr, Eugene Bleecker, Stephanie A. Christenson, David Couper, Jeffrey L. Curtis, Natalia A. Gouskova, et al. 2016. "Clinical Significance of Symptoms in Smokers with Preserved Pulmonary Function." *The New England Journal of Medicine* 374 (19): 1811–21. https://doi.org/10.1056/NEJMoa1505971

Xie, Min, Xiansheng Liu, Xiaopei Cao, Mingzhou Guo, and Xiaochen Li. 2020. "Trends in Prevalence and Incidence of Chronic Respiratory Diseases from 1990 to 2017." *Respiratory Research* 21 (1): 1–13. https://doi.org/10.1186/s12931-020-1291-8.

The Future of Treating Hyperinflation in Emphysema

17

Justin L. Garner and Pallav L. Shah

INTRODUCTION

Management of severe hyperinflation of end-stage emphysema has been transformed since the advent of lung volume reduction (LVR) in 1957 (1). The objectives and the benefits are undoubted: improved lung function, exercise capacity, quality of life, and survival have been achieved with a variety of techniques in numerous clinical trials (2, 3). Surgery initially was a heroic endeavour in individuals selected from a very sick population. The challenge to improve the safety and widen the eligibility for the procedure has in the past two decades ushered in a wave of innovations (see Chapter 12). These and those in prospect are discussed in this chapter.

DIAGNOSTICS

Patient selection is key and informed by an array of metrics derived from lung function, imaging, exercise capacity, and predictive models. A drive towards less invasive and onerous testing paradigms in individuals who have significant physiological compromise is likely to be embraced.

Lung function testing

Spirometry, whole body plethysmography, and gas transfer measurements are well-established conventions in clinical medicine. Spirometry, however, necessitates a maximally forced manoeuvre which is difficult for emphysematous hyperinflated patients to achieve (4). Moreover, the recognition of chronic

DOI: 10.1201/9781003251439-17

obstructive pulmonary disease (COPD) as a disease of small airways, largely invisible to spirometry, ha exposed the fallibility of dependence on this test (5). An alternative to spirometry is impulse oscillom etry, a validated technique independent of patient effort, utilising the fluctuating pressure/flow response to a mix of sound wave frequencies (5–30Hz) imposed on tidal flow to extract information on airway mechanics, especially those of the smaller airways (6). It is a much less taxing tidal breathing techniqu that is quick to perform over several minutes compared with spirometry and more sensitive to and infor mative of the small airways and their response to therapeutic intervention (7).

Cardiopulmonary exercise testing (CPET) on a cycle ergometer is the gold-standard physiologi cal assessment in patients with COPD (8). However, the expense of the equipment and the expertis demanded for laboratory based CPET limits its accessibility. The most frequently employed method eval uating endurance is the field test, including the six-minute walk test (6MWT), incremental shuttle walk ing test (ISWT), and endurance shuttle walking test (ESWT), and which have been shown to be valid reliable, and responsive to change (9). It is affordable but does yield rather less physiological informatio (10, 11). The four-metre gait speed (4MGS) is a simple and quick functional assessment tool used in th community for older adults and correlates with exercise capacity, dyspnoea, and health-related quality o life with a MCID of 0.11 m/s (12, 13). The one-minute sit-to-stand (STS) test is a promising alternativ with a MCID of three repetitions (14).

Imaging

Computed tomography

Computed tomography (CT) has been in routine use since 1972 and is the cornerstone of imag ing in COPD (15). Reconstruction of axial slices down to 0.5 mm thickness generates detailed three dimensional representations of the lung, notably the parenchyma, tracheobronchial tree, and vasculature

The importance of assessing emphysema severity and distribution was exemplified by the Nationa Emphysema Treatment Trial (NETT): Patients with heterogeneous upper zone predominant involvemen and low baseline exercise capacity undergoing lung volume reduction surgery (LVRS) were shown to hav improved survival compared with those receiving standard-of-care treatment (16). Quantitative CT (qCT is used to determine eligibility for LVR procedures such as endobronchial valve implantation – in additio to objective emphysema characterisation at −950 Hounsfield units (HU), reports include measurement o fissure integrity, a surrogate for the absence of collateral ventilation. However, the resolution of conven tional volumetric CT is unable to capture the small airways, those less than 2 mm internal diameter, th principal site of pathology and obstruction in COPD (5). Micro-CT provides exceptionally high resolutio (1 μm per voxel) of lung architecture equivalent to microscopic histological evaluation, but high radiatio doses limit its application to excised specimens (17, 18).

Advanced imaging modalities permit simultaneous regional evaluation of structural and functiona (i.e., ventilation and/or perfusion) abnormalities, for example, parametric response mapping (19), xeno ventilation CT using a dual-energy technique (20, 21), dual-energy perfusion CT (22), and respiratory gated 4D-CT that produces a video (23) – employment of these novel techniques is likely to increase i the coming years.

Nuclear medicine

Single-photon emission computed tomography (SPECT) utilises radioisotopes to generate a high resolution regional map of ventilation and perfusion comparing favourably with traditional planar lung scintigraphy (24–27). Emerging data support its value in pre-operative planning (28) and in predicting post-operative pulmonary reserve (29, 30).

Magnetic resonance imaging

Magnetic resonance imaging (MRI) eliminates the need for ionising radiation, but the low density of hydrogen ions within the lung has translated to images of low signal intensity and poor signal-to-noise ratio (31). Hyperpolarised Xenon-129 (32), helium-3 (33–35), and oxygen-enhanced MRI (36) have been developed to overcome these limitations and show promise as imaging adjuncts for LVR.

Biomarkers

A robust biomarker of disease severity that can reliably predict and evaluate the response to LVR remains elusive. A number have been studied (37). A current promising candidate is the bronchoalveolar lavage fluid neutrophil-derived microvesicle, levels of which have been shown to correlate with a number of key functional and clinically relevant disease severity indices compared with Th1- cytokines (38). It remains to be seen whether a point-of-care test for this and other biomarkers could eventually be translated to the outpatient setting.

THERAPEUTICS

Surgical techniques

LVRS has undergone significant advances in procedural technique. In NETT, bilateral LVRS was performed via median sternotomy (MS; 70%) or multiport video-assisted thoracoscopic surgery (VATS; 30%) (16). Functional outcomes, morbidity, and mortality were comparable, but VATS was associated with an earlier post-operative recovery at reduced costs (39), and is now the preferred approach (40). Future developments in the field are summarised below.

Uniportal VATS

The uniportal VATS (uVATS) approach progresses the concept of minimally invasive surgery with a single 3-4 cm incision (41). With improved cosmesis, less operative pain, and paraesthesia, its use is gaining in worldwide popularity. Adopting a sub-xiphoid entry point affords access to both thoracic cavities to perform bilateral lung resections in a single session (42) with potentially reduced post-operative pain and early mobilisation (43).

Robotic-assisted thoracic surgery

Robotic-assisted thoracic surgery (RATS) has been developed to overcome the limitations of standard thoracoscopy, notably acquisition of a stable three-dimensional field of view, precise wristed movements with greater degrees of freedom, and optimised ergonomics for the operator. The most commonly used platform, da Vinci (Intuitive Surgical, Sunnyvale, CA, USA), requires three to five access ports; single-port deployed devices are currently in development (44). A propensity score-matched analysis comparing RATS with uVATS for non-small cell lung cancer (NSCLC) showed similar peri-operative outcomes for procedural time, length of hospital stays, and complication rates; interestingly, RATS was associated with less intraoperative blood loss and more dissected lymph node stations (45). RATS has also been shown to be a cost-effective strategy for lobectomy in patients with lung malignancy in higher volume centres (46).

Extrapolating from the work undertaken in the field of lung cancer, RATS is likely to have an increasingl prominent role in LVRS.

Natural orifice trans-luminal endoscopic surgery

Natural orifice trans-luminal endoscopic surgery (NOTES) via an oral or umbilical approach, while con ceptual, is an attractive strategy that has mainly been studied in animal models (47) – its translation to the clinical arena will require substantial advances in flexible robotic endoscopes with multifunctiona instrumentation including in traction and countertraction to safely achieve resection margins (48, 49).

Awake surgery

In a randomised controlled trial, awake non-resectional LVRS (performed under thoracic epidural with a non-cutting endostapler reducing lung volume by 20 to 30%) was associated with a greater proportion o early discharges compared with non-awake resectional LVRS via multiport VATS (50). Refinement of thi technique with uniportal access results in less post-operative pain than a multiport approach (51) and is a potential choice for infirm and elderly patients.

Chest drainage

Digital drainage devices such as Thopaz provide objective quantification of air leak to facilitate earlie thoracostomy tube removal, ambulation, and discharge (± with Heimlich valve) compared with a standar underwater-seal system (52).

Enhanced recovery protocols

In parallel with honed surgical techniques, perioperative care has evolved with multimodal analgesia early feeding, mobilisation, chest drain removal, and implementation of pulmonary rehabilitation befor and after surgery (53, 54).

Transplantation

Lungs declined for transplantation, reconditioned with ex vivo lung perfusion, are a potential source fo increasing the donor pool (55, 56). Transplantation of bioengineered lung (BEL) in a porcine model, a structure of autologous stem cells on an acellular scaffold, shows early promise (57).

Bronchoscopic techniques

Minimally invasive bronchoscopic techniques offer a number of advantages over surgery: (1) safety with a short general anaesthesia or moderate sedation; (2) natural orifice access; and (3) more rapid turnaroun of patients and improved cost-effectiveness. Current technologies and their future development are con sidered below.

Unidirectional valves

One-way valves induce lobar atelectasis, occluding the segmental bronchi during inspiration, permitting evacuation of air and mucus in expiration. The endobronchial valve (EBV) by Pulmonx, a duck-bill mech anism formed in silicone mounted on a nitinol frame, has been shown to improve not only lung function and exercise capacity but, importantly, quality of life and survival in selected individuals and has been approved by the National Institute of Clinical Excellence (NICE) and the Food and Drug Administration (FDA) for severe emphysema and hyperinflation (58).

Tackling pneumothorax
The most common complication is pneumothorax, in fact, a sign of technical success, occurring in up to 34.4% of individuals and mandating at least a 72-hour in-hospital stay post-procedure (59, 60). The mechanism is speculated to be a tear in the adjoining untreated lobe, which is at increased risk with greater emphysematous destruction (61, 62). To mitigate this complication, some operators have employed pre-emptive chest drain insertion following EBV implantation to allow early discharge home (63) – pneumothorax may occur at any time but is likely to be most impactful in the immediate post-operative period, and this may be an appropriate strategy in selected high-risk individuals in whom the most diseased lobe is not treated *and* the contralateral destruction score is >60% (64). The integration of programmable servomotors into the valvular mechanism may permit more graduated atelectasis avoiding the rapid architectural changes frequently encountered (65).

Smaller devices for subsegmental deployment
A targeted subsegmental approach using smaller valvular devices compared with a pan-lobar occlusion strategy may preserve relatively functioning compressed parenchyma and potentially minimise the occurrence of pneumothorax (and also of respiratory failure) and could be used to treat multi-lobar disease more effectively. The utilisation of navigation bronchoscopy platforms (± robotic assistance) may facilitate more precise delivery and deployment to the smaller airways (66–68).

Improving biocompatibility
The nitinol frame is designed with biocompatibility in mind (69). Inevitably, implants are subject to biofilm formation and are particularly vulnerable in airways colonised with microorganisms including pseudomonas (70). Advances in material science may make it possible to coat or impregnate implants with a pathogen-repellent layer to combat mucus accumulation, microbial aggregation, and acute infection (71). The contribution of metallurgy developing novel biocompatible alloys for implantable devices with similar properties to nitinol, notably shape memory and super-elasticity, will be welcomed for individuals allergic to nickel and/or titanium (72, 73).

Predictive modelling
Modelling and simulation technologies have revolutionised many industries, notably the field of aerospace. Computed tomography structural modelling of the mechanical forces at play within the lung before and after device implantation could be hugely valuable to help predict the effects on surrounding structures and the likelihood of developing complications such as pneumothorax, or rarely, hilar torsion (74). Indeed, the latter has been attributed to the unforeseen deleterious impact of combined right upper and middle lobe treatments in a small proportion of individuals.

Broadening eligibility in the presence of collateral ventilation
Unidirectional valves induce lobar atelectasis, provided there is satisfactory occlusion of the supplying segmental bronchi and absence of collateral ventilation (CV). The TRANSFORM and LIBERATE studies identified 16.5% (59) and 9.2% (60) of individuals, respectively, who were CV positive at the time of Chartis evaluation. Strategies to increase fissure integrity would be expected to broaden the eligibility in individuals with limited therapeutic options, especially in those who may not be robust candidates for lobectomy. Strategies under evaluation include the instillation of sealant, biological (NCT04256408) or synthetic (NCT04559464), and stapling of the incomplete lobar boundary via a VATS approach (75).

Endobronchial coils

Delivered in a straight wire configuration to assume a two-turn spiral on deployment in the middle third of the lung, endobronchial coils shrink the treated lobe and are thought to restore elastic recoil and tether the bronchi, maintaining their patency. Studies looked promising (76–80). Unfortunately, manufacture has been discontinued by market forces. A variety of generic coil sizes were designed for use. With the development of engineering-based software platforms for segmenting the airway tree and predictive modelling of the parenchymal mechanical forces at play, it is envisioned that customisable devices will be manufactured to optimise lung volume reduction while offsetting the risk of complications, for example pneumothorax. Made from nitinol, improvements in biocompatibility may permit their use in individuals with microbial colonisations (81) and/or allergies to the alloy constituents. Lastly, coils are considered permanent devices – the integration of mechanics within the shaft to permit adjustable conformational changes via the bulbar tip offers the ability to remove the device in the context of recurrent infective exacerbations or haemoptysis.

Transbronchial stents

Designed with the intent of maximising gaseous deflation on expiration, transbronchial stents frequently suffered from luminal occlusion by granulation tissue despite paclitaxel impregnation, counteracting the pronounced physiological benefits observed shortly after implantation (82, 83). Advances in surface repellent materials to avoid this complication would make this a valuable adjunct to the therapeutic armamentarium.

Steam

The benefits of bronchoscopic thermal vapour ablation (BTVA) in individuals with the presence of CV are countered by the inflammatory side effects of COPD exacerbation (24%), pneumonia/pneumonitis (18%) and haemoptysis (requiring bronchoscopic tamponade; 2%) (84). A reduced calorific volume may assist with minimising these complications.

Sealant (synthetic and biological)

Similar to steam therapy, the synthetic sealant, AeriSeal, is associated with an increased risk of causing COPD exacerbation (85). Smaller volume instillations are currently under investigation in an attempt to mitigate the potential for inflammatory fallout. While biocompatibility is not an issue with autologous blood instillation, the risk of infection exists, and the use of synthetic sterile sealant may minimise this.

Endobronchial "drawstring" lung volume reduction

Bronchus Technologies Inc. submitted a patent in 2006 describing a method for lung volume reduction employing a plurality of anchors placed peripherally in the target lobe and their respective cords retracted via a proximal lockable connector thus collapsing the parenchyma, akin to a drawstring mechanism (US6997189B2). The novel technique has yet to be evaluated in a clinical trial.

Enhanced recovery protocols

Improvements in perioperative care including the implementation of pulmonary rehabilitation before and shortly after intervention (60) will help capitalise on treatment gains in the longer term.

Hybrid approaches

The development of multimodality therapeutic algorithms will afford a more versatile and bespoke approach to the individual, for example, unilateral or bilateral LVR (surgically and/or bronchoscopically achieved) in combination with novel airway treatments such as targeted lung denervation (86) and metered radial cryospray (87).

CONCLUSION

The field of lung volume reduction is rapidly evolving with the development and translation of novel technologies in both surgical and bronchoscopic arenas. Undoubtedly, the direction of travel will continue towards exploration of minimal invasive access approaches and tissue disruptive techniques performed as day case admissions. The future of treating hyperinflation is bright.

ABBREVIATIONS

BEL: Bioengineered lung
BTVA: Bronchoscopic thermal vapour ablation
COPD: Chronic obstructive pulmonary disease
CPET: Cardiopulmonary exercise test
CT: Computed tomography
CV: Collateral ventilation
EBV: Zephyr® Endobronchial Valve by Pulmonx
ESWT: Endurance shuttle walking test
FDA: Food and Drug Administration
HU: Hounsfield units
LVR: Lung volume reduction
LVRS: Lung volume reduction surgery
MCID: Minimal clinically important difference
MRI: Magnetic resonance imaging
NICE: National Institute of Clinical Excellence
NOTES: Natural orifice trans-luminal endoscopic surgery
qCT: Quantitative computed tomography
RATS: Robotic-assisted thoracic surgery
SPECT: Single-photon emission computed tomography
STS: Sit-to-stand test
VATS: Video-assisted thoracoscopic surgery
4MGS: Four-metre gait speed
6MWT: Six-minute walk test

REFERENCES

1. Brantigan OC, Mueller E. Surgical treatment of pulmonary emphysema. *The American Surgeon.* 1957;23(9):789–804.
2. Shah PL, Herth FJ, van Geffen WH, et al. Lung volume reduction for emphysema. *The Lancet Respiratory Medicine.* 2017;5(2):147–56.
3. van Geffen WH, Slebos DJ, Herth FJ, et al. Surgical and endoscopic interventions that reduce lung volume for emphysema: a systemic review and meta-analysis. *The Lancet Respiratory Medicine.* 2019;7(4):313–24.
4. Pride NB. Tests of forced expiration and inspiration. *Clinics in Chest Medicine.* 2001;22(4):599–622, vii.
5. Hogg JC, Macklem PT, Thurlbeck WM. Site and nature of airway obstruction in chronic obstructive lung disease. *The New England Journal of Medicine.* 1968;278(25):1355–60.

6. Brashier B, Salvi S. Measuring lung function using sound waves: role of the forced oscillation technique and impulse oscillometry system. *Breathe* (Sheffield, England). 2015;11(1):57–65.

7. Garner JL, Biddiscombe MF, Meah S, et al. Endobronchial valve lung volume reduction and small airway function. *American Journal of Respiratory and Critical Care Medicine*. 2021;203(12):1576–9.

8. Boutou AK, Zafeiridis A, Pitsiou G, et al. Cardiopulmonary exercise testing in chronic obstructive pulmonary disease: an update on its clinical value and applications. *Clinical Physiology and Functional Imaging*. 2020;40(4):197–206.

9. Holland AE, Spruit MA, Troosters T, et al. An official European Respiratory Society/American Thoracic Society technical standard: field walking tests in chronic respiratory disease. *The European Respiratory Journal*. 2014;44(6):1428–46.

10. Puente-Maestu L, Palange P, Casaburi R, et al. Use of exercise testing in the evaluation of interventional efficacy: an official ERS statement. *The European Respiratory Journal*. 2016;47(2):429–60.

11. Zeng Y, Jiang F, Chen Y, et al. Exercise assessments and trainings of pulmonary rehabilitation in COPD: literature review. *International Journal of Chronic Obstructive Pulmonary Disease*. 2018;13:2013–23.

12. Kon SS, Patel MS, Canavan JL, et al. Reliability and validity of 4-metre gait speed in COPD. *The European Respiratory Journal*. 2013;42(2):333–40.

13. Kon SS, Canavan JL, Nolan CM, et al. The 4-metre gait speed in COPD: responsiveness and minimal clinically important difference. *The European Respiratory Journal*. 2014;43(5):1298–305.

14. Crook S, Büsching G, Schultz K, et al. A multicentre validation of the 1-min sit-to-stand test in patients with COPD. *The European Respiratory Journal*. 2017;49(3).

15. Pan X, Siewerdsen J, La Riviere PJ, Kalender WA. Anniversary paper. Development of x-ray computed tomography: the role of medical physics and AAPM from the 1970s to present. *Medical Physics*. 2008;35(8):3728–39.

16. Fishman A, Martinez F, Naunheim K, et al. A randomized trial comparing lung-volume-reduction surgery with medical therapy for severe emphysema. *The New England Journal of Medicine*. 2003;348(21):2059–73.

17. Watz H, Breithecker A, Rau WS, Kriete A. Micro-CT of the human lung: imaging of alveoli and virtual endoscopy of an alveolar duct in a normal lung and in a lung with centrilobular emphysema–initial observations. *Radiology*. 2005;236(3):1053–8.

18. Hogg JC, McDonough JE, Suzuki M. Small airway obstruction in COPD: new insights based on micro-CT imaging and MRI imaging. *Chest*. 2013;143(5):1436–43.

19. Bhatt SP, Soler X, Wang X, et al. Association between functional small airway disease and FEV1 decline in chronic obstructive pulmonary disease. *American Journal of Respiratory and Critical Care Medicine*. 2016;194(2):178–84.

20. Chae EJ, Seo JB, Goo HW, et al. Xenon ventilation CT with a dual-energy technique of dual-source CT: initial experience. *Radiology*. 2008;248(2):615–24.

21. Park EA, Goo JM, Park SJ, et al. Chronic obstructive pulmonary disease: quantitative and visual ventilation pattern analysis at xenon ventilation CT performed by using a dual-energy technique. *Radiology*. 2010;256(3):985–97.

22. Chae EJ, Kim N, Seo JB, et al. Prediction of postoperative lung function in patients undergoing lung resection: dual-energy perfusion computed tomography versus perfusion scintigraphy. *Investigative Radiology*. 2013;48(8):622–7.

23. Ley-Zaporozhan J, Ley S, Mews J, et al. Changes of emphysema parameters over the respiratory cycle during free breathing: preliminary results using respiratory gated 4D-CT. *COPD*. 2017;14(6):597–602.

24. Suga K, Kawakami Y, Zaki M, et al. Clinical utility of co-registered respiratory-gated 99mTc-Technegas MAA SPECT-CT images in the assessment of regional lung functional impairment in patients with lung cancer. *European Journal of Nuclear Medicine and Molecular Imaging*. 2004;31(9):1280–90.

25. Suga K, Kawakami Y, Koike H, et al. Lung ventilation-perfusion imbalance in pulmonary emphysema: assessment with automated V/Q quotient SPECT. *Annals of Nuclear Medicine*. 2010;24(4):269–77.

26. Jögi J, Ekberg M, Jonson B, et al. Ventilation/perfusion SPECT in chronic obstructive pulmonary disease: an evaluation by reference to symptoms, spirometric lung function and emphysema, as assessed with HRCT. *European Journal of Nuclear Medicine and Molecular Imaging*. 2011;38(7):1344–52.

27. Jogi J, Markstad H, Tufvesson E, et al. The added value of hybrid ventilation/perfusion SPECT/CT in patients with stable COPD or apparently healthy smokers. Cancer-suspected CT findings in the lungs are common when hybrid imaging is used. *International Journal of Chronic Obstructive Pulmonary Disease*. 2015;10:25–30.

28. Wechalekar K, Garner J, Gregg S. Pre-surgical evaluation of lung function. *Seminars in Nuclear Medicine*. 2019;49(1):22–30.

29. Sudoh M, Ueda K, Kaneda Y, et al. Breath-hold single-photon emission tomography and computed tomography for predicting residual pulmonary function in patients with lung cancer. *The Journal of Thoracic and Cardiovascular Surgery*. 2006;131(5):994–1001.

30. Inmai T, Sasaki Y, Shinkai T, et al. Clinical evaluation of 99mTc-Technegas SPECT in thoracoscopic lung volume reduction surgery in patients with pulmonary emphysema. *Annals of Nuclear Medicine.* 2000;14(4):263–9.

31. Milne S, King GG. Advanced imaging in COPD: insights into pulmonary pathophysiology. *Journal of Thoracic Disease.* 2014;6(11):1570–85.

32. Dregely I, Mugler JP, 3rd, Ruset IC, et al. Hyperpolarized Xenon-129 gas-exchange imaging of lung microstructure: first case studies in subjects with obstructive lung disease. *Journal of Magnetic Resonance Imaging: JMRI.* 2011;33(5):1052–62.

33. Kirby M, Mathew L, Wheatley A, et al. Chronic obstructive pulmonary disease: longitudinal hyperpolarized (3)He MR imaging. *Radiology.* 2010;256(1):280–9.

34. Kirby M, Mathew L, Heydarian M, et al. Chronic obstructive pulmonary disease: quantification of bronchodilator effects by using hyperpolarized ^{3}He MR imaging. *Radiology.* 2011;261(1):283–92.

35. Kirby M, Heydarian M, Wheatley A, et al. Evaluating bronchodilator effects in chronic obstructive pulmonary disease using diffusion-weighted hyperpolarized helium-3 magnetic resonance imaging. *Journal of Applied Physiology* (Bethesda, MD: 1985). 2012;112(4):651–7.

36. Ohno Y, Iwasawa T, Seo JB, et al. Oxygen-enhanced magnetic resonance imaging versus computed tomography: multicenter study for clinical stage classification of smoking-related chronic obstructive pulmonary disease. *American Journal of Respiratory and Critical Care Medicine.* 2008;177(10):1095–102.

37. Mannino DM. Biomarkers for chronic obstructive pulmonary disease diagnosis and progression: insights, disappointments and promise. *Current Opinion in Pulmonary Medicine.* 2019;25(2):144–9.

38. Soni S, Garner JL, O'Dea KP, et al. Intra-alveolar neutrophil-derived microvesicles are associated with disease severity in COPD. *American Journal of Physiology Lung Cellular and Molecular Physiology.* 2021;320(1):L73–183.

39. McKenna RJ Jr, Benditt JO, DeCamp M, et al. Safety and efficacy of median sternotomy versus video-assisted thoracic surgery for lung volume reduction surgery. *The Journal of Thoracic and Cardiovascular Surgery.* 2004;127(5):1350–60.

40. McKenna RJ, Jr. Thoracoscopic lung volume reduction surgery. *Operative Techniques in Thoracic and Cardiovascular Surgery.* 2007;12(2):141–9.

41. Ng CSH, Rocco G, Wong RHL, et al. Uniportal and single-incision video-assisted thoracic surgery: the state of the art. *Interactive Cardiovascular and Thoracic Surgery.* 2014;19(4):661–6.

42. Chiu CH, Chao YK, Liu YH. Subxiphoid approach for video-assisted thoracoscopic surgery: an update. *Journal of Thoracic Disease.* 2018;10(Suppl 14):S1662–s5.

43. Lemaitre PH, Stanifer BP, Sonett JR, Ginsburg ME. Technical aspects of lung volume reduction surgery including anesthetic management and surgical approaches. *Thoracic Surgery Clinics.* 2021;31(2):129–37.

44. Simaan N, Bajo A, Reiter A, et al. Lessons learned using the insertable robotic effector platform (IREP) for single port access surgery. *Journal of Robotic Surgery.* 2013;7(3):235–40.

45. Yang S, Guo W, Chen X, et al. Early outcomes of robotic versus uniportal video-assisted thoracic surgery for lung cancer: a propensity score-matched study. *European Journal of Cardio-Thoracic Surgery: Official Journal of the European Association for Cardio-thoracic Surgery.* 2018;53(2):348–52.

46. Nguyen DM, Sarkaria IS, Song C, et al. Clinical and economic comparative effectiveness of robotic-assisted, video-assisted thoracoscopic, and open lobectomy. *Journal of Thoracic Disease.* 2020;12(3):296–306.

47. Liu YH, Chu Y, Wu YC, et al. Natural orifice surgery in thoracic surgery. *Journal of Thoracic Disease.* 2014;6(1):61–3.

48. Fuchs KH, Breithaupt W. Transgastric small bowel resection with the new multitasking platform EndoSAMURAI™ for natural orifice transluminal endoscopic surgery. *Surgical Endoscopy.* 2012;26(8):2281–7.

49. Perretta S, Dallemagne B, Barry B, Marescaux J. The ANUBISCOPE® flexible platform ready for prime time: description of the first clinical case. *Surgical Endoscopy.* 2013;27(7):2630.

50. Pompeo E, Rogliani P, Tacconi F, et al. Randomized comparison of awake nonresectional versus non-awake resectional lung volume reduction surgery. *The Journal of Thoracic and Cardiovascular Surgery.* 2012;143(1):47–54.e1.

51. Mineo TC, Fabbi E, Ambrogi V. Nonintubated uniportal nonresectional videothoracoscopic lung volume reduction surgery. *Video-Assisted Thoracic Surgery.* 2017;2(9).

52. Toth JW, Reed MF, Ventola LK. Chest tube drainage devices. *Seminars in Respiratory and Critical Care Medicine.* 2019;40(3):386–93.

53. Dumans-Nizard V, Guezennec J, Parquin F, et al. Feasibility and results of a fast-track protocol in thoracic surgery. *Minerva Anestesiologica.* 2016;82(1):15–21.

54. Zhang M, Zhang H, Wu W, et al. Uniportal thoracoscopic lung volume reduction surgery using enhanced recovery protocol for patients with diffuse emphysema: a midterm follow-up. *International Journal of Clinical and Experimental Medicine.* 2019;12(1):923–9.

55. Cypel M, Yeung JC, Liu M, et al. Normothermic ex vivo lung perfusion in clinical lung transplantation. *The New England Journal of Medicine*. 2011;364(15):1431–40.
56. Cypel M, Yeung JC, Machuca T, et al. Experience with the first 50 ex vivo lung perfusions in clinical transplantation. *The Journal of Thoracic and Cardiovascular Surgery*. 2012;144(5):1200–6.
57. Nichols JE, La Francesca S, Niles JA, et al. Production and transplantation of bioengineered lung into a large animal model. *Science Translational Medicine*. 2018;10(452).
58. Garner JL, Shah PL. Endobronchial treatment of severe asthma and severe emphysema with hyperinflation. *Current Opinion in Pulmonary Medicine*. 2022;28(1):52–61.
59. Kemp SV, Slebos DJ, Kirk A, et al. A multicenter randomized controlled trial of zephyr endobronchial valve treatment in heterogeneous emphysema (TRANSFORM). *American Journal of Respiratory and Critical Care Medicine*. 2017;196(12):1535–43.
60. Criner GJ, Sue R, Wright S, et al. A multicenter randomized controlled trial of zephyr endobronchial valve treatment in heterogeneous emphysema (LIBERATE). *American Journal of Respiratory and Critical Care Medicine*. 2018;198(9):1151–64.
61. Valipour A, Slebos DJ, de Oliveira HG, et al. Expert statement: pneumothorax associated with endoscopic valve therapy for emphysema–potential mechanisms, treatment algorithm, and case examples. *Respiration; International Review of Thoracic Diseases*. 2014;87(6):513–21.
62. Gompelmann D, Lim HJ, Eberhardt R, et al. Predictors of pneumothorax following endoscopic valve therapy in patients with severe emphysema. *International Journal of Chronic Obstructive Pulmonary Disease*. 2016;11:1767–73.
63. Fitzmaurice GJ, Lau K, Redmond KC. The LIBERATE trial: options to reduce the risk of post-procedural pneumothorax and length of stay. *American Journal of Respiratory and Critical Care Medicine*. 2018;198(12):1586–7.
64. Criner GJ, Sue R, Sciurba FC, Slebos DJ. Reply to Fitzmaurice et al.: the LIBERATE trial: options to reduce the risk of post-procedural pneumothorax and length of stay. *American Journal of Respiratory and Critical Care Medicine*. 2018;198(12):1587–8.
65. Niimi Y, Murata S, Mitou Y, Ohno Y. Use of a novel drainage flow servo-controlled CPB for mitral valve replacement in a Jehovah's Witness. *Perfusion*. 2018;33(6):490–2.
66. Folch EE, Pritchett MA, Nead MA, et al. Electromagnetic navigation bronchoscopy for peripheral pulmonary lesions: one-year results of the prospective, multicenter NAVIGATE Study. *Journal of Thoracic Oncology*. 2019;14(3):445–58.
67. Cheng GZ, Liu L, Nobari M, et al. Cone beam navigation bronchoscopy: the next frontier. *Journal of Thoracic Disease*. 2020;12(6):3272–8.
68. Folch E, Mittal A, Oberg C. Robotic bronchoscopy and future directions of interventional pulmonology. *Current Opinion in Pulmonary Medicine*. 2022;28(1):37–44.
69. Wadood A. Brief overview on nitinol as biomaterial. *Advances in Materials Science and Engineering*. 2016;2016:4173138.
70. Maurice NM, Bedi B, Sadikot RT. Pseudomonas aeruginosa biofilms: host response and clinical implications in lung infections. *American Journal of Respiratory Cell and Molecular Biology*. 2018;58(4):428–39.
71. Song K, Min T, Jung JY, et al. A superhydrophilic nitinol shape memory alloy with enhanced anti-biofouling and anti-corrosion properties. *Biofouling*. 2016;32(5):535–45.
72. Kim H, Johnson JW. Corrosion of stainless steel, nickel-titanium, coated nickel-titanium, and titanium orthodontic wires. *The Angle Orthodontist*. 1999;69(1):39–44.
73. Chakravarthi S, Padmanabhan S, Chitharanjan AB. Allergy and orthodontics. *Journal of Orthodontic Science*. 2012;1(4):83–7.
74. Burrowes KS, Doel T, Brightling C. Computational modeling of the obstructive lung diseases asthma and COPD. *Journal of Translational Medicine*. 2014;12(2):S5.
75. Majid A, Ospina-Delgado D, Kheir F, et al. Thoracoscopic surgical stapling as salvage therapy for failed endobronchial valve treatment in patients with incomplete lobar fissures: initial experience. *Journal of Bronchology & Interventional Pulmonology*. 2022;29(1):e4–e7.
76. Shah PL, Zoumot Z, Singh S, et al. Endobronchial coils for the treatment of severe emphysema with hyperinflation (RESET): a randomised controlled trial. *The Lancet Respiratory Medicine*. 2013;1(3):233–40.
77. Deslee G, Mal H, Dutau H, et al. Lung volume reduction coil treatment vs usual care in patients with severe emphysema: the REVOLENS randomized clinical trial. *JAMA*. 2016;315(2):175–84.
78. Deslee G, Leroy S, Perotin JM, et al. Two-year follow-up after endobronchial coil treatment in emphysema results from the REVOLENS study. *The European Respiratory Journal*. 2017;50(6).
79. Sciurba FC, Criner GJ, Strange C, et al. Effect of endobronchial coils vs usual care on exercise tolerance in patients with severe emphysema: the RENEW randomized clinical trial. *JAMA*. 2016;315(20):2178–89.

80. Klooster K, Valipour A, Marquette CH, et al. Endobronchial coil system versus standard-of-care medical management in the treatment of subjects with severe emphysema. *Respiration; International Review of Thoracic Diseases.* 2021;100(8):804–10.
81. Orton CM, Garner JL, Desai SR, et al. Aspergillus cavitation complicating endobronchial lung volume reduction coil placement. *American Journal of Respiratory and Critical Care Medicine.* 2020;201(3):e8–e9.
82. Shah PL, Slebos D-J, Cardoso PFG, et al. Design of the exhale airway stents for emphysema (EASE) trial: an endoscopic procedure for reducing hyperinflation. *BMC Pulmonary Medicine.* 2011;11(1):1.
83. Shah PL, Slebos DJ, Cardoso PF, et al. Bronchoscopic lung-volume reduction with Exhale airway stents for emphysema (EASE trial): randomised, sham-controlled, multicentre trial. *Lancet* (London, England). 2011;378(9795):997–1005.
84. Shah PL, Gompelmann D, Valipour A, et al. Thermal vapour ablation to reduce segmental volume in patients with severe emphysema: STEP-UP 12 month results. *The Lancet Respiratory Medicine.* 2016;4(9):e44–e5.
85. Come CE, Kramer MR, Dransfield MT, et al. A randomised trial of lung sealant versus medical therapy for advanced emphysema. *The European Respiratory Journal.* 2015;46(3):651–62.
86. Valipour A, Shah PL, Herth FJ, et al. Two-year outcomes for the double-blind, randomized, sham-controlled study of targeted lung denervation in patients with moderate to severe COPD: AIRFLOW-2. *International Journal of Chronic Obstructive Pulmonary Disease.* 2020;15:2807–16.
87. Garner JL, Shaipanich T, Hartman JE, et al. A prospective safety and feasibility study of Metered CryoSpray (MCS) for patients with chronic bronchitis in COPD. *European Respiratory Journal.* 2020:2000556.

Index